Professionalism
Across
Occupational
Therapy Practice

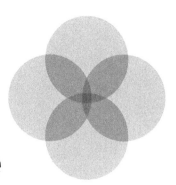

Professionalism
Across
Occupational Therapy Practice

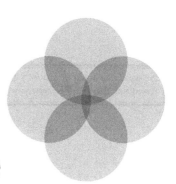

Elizabeth D. DeIuliis, OTD, OTR/L
Assistant Department Chair, Director of Community & Clinical
Education, Academic Fieldwork Coordinator
Department of Occupational Therapy
John G. Rangos Sr. School of Health Sciences
Duquesne University
Pittsburgh, Pennsylvania

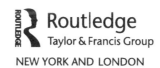
Routledge
Taylor & Francis Group

NEW YORK AND LONDON

Professionalism Across Occupational Therapy Practice includes ancillary materials specifically available for faculty use, including PowerPoint Slides. Please visit http://www.routledge.com/9781630910914 to obtain access.

First published in 2017 by SLACK Incorporated

Published 2024 by Routledge
605 Third Avenue, New York, NY 10158

and by Routledge
4 Park Square, Milton Park, Abingdon, Oxon OX14 4RN

Routledge is an imprint of the Taylor & Francis Group, an informa business

Library of Congress Cataloging-in-Publication Data

Names: DeIuliis, Elizabeth D., 1981- author.
Title: Professionalism across occupational therapy practice / Elizabeth D.
    DeIuliis.
Description: Thorofare, NJ : SLACK Incorporated, [2017] | Includes
    bibliographical references.
Identifiers: LCCN 2017004017 (print) | ISBN 9781630910914 (alk. paper)

Subjects: | MESH: Occupational Therapists | Professionalism | Occupational
    Therapy--ethics
Classification: LCC RM735 (print) | NLM W 21 | DDC
    615.8/515024--dc23
LC record available at https://lccn.loc.gov/2017004017

ISBN: 9781630910914 (pbk)
ISBN: 9781003526018 (ebk)

DOI: 10.4324/9781003526018

DEDICATION

This book is dedicated to my father, Brian L. Dwyer, who instilled in me, at an early age, the importance and power of attitude. Thank you for being my greatest role model of what a true professional is.

Contents

Acknowledgments

I would like to express sincere gratitude to my family, colleagues, and students who contributed to this project.

I would like to particularly mention my husband, Alessio; my parents, Brian and Maureen Dwyer; my children, Grace and Enzo; and extended family and friends for their constant support, motivation, and drive.

My faculty team at Duquesne University including Department Chairperson Dr. Jaime Muñoz, Dr. Elena Donoso Brown, Dr. Kim Szucs, Dr. Jeryl Benson, Dr. Ann Cook, Dr. Ann Stuart, and Mrs. Adriana Pearson—for their wisdom, encouragement, and inspiration in bringing a personal passion to fruition.

A special note of consideration given to the contributing authors, Dr. Leesa DiBartola, Dr. Andrea Fairman, and Dr. Sarah Wallace who provided their valuable input and expertise regarding interprofessional professionalism and ethics and scholarship.

A number of students/alumni at Duquesne University also deserve special recognition, including Grace Monroe, Chase Ratliff, Meredith Karavolis, Renae Fitcher, and Abby Catalano for their unwavering assistance, in literature searches and analyses and formatting.

Appreciation is extended to Brien Cummings at SLACK Incorporated for seeking me out for this opportunity and for his continued flexibility and support through this process.

ABOUT THE AUTHOR

Elizabeth D. DeIuliis, OTD, OTR/L, is the Assistant Department Chair, Director of Community & Clinical Education, and Academic Fieldwork Coordinator within the Department of Occupational Therapy, John G. Rangos Sr. School of Health Sciences at Duquesne University in Pittsburgh, Pennsylvania.

As a teaching-scholar, Dr. DeIuliis's teaching philosophy includes the use of a variety of instructional methods to foster self-directed, and active learning of her student cohorts within the adult physical disability curricula such as the flipped classroom model and simulated-learning. She actively participates in the University's Interprofessional Education Collaborative (IPEC) Committee, focusing on the advance of interprofessional education and practice in the University. Furthermore, Dr. DeIuliis was awarded the 2014 Creative Teaching Award through Duquesne University's Center for Teaching Excellence, the 2015 Dean's Award for Excellence in Teaching, and the 2016 recipient of the University's Student Learning Outcome Assessment Award. Dr. DeIuliis has developed a strong passion and connection with the fieldwork education process and has continued to be an advocate for fieldwork education and overall student learning development within the department, school, and occupational therapy profession. Dr. DeIuliis has received a certificate of completion from the AOTA Fieldwork Educator Course, serves on the Greater Pittsburgh Fieldwork Council, and has presented at various conferences on fieldwork education.

In addition, Dr. DeIuliis has upheld both clinical and administrative positions within various hospitals within the local Pittsburgh area. Dr. DeIuliis is an active member of the Pennsylvania Occupational Therapy Association, in addition to District II Delegate to the Board, member of the American Occupational Therapy Association, and received an appointment to the NBCOT Certification Examination Validation Committee in 2012.

In addition, she maintains clinical practice, at Centers for Rehab Services—UPMC Shadyside Hospital, in Pittsburgh, Pennsylvania. Her clinical experience is primarily acute-care, hospital-based rehabilitation, and she created an evidenced-based occupational therapy program for individual's status-post a breast-cancer related surgery during her clinical occupational therapy doctorate program from Chatham University.

Contributing Authors

Leesa M. DiBartola, EdD, DPT, PT, MCHES (Chapter 3)
Assistant Chair, Director of Clinical Education, Department of Physical Therapy
John G. Rangos Sr. School of Health Sciences
Duquesne University, Pittsburgh, Pennsylvania

Andrea D. Fairman, PhD, OTR/L, CPRP (Chapter 15)
Associate Professor, Department of Occupational Therapy
School of Health and Rehabilitation Sciences
MGH Institute of Health Professions, Boston, Massachusetts

Sarah E. Wallace, PhD, CCC-SLP (Chapter 3)
Associate Professor, Department of Speech-Language Pathology
Duquesne University, Pittsburgh, Pennsylvania

INTRODUCTION

The purpose of this text is to provide an overview of the wide-ranging professional knowledge, skills, and attitudes that encompass professionalism across the occupational therapy profession. Professionalism can be described as the attributes, characteristics, or behaviors that are not explicitly part of the profession's core of knowledge and technical skills, but are nevertheless required for success in the profession. The heart of the occupational therapy profession is embedded in a commitment to uphold ethical, moral, legal, and social principles. Socialization toward this concept of professionalism in the occupational therapy profession occurs during three main phases. First, formal academic education, then, fieldwork education, and finally, clinical practice. Professional socialization is an active process and includes a variety of participants including the students themselves; the socializing agents, or role models such as mentors, and fieldwork and academic educators and managers; the students' peers; and the clients with whom the students interact. The focus on professional behaviors is especially crucial now as occupational therapy education continues the discussion regarding transitioning to a doctoring profession with an entry-level degree and changes in the health care environment due to health care reform

While the subject of professionalism has been addressed in components of other occupational therapy text books in past years, this is the first occupational therapy book in more than a decade designed with a direct focus on professionalism from the perspective of the classroom, the clinic, and more. The primary intended audience is occupational therapy students in the classroom, occupational therapy fieldwork students, and all levels of occupational therapy practitioners. However, occupational therapy academic educators, leaders, managers, supervisors, and fieldwork educators may also benefit from the content of this text as a best practice resource to use with their colleagues, employees, and students.

When most people think of professionalism, ethics, or moralism, they often think of a set of rules for distinguishing between right and wrong, such as the proverbial Golden Rule, or the ethic of reciprocity ("Do unto others as you would have them do unto you"), or a code of professional conduct such as the Hippocratic Oath: "First of all, do no harm" (Tyson, 2001). However, the true definition of professionalism is not an easy one, and it not necessarily black and white nor about being perfect. In fact, it could be argued that it is often easier to describe what is not professional versus what is professional behavior/conduct. However, it could also be disputed that although professionalism can be recognized when you see it, you may not necessarily be able to put your finger on what "it" is exactly. Simply working in an identified profession, such as medicine, nursing, or occupational therapy does not automatically make one a professional. In fact, the specific context or environment that an individual is in may have a direct impact on expectations of the profession. For example, it may be acceptable to wear jeans in a private outpatient pediatric practice, but not acceptable to wear jeans in a physician-owned private practice. While professionalism may look different among various professions or settings, the core elements are relatively the same. This text will discuss these various expectations in the collegial/academic setting, the clinic, and workplace, and in general society.

There is a considerable amount of literature that argues that professionalism is something that is innate, something learned, or that it is a byproduct of one's generation. This text will discuss how expectations of professionalism have evolved generation to generation, specifically examining Generation "Y" or the Millennials, beause this is the stereotypical description for the majority of undergraduate/graduate occupational therapy students today. This generation is also the largest generation, after the Baby Boomers, and the future of the occupational therapy profession.

Part I of this text will identify and define several key words and themes associated with professionalism including professional ethics, professional responsibility, professional competency, and professional behaviors. Professionalism among other health care professions, such as physical therapy, nursing, and medicine, will be compared and contrasted with the expectations of the occupational therapy profession. In fact, some health care professions identify a specific definition of professionalism to guide their students and practitioners. At this time, there is no formal definition of professionalism in occupational therapy practice, yet the author will provide suggestions to serve as a blueprint for use.

Figure I-1. Combination of intrinsic and extrinsic qualities.

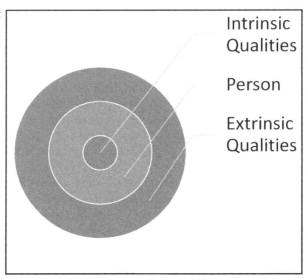

Intrinsic Qualities

Person

Extrinsic Qualities

This text will inform you that professionalism isn't just one thing, but a unique combination of intrinsic and extrinsic qualities. Intrinsic value has traditionally been thought to lie at the heart of ethics. Intrinsic qualities of professionalism can include those attributes that come from within one's self such as knowledge, skills, and attitudes. Examples may include initiative, motivation, and self-directedness. It is contrasted with extrinsic value, the value of which depends on how much it generates intrinsic value, and is displayed outward such as such as one's behaviors, actions, and contributions. Examples may include: professional image, interpersonal and communication skills, and teamwork (Figure I-1).

Part II of this text will provide an overview on professionalism for the occupational therapy student and educator in the classroom (didactic) environment. Professionalism is a core value and expectation of all health care provider educational programs, including occupational therapy. A review of current educational pedagogies and teaching approaches, as well as methods to foster occupational therapy students to professional expectations will be addressed. In addition, vignettes will be used to depict common professional behavior blunders and how to handle them.

Part III will focus on professionalism during occupational therapy fieldwork education. An overview of level I and level II fieldwork and doctoral experiential component expectations, as well as similarities and differences among fieldwork settings, supervision models, and fieldwork educator qualities will be examined. Vignettes will be provided to illustrate common professional behavior problems in fieldwork education, and strategies to prevent and handle them.

Professional development and growth merely begins at entry-level education and fieldwork and then extends throughout an individual's career. Part IV is intended to support the continued development and enhancement of professionalism throughout the continuum of clinical practice, aimed for a new graduate, and all levels of clinical practice. This section will cover various professional responsibilities and expectations of novice to expert occupational therapy practitioners such as preparation for the NBCOT exam, building a professional résumé and portfolio, job search process and interview skills. In addition, the importance of continued competency, and engaging in professional service will be discussed. Lastly, professionalism and ethics in research and scholarship will also be discussed in this section. In summary, this textbook will illustrate that professionalism is not just one thing, but a unique and sophisticated combination of an individuals' values, beliefs, attitudes, conduct, and performance.

Ancillary materials are provided for the occupational therapy student, educator, and manager via routledge.com/9781630910914. Supplemental materials include lecture materials such as basic PowerPoint lectures and additional learning activities to enhance teaching and learning regarding the various topics discussed in this text.

This textbook will use a developmental approach to teaching and learning, paralleling the Revised Bloom's taxonomy (Anderson & Krathwohl, 2001). This classification system provides a graded, holistic methodology to human teaching and learning. The concept of professionalism will be exemplified by using both a knowledge-based approach (factual) to subject matter requiring higher-level learning such as metacognition, which is a crucial component of professionalism. The chapter objectives, learning activities and ancillary materials will challenge the reader to recall, comprehend, apply analyze, synthesize, evaluate, and create knowledge directly to their context.

References

Anderson, L. W., & Krathwohl, D. (Eds.). (2001). *A taxonomy for learning, teaching, and assessing: A revision of Bloom's taxonomy of educational objectives.* New York, NY: Longman.

Tyson, P. (2001, March 27). The Hippocratic Oath today. Retrieved from http://www.pbs.org/wgbh/nova/body/hippocratic-oath-today.html

Elizabeth D. DeIuliis, OTD, OTR/L
Assistant Department Chair
Director of Community & Clinical Education,
Academic Fieldwork Coordinator
Department of Occupational Therapy
John G. Rangos Sr. School of Health Sciences
Duquesne University
Pittsburgh, Pennsylvania

Part I

What Is Professionalism?

Chapters 1 to 4 are designed to increase the reader's knowledge and understanding of basic terminology associated with professionalism, the process of professionalization in health care disciplines, and specific influences in the occupational therapy profession.

Definitions of Professionalism

Elizabeth D. DeIuliis, OTD, OTR/L

INTRODUCTION

This chapter will provide various definitions to terminology associated with professionalism, as well as introduce some of the general attributes and traits of professionalism and professional behavior.

KEY WORDS

Behavior: An individual's externally observable actions, which are influenced by character, attitudes, and values

Competency: A measure of an individual's skill level, competency is attaining and maintaining an adequate level of knowledge and skill, and the application thereof

Professional: An individual who possesses the knowledge, skill, training, and education to successfully and competently practice in a given profession

Professionalism: Conformation to the standards and norms of a given profession; a behavior exhibited by a professional that conveys an appropriate and consistent attitude for their role

Professionalization: The sociological phenomenon or deliberate process by which an occupation or vocation transforms itself into a regulated profession of high integrity and competence

Responsibility: A state of accountability to adhere to the set beliefs and values of the profession; responsibility exists between oneself, colleagues, consumers, and society

DeIuliis, E.D.
Professionalism Across Occupational Therapy Practice (pp 3-42).
© 2017 Taylor & Francis Group.

OBJECTIVES

By the end of reading this chapter and completing the learning activities, the reader should be able to:

1. Define and differentiate basic terminology including profession, professional, professionalism, and professionalization

2. Compare and contrast various definitions of professionalism

3. Describe four common elements of professionalism: ethics, responsibility, competency, and behavior

4. Explain the relationship between intrinsic and extrinsic qualities of professionalism

There is historic difficulty among the occupational therapy profession and among non-occupational therapists including other health care professions and stakeholders, such as third-party payers, articulating the unique role and professional identity of occupational therapy practitioners (Bannigan, 2000; Boutin-Lester & Gibson, 2002; Dickinson, 2003; Gripper, 2008; Pattison, 2006; Wilding & Whiteford, 2008; Withers & Shann, 2008). In the early 1900s, when the field of occupational therapy was emerging, scientific methods were becoming the focus of American medicine. During this time, occupational therapists continued to voice the humanistic influence on the health and well-being of the person. The occupational therapy profession has since struggled with "balancing the scientific and humanistic trends inherent in occupational therapy, of finding occupational therapy's place in American medicine, and of meeting the aims of scientific medicine" (Quiroga, 1995, p. 14). Now, more than a century later, occupational therapists still have difficulty maintaining a unique identity and incorporating the profession's founding principles and language. Due to the complexity of occupational therapy, many therapists have found it difficult to articulate exactly what we do (Fisher, 1998). Cooper (2012) supports this by stating that "We are a profession that has been difficult to describe. Each us of has had the challenge of explaining to a member of the general public what an occupational therapy practitioner does, often with limited success" (p. 205).

The role of occupational therapy is often misunderstood as only pertaining to vocational therapy due to the word occupational being mainly associated with work in the United States. It is not uncommon for patients to wrongly assume they don't fall under the scope of services an occupational therapy practitioner provides with phrases such as "Oh, I am retired, I don't have a job," associating occupational therapy with helping people recover for their jobs. Although there are occupational therapy practitioners who do work in vocational counseling, the field of occupational therapy is significantly more diverse. This instance is just a small example that shows that there needs to be a stronger distinction of the occupational therapy role, professional identity, and related terminology.

In 2003, the American Occupational Therapy Association (AOTA) began a pursuit to create a Centennial Vision, commemorating the profession's 100th anniversary, which will take place in 2017 (AOTA, 2007a). During the planning phases, the committee identified issues such as raising public awareness, preventing professional encroachment, and identifying new knowledge and skills of occupational therapy practitioners. One of the major barriers identified in the strategic plan for the Centennial Vision was "unclear professional language and terminology" (AOTA, 2007a, p. 614). The very fact that one of the profession's leading organizations identified this concern, and that the Centennial Vision was intentionally written to address this barrier, gives further recognition to the struggle of defining and using occupational therapy–specific terminology. More recently, the AOTA has branded an effort in promoting the Distinct Value of Occupational Therapy. Lamb and Metzler (2014) state that "occupational therapy professionals must link the value of occupational therapy to the needs emerging within the greater health care system" (p. 9). Although this current brand directly focuses on the advocacy needed to survive in the changing

---

Box 1-1

Wilding and Whiteford (2008) found that the language that we use changes our sense of identity. For example, instead of using the term functional abilities, we can use occupational performance.

Summary of Authors' Findings:

- Initial difficulty explaining occupational therapy (gap between what they said and what they meant)
- Once changed language → became more confident, articulate, more assertive
- Transformation from unconfident/unclear to self-assured and articulate

Whereas the Occupational Therapy Practice Framework: Domain and Process, 3rd edition helps the profession to establish discipline-specific language in the context of service delivery, it can be a challenge to use in everyday practice. By using the terminologies of occupation, we are validating our professional representation and our identity.

---

health care arena, this association Lamb and Metzler recommend also needs to involve the basic core values of the occupational therapy profession that are not universally defined, such as professionalism.

One of the strategies recommended to promote the distinct value of occupational therapy is via terminology (Lamb & Robosan-Burt, n.d.). This resource developed by Lamb and Robosaun-Burt highlights the importance of using occupational therapy–specific language such as "occupation and occupational performance" as a means to educate others regarding the power of occupation. This notion regarding the importance of language and word choice as a vehicle to promote identity is not new, and is in fact under-recognized. Wilding and Whiteford (2008) performed a qualitative study investigating how the use of language transforms occupational therapy practitioners' sense of identity (Box 1-1). If we can further define what professionalism means for the occupational therapy profession, will we be better suited to model, teach, and enforce it for the future?

Robinson, Tanchuck, and Sullivan (2012) explored the perspectives of occupational therapy faculty members and students on the meaning of professionalism. The researchers investigated questions such as What is professionalism? What is not professionalism? How is professionalism different in other health professions—for example, medicine? In the context of occupational therapy, what are the most important and relevant aspects of professionalism? The themes across the faculty member focus groups included professional responsibility, professional awareness, and the context-specific nature of professionalism. Across the student group, the themes included uncertainty toward professional expectations, a search for answers in concrete concepts, and a general awareness of context-specific differences in professionalism. It is suggested that both understanding and enacting professionalism may be a part of a developmental process that exists on a continuum.

In response to the strategic plan of the AOTA Centennial Vision, this text aims to serve as a blueprint of best practice for professionalism across the occupational therapy profession. First, it is important to provide distinction between various terms associated with professionalism. This process of professional differentiation is complex. To begin, how would you classify the field of occupational therapy? Is it a profession, occupation, career, or a job? How would you describe individuals who work in the field of occupational therapy? Are they practitioners, employees, members of a workforce, or professionals? If the field of occupational therapy is a profession, are all occupational therapy practitioners "professionals?" If you are a professional, do you instinctively portray professionalism? These are all complex questions. An occupational therapy practitioner

Box 1-2
Because knowledge and understanding of the roles, responsibilities, and values of other disciplines is essential to being an occupational therapy professional, the professionalization of these and other allied health professions will be discussed in Chapter 3.

could have superb technical skills, specialized knowledge, and service competency but none of these characteristics exemplify their level of professionalism, or professional behaviors. Many of these above terms can appear to be ambiguous and confusing not only to occupational therapy professionals, but also to outsiders as well. Let's explore some of these terms' connotations, as well as some additional insight into professionalism.

The words occupation and profession are often used interchangeably, but their definitions are clearly different. An occupation, outside of occupational therapy jargon, can be defined as a job, vocation, or regular activity that is performed for payment ("Occupation," 2017). A profession, as opposed to an occupation, is a vocation that requires extensive education and specialized training, and has a body of specific knowledge and skills put into service for the good of others ("Profession," 2017). Professions typically have sets of stated values and codes of ethics to guide their practice and to help articulate their professional identity (Box 1-2). For example, the AOTA, the American Physical Therapy Association (APTA) and the American Speech-Language-Hearing Association (ASHA) all include information regarding their core values and their codes of ethics on their respective websites (see Box 1-2) (AOTA, 2015; APTA, 2010, 2013; ASHA, 2016).

Therefore, disciplines such as medicine, law, and occupational therapy would meet these criteria and be considered professions. There is a specialized, complex, and at times uncertain nature of the expertise associated with the title of 'profession' which confers some form of autonomy, indicating that a profession is expected to regulate itself. Sauter-Davis (2014) indicates that a "profession includes shared perspectives in knowledge, attitudes, and behaviors" (p. 647). The practice of specialized expertise and the ethical obligations associated with said practice are two key factors that differentiate a profession from other occupations (Ozar, 2004). This suggests that it is the profession itself that dictates the principles by which it is governed and held to. Decisions are made and actions are taken based on a professional's expertise, knowledge, and reason. Therefore, the principles that govern disciplines such as medicine, law, and occupational therapy may have some similarities, yet significant differences, as they are each a singular profession. While the occupational therapy profession has definite ethical principles to guide practice, there is currently no official document or statement devoted to defining and describing professionalism or professional behaviors in the discipline of occupational therapy.

Next, it is important to highlight the clear distinction between a professional, a practitioner, and an employee. The term professional is used so widely in society that its meaning and connotation can be taken for granted. Dictionary.com (2017) defines a professional as "a person who belongs to one of the professions, especially one of the learned professions." The World Health Organization states that a "professional is an all-encompassing term that includes individuals with the knowledge and/or skills to contribute to the physical, mental and social well-being of a community" (2010, p. 13). A professional displays a commitment to competence, and is skillful due to specialized training and/or education received. This contrasts with the definition of employee or worker, which indicates a person who is employed for wages or salary, especially at a nonexecutive level ("Employee," 2017). A practitioner is defined as a "person engaged in the practice of a profession, occupation, etc." and someone "who practices something specified" such as a medical practitioner ("Practitioner," 2017). Often the medical and social care professions use these titles to distinguish the level of qualifications, competency, and training which a practitioner undertakes. Throughout literature, there have been various terms used to describe this novice-to-expert continuum

	TABLE 1-1	
	COMPETENCE LEVELS	
LEVEL OF COMPETENCE	DESCRIPTION	EXAMPLE
Entry-Level Occupational Therapist	Working on initial skill development (new graduate) OR entering new practice Skill set is still developing for a given setting.	An occupational therapy practitioner who has been practicing for 10 years in mental health and is now moving into school-based practice would be considered entry level in the school-based setting.
Intermediate Level Occupational Therapist	Working on increased skill development and mastery of basic role functions Demonstrates ability to respond to situations based on experience	An occupational therapy practitioner who has been working in a pediatric out-patient setting for 5 years may decide to pursue a specialization to advance their knowledge and skill set, such as board certified in pediatrics or specialty training in feeding and swallowing.
Advanced Level Occupational Therapist	Refining specialized skills with the ability to understand complex issues enter into practice This may involve taking on additional responsibilities such as service, leadership, mentoring, or administration	An occupational therapy practitioner who has been working in the home health setting for 8 years may be promoted to a middle-level manager, which requires additional responsibilities such as supervision of staff, program development, and fiscal responsibilities, such as managing payroll.

Adapted from American Occupational Therapy Association. (1993). Occupational therapy roles. *American Journal of Occupational Therapy, 47*(12), 1087-1099.

regarding service competency (skill level), experience level related to clinical reasoning (problem solving), and supervisory responsibilities (the overseeing of other individuals in the field). For example, in the occupational therapy profession, there are typically three main levels to indicate an occupational therapy practitioner's competence: entry-level, intermediate and advanced. These levels are not based upon years of clinical experience, but rather performance and skill set, which is attained by work experience, training, and professional socialization.

Competence can be defined as the quality or state of being functionally adequate or having sufficient knowledge, judgment skill, or strength (Table 1-1) ("Competence," 2016).

Competence can also be used to describe levels in supervisory roles (Table 1-2). Although entry-level registered occupational therapists are not required to have supervision, it may be recommended dependent upon the setting, population, or skill set of the new practitioner.

TABLE 1-2 EXPERIENCE LEVELS	
Entry-Level Practitioner	Less than 1 year of experience
Intermediate-Level Practitioner	1-3 years of experience
Advanced-Level Practitioner	3 or more years of experience

Adapted from American Occupational Therapy Association. (1993). Occupational therapy roles. *American Journal of Occupational Therapy, 47*(12), 1087-1099.

According to the AOTA (1999), close supervision by an intermediate or advanced practitioner is recommended. Furthermore, supervision and mentorship from a more experienced practitioner can result in professional development and growth as a professional (Brayman et al., 2009).

THEORETICAL FRAMEWORK FOR PROFESSIONAL GROWTH AND DEVELOPMENT

Conceptually, two commonly mentioned models related to the development of competence and skill in health care are the Dreyfus and Dreyfus Skill Acquisition Model and the Benner Model.

Dreyfus and Dreyfus Skill Acquisition Model

Dreyfus and Dreyfus (1980) were brothers who created a hierarchy of human skill acquisition to model how individuals acquire skills through formal instruction and practicing skills. Their research was based upon studies of airplane pilots, chess players, automobile drivers, and adults who learned a second language, and investigated how professionals attain and master skills. This model describes a stepwise manner for the mental processing, logic, and principles that guide reasoning as one advances through the various stages of skill attainment. Dreyfus and Dreyfus propose four stages: novice, competence, proficiency and expertise. This can be useful to keep in mind as we begin to define the process of developing professionalism (Table 1-3).

Benner Stages of Clinical Competence

In the 1980s, Patricia Benner built upon the work of Dreyfus and Dreyfus, specific to the field of nursing (Benner, 1984). She reinvented this framework based upon on the narratives of newly qualified as well as expert nurses, which captured their clinical and ethical judgments. These experiences and comprehensions of nurses were related to their clinical practice knowledge and to the development of their professionalism and leadership skills. Benner introduced the "Novice to Expert" concept that expert nurses develop skills and understanding of patient care over time, through a sound educational base as well as a multitude of experiences. She proposed that one could gain knowledge and skills ("knowing how") without ever learning the theory ("knowing that"). She further explains that the development of knowledge in applied disciplines such as medicine and nursing is composed of the extension of practical knowledge (know how) through research and the characterization and understanding of the "know how" of clinical experience. Benner's model (1984), which was written in *From Novice to Expert: Excellence and Power in*

TABLE 1-3
DREYFUS AND DREYFUS SKILL LEVELS

STAGE	DEFINITION
Novice	In this stage, a person follows rules that are context-free and feels no responsibility for anything other than following the rules.
Competence	This stage develops after an individual has considerable experience.
Proficiency	This stage is shown in individuals who use intuition in decision-making and develop their own rules to formulate plans.
Expertise	This stage is characterized by a fluid performance that happens unconsciously, automatically, and no longer depends upon explicit knowledge.

Adapted from Dreyfus, H., & Dreyfus, S. (1980). *A five-stage model of mental activities involved in directed skill acquisition.* Berkeley, CA: Operations Research Center, University of California.

Clinical Nursing Practice also frames skill acquisition as moving through various stages, in a more expressive manner. The five stages are: novice, advanced beginner, competency, proficiency, and expert (Table 1-4).

Following the Benner model, occupational therapists at the novice stage are still in school. Occupational therapists at the advanced beginner stage use learned procedures and rules to determine what actions are required for the immediate situation, which could be fieldwork and entry-level practice. Competent occupational therapists are task-oriented and deliberately structure their work in terms of plans for goal achievement. These competent therapists can respond to many clinical situations, but lack the ability to recognize situations in terms of an overall picture. Proficient occupational therapists perceive situations as a whole and have more ability to recognize and respond to changing circumstances. Expert occupational therapists recognize unexpected clinical responses and can alert others to potential problems before they occur. Experts have an intuitive grasp of whole situations, and are able to accurately diagnose and respond without wasteful consideration of ineffective possibilities. Due to their superior performance, expert occupational therapists are often consulted by others and are relied upon to be educators, mentors and/or leaders (Benner, 1984).

HOW CAN WE RELATE THESE TWO FRAMEWORKS TO PROFESSIONALISM?

Using the Dreyfus and Dreyfus model, professional skill is not primarily context-free but context-dependent. With progression through the stages of skill acquisition, the significance of context and professional skill development becomes more evident. Things change as you move from novice to expert. It is more than just knowing more, or gaining skill. You have a difference in how you perceive, how you approach problem solving, and how you make decisions. Benner's theory states that over time, nurses develop skills and knowledge through sound education and experience.

TABLE 1-4 BENNER'S MODEL OF SKILL DEVELOPMENT	
STAGE	**DESCRIPTION**
Novice	Beginner with no experience, taught general rules to help perform tasks, i.e. "Tell me what to do and I'll do it"; learners focus on learning the rules of a particular skill.
Advanced Beginner	Demonstrates acceptable performance; has gained prior experience in actual situations to recognize recurring components; principles are based more on experience. Learners focus on applying the rules of a skill in specific situations that become increasingly dependent on the particular context of the situation.
Competency	More aware of long-term goals, gains perspective from planning own actions based on conscious, abstract, and analytical thinking, and helps to achieve greater efficiency and organization. Learners see actions in terms of long-range goals or plans and are consciously aware of their skills.
Proficiency	More holistic understanding; improved decision-making; learns from experiences what to expect in certain situations; and how to modify plans. Learners perceive situations as "wholes" rather than "aspects," and their performance is guided by intuitive behavior.
Expert	No longer relies on principles, rules or guidance to connect situations and determine actions; has intuitive grasp of situations. Performance is now fluid, flexible and highly proficient. Learners integrate mastered skills with their own personal styles (Driscoll, 2002; Leach, 2002).

Adapted from Benner, P. (1984). *From novice to expert: Excellence and power in clinical nursing practice*. Menlo Park, NJ: Addison-Wesley; Benner, P. A. (2004). Using the Dreyfus model of skill acquisition to describe and interpret skill acquisition and clinical judgment in nursing practice and education. *Bulletin of Science, Technology, & Society, 24*(3), 188-199.

It differentiates the practical, "knowing how," and theoretical, "knowing that," categories of knowledge in nursing practice (Brykczynski, 2010). Her theory was one of the first to characterize the learning process of nursing, from a clinical and professional standpoint. Developing skills through a situational experience is a prerequisite for expertise (i.e. develop clinical and professional skills through occupational therapy fieldwork education). Benner states that "expertise develops when the clinician tests and refines propositions, hypotheses, and principle-based expectations in actual practice situations. Experience is therefore a requisite for expertise" (1984, p. 3).

It is evident that both professionals and practitioners are required to demonstrate a level of expertise; however, it is the responsibility of a professional to maintain this expectation. In short, becoming a professional does not happen overnight, nor is it automatic when you graduate, pass your board certification exam, or receive licensure. As occupational therapy practitioners, we are "considered" professionals. We hold a professional license, various credentials, and possess specific skills that make us a unique entity in the workplace. But being a professional is different than acting like a professional. Professionalism is not just a list of traits, but a mindset; it's a way of approaching the work and the challenges, which demonstrates not only clinical and technical skills, but character traits as well. This unique skill set is derived from many hours of study, learning, preparation, and self-reflection. Therefore, all occupational therapists and occupational therapy assistants are practitioners, yet not all occupational therapy practitioners are professional, nor demonstrate professionalism.

The term professionalism means "conforming to the standards of a profession," and this does not simply imply the technical standards ("Professionalism," 2016). Merriam-Webster describes professionalism as a "set of attitudes, judgments and behaviors believed to be appropriate to a particular occupation" ("Professionalism," 2016). While these definitions of professionalism define the word, it does little to help one to understand which qualities and characteristics are important, or how one can become a recognized professional in his or her field. Professionals should aspire to exhibit behaviors consistent with their profession. However, the exact nature of such behaviors has not been clearly defined in the field of occupational therapy.

Being professional is the act of behaving in a manner defined and expected by the chosen profession. Hill (2000) describes professionalism as the "active demonstration of the traits of a professional" (p. 96). The concept of professionalism is multifaceted, and generally comprised by a combination of values, beliefs, attitudes and behaviors. Epstein and Hundert's (2002) definition of professionalism is a very useful one: "the habitual and judicious use of communication, knowledge, technical skills, clinical reasoning, emotions, values, and reflection in daily practice for the benefit of the individual and community being served." This statement is suitable in that it encapsulates the multi-dimensions of professionalism. Newkirk (1982) defined professionalism as "the quality of an individual to overtly display characteristics that positively represent the standards of one's profession and a commitment to advancing the program or activity of the profession" (n.p.). The act employing these professional beliefs, attitudes and behaviors could serve as a definition for professionalism, or, as Sauter-Davis (2014) indicates, professionalization.

Professionalization is the sociological phenomenon or deliberate process by which an occupation or vocation transforms itself into a true "profession of the highest integrity and competence" ("Professionalization," 2016). Becoming a professional involves determining suitable qualifications (creating some degree between those that are qualified and unqualified) identifying roles and role functions, and forming a professional body or association in charge of the conducts of the profession. Wilensky (1964), a well written sociologist, discusses this notion of professionalization and identified the following traits as those that indicate a profession: "specialization, ultimate application of theory, stability of employment and the existence of work rules," or professional norms (p. 138). Factors influencing the professionalization of various health care disciplines will be discussed in Chapter 3.

For instance, the birth of moral treatment in the twentieth century and the return of soldiers who were wounded at the end of World War I, was the beginning of the professionalization of occupational therapy, members of which were first labeled as reconstruction aides (Low, 1992). During this time, full-time employment of occupational therapists was recognized, in addition to the establishment of the National Society for the Promotion of Occupational Therapy in 1917. This organization was later renamed as the American Occupational Therapy Association, the national organization for the field of occupation therapy. A discussion on the evolution of professionalism in the occupational therapy discipline will be discussed in Chapter 4.

Figure 1-1. Schematic of professionalism components.

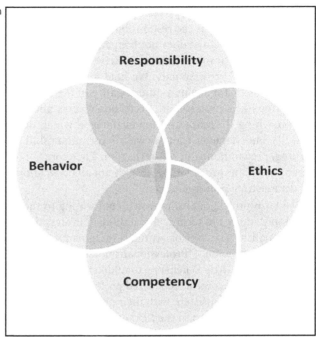

GENERAL COMPONENTS OF PROFESSIONALISM

There is an abundance of literature that discusses professionalism. Although the "recipe" may be different from discipline to discipline, the general "ingredients" that make up a professional are shared. These four common ingredients are: professional ethics, professional responsibility, professional behavior and professional competency. Each of these important components of professionalism will be discussed next (Figure 1-1).

Professional Ethics

Ethics and morality are two terms that are integrally linked with the concept of professionalism. Professionalism is foundational for a profession's fulfillment of its social and ethical responsibility to society. All social and health care professionals are required to understand and practice the ethics of care because they aim to serve the public, and members of the public have great personal needs that they give over to professionals in their time of need (Mootz, Coulter, & Schultz, 2005). Ethics is a branch of philosophy that guides ways of understanding and examining a moral life (Beauchamp & Childress, 2012). Ethics is a code of morality, and a system of principles governing the appropriate conduct for a person or group. Integrity, honesty, diligence, loyalty, respect and commitment are all part of an ethical character which in turn exemplifies professionalism. Every aspect of human behavior is influenced by personal values, but values are not easily defined or achieved. Professionals are driven by a code of ethics. They have a strong sense of right and wrong. Their integrity ensures that they adhere strongly to a set of values about how they do their work. Integrity leads others to trust the professional. They say what they will do and do what they say. Therefore, professional ethics refers to principles or rules intended to express the particular values and standards of behavior of a profession that serve as guidelines for professional behavior. They help to explain the profession to people served, and serve as a code of conduct to the belonging professionals. Most professions have internally enforced codes of practice that members of the profession must follow to prevent exploitation of the client and to preserve the integrity of the profession.

These rules ensure our client's best interest and protect the profession itself and its position in the public mind. More information on ethics and occupational therapy will be discussed in Chapter 4.

Professional Responsibility

The term responsibility indicates a state of or fact of accountability, concern for, obligation, or a sense of having control ("Responsibility," 2016). Professional responsibility is a term associated quite frequently with the law profession. Professional responsibility dictates that a professional displays morality and in many cases legal accountability for their actions, upholds the principles of the profession (as well as any stipulations mandated by federal or state authorities such as the Health Insurance Portability and Accountability Act or the American Disabilities Act) and demonstrates high standards of quality care. This sense of responsibility symbolizes a contract to adhere to the set beliefs and values of the profession between oneself, colleagues, consumers, and/ or society. A health care professional deliberately puts the interest of its consumers ahead of their own. Professionals embody a strong sense of empathy, a desire to do good, responsible attitude, and adherence to the governing law. It is also a professional's responsibility to display unwavering commitment to excellence and lifelong learning, as it is imperative that a professional stays current in their field. This means that a professional is committed to continued training and development. This concept of commitment to learning will be further discussed under professional competency.

Professional Behavior

Behavior or conduct is defined as the way of acting or the way in which one behaves. Behavior refers to one's actions or reactions ("Behavior," 2016). As noted previously, although you know it when you see it (or don't see it), it is often easier to describe unprofessional behavior as opposed to professional behavior, due to variances between professions. Unprofessional behavior could be defined as "not conforming to the standards of a profession." In other words, professional behavior is an appropriate reflection of professionalism (Yusoff, 2009). Therefore, professionalism is manifested by a combination of physical, observable behaviors (extrinsic) and an individual's personal mindset, values and knowledge (intrinsic). Some examples of these behaviors and mentality include appropriate professional presentation, timeliness, interpersonal skills, reliability, dependability, and self-motivation. These factors and more will be discussed in greater detail later in this chapter.

Professional Competency

Competency means attaining and maintaining an adequate level of knowledge and skill, and application of that knowledge and skill ("Competence," 2016). Competence also includes the wisdom to recognize the limitations of that knowledge and when consultation with other professionals is appropriate or referral to other professionals necessary. Similar to professional responsibility, demonstrating professional competence indicates a continuing commitment to learning and professional improvement in order to maintain the knowledge and skill to provide services in a competent manner. Professional competency implies that professionalism is something which can be taught, developed, measured, and assessed, though it can be argued whether professionalism is something innate or learned. Professionals have high levels of expectations both of themselves and others and engage in professional growth to maintain the knowledge and skill set necessary to provide services competently. In so many words, professionals are determined to always do the right thing and to do the right thing well.

The best way to understand the concept of professionalism is to think of occupations differing as to the degree that they are professional. Therefore, even though medicine, law and occupational therapy are all professions, there are paramount differences which make each unique. The degree to which an occupation meets the definition of a profession should be assessed by measuring

Figure 1-2. Balance of intrinsic and extrinsic factors of professionalism.

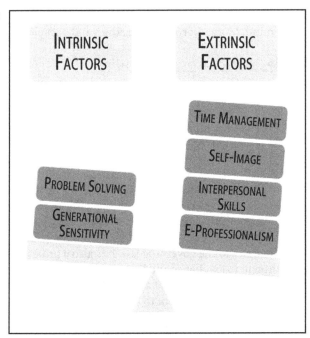

the occupation on certain key characteristics. Paralleling one of the foundational principles of the occupational therapy profession, professionalism is a holistic construct, encompassing both intrinsic and extrinsic qualities (Figure 1-2). These intrinsic and extrinsic qualities are what helps shape one's professional identity and are both personally and socially constructed. Bierema (2011) describes professionalization as the "building of specialized knowledge and skills, incorporating a sense of occupational identity, internalizing the norms of the profession, and adapting the values and norms into individual behavior and self-concept" (p. 29). In order to be a professional, there needs to be a sense of balance among these internal and external attributes.

INTRINSIC QUALITIES OF PROFESSIONALISM

Intrinsic qualities of professionalism can include those attributes that come from within one's ethos, personal character or moral disposition, such as an individual's knowledge, skills and attitudes (Zimmerman, 2014). During her Eleanor Slagle Lectureship, Suzanne Peloquin (2005) accentuated the importance of a human's ethos, or essence, in the makeup of an individual's character, or moral disposition. In many ways, various factors of professionalism can be attributed to one's mindset, or personal conscience, which is an internal by-product of their personal values and moral beliefs that are integral to their overall inner character. Examples of intrinsic qualities of professionalism can include:

- Self-management
- Problem solving and critical reasoning skills
- Integrity and honesty
- Dependability and reliability
- Generational and cultural sensitivity

Self-Management

Self-management is used to encompass various elements of intrinsic professionalism such as self-motivation, self-discipline, initiative, self-reliance, pro-active approach, self-awareness, and autonomy. You may have heard a person who exhibits excellent self-management characterized as a "self-starter" or a "driver," meaning that he or she, without exception, exhibit the desire to change, grow, and take risks in order to improve his or her self. They take initiative, act independently, and self-motivate. Furthermore, on the Myers-Briggs Personality Type instrument, there is a personality type listed as a "driver," describing it as a "go-get-it-done," "can-do mentality," "whatever-it-takes personality," or an individual who is result-focused (The Myers & Briggs Foundation, n.d.). A professional also demonstrates self-awareness, by demonstrating mindfulness of his or her own values, motivations, and emotions. However, professionals are not only intuitive to their own strengths and areas of need, yet are also perceptive of interactions with others. Some literature defines this sense of awareness as having emotional intelligence, which is a term used to describe the ability to "manage oneself and his or her relationships effectively" ("Emotional Intelligence," 2017). Self-management also can denote one's ability to self-regulate—or maintain emotional stability, even under pressure—during unanticipated or anticipated events. In today's society, which seems to be in a constant era of change, having this sense of stability is critical.

Autonomy is a crucial component of professionalism and self-management, and is often noted as an ethical principle or value in many official documents relating to ethics. Professional autonomy is defined as having a high degree of control over one's professional affairs ("Profession," 2017). An individual who exhibits autonomy is responsible for making their own decisions regarding their own actions, as well as in the care of others, such as consumers. For example, it is a right of clients receiving occupational therapy services to be fully informed regarding the benefits, risks, and potential outcomes of interventions. As treating occupational therapists, it is our professional responsibility to respect the client's right to refuse services.

Problem Solving and Critical Reasoning Skills

The next intrinsic quality of professionalism that will be discussed is problem solving and critical thinking skills. Problem solving and critical thinking refer to the ability to use knowledge, facts, and data to effectively solve problems. This doesn't mean you need to have an immediate answer at all times; it means you have the ability to think on your feet, assess problems, and find and develop a well thought-out solution within a reasonable time frame. Good problem solving skills empower individuals in their educational, professional, and personal lives. The current structure of health care and health care environments requires a strong skill set of problem solving, as well as the ability to think and be productive in fast-paced settings. The ability to think critically in a range of contexts is essential for the development of knowledge, understanding, and performance. Within occupational therapy clinical practice, critical reasoning is characterized as clinical or professional reasoning. Professional reasoning is a complex, multidimensional, whole-body thought process which involves problem solving on multiple levels. These levels include human reasoning of societal morals and values, as well as one's individual set of values and system of beliefs. Professional reasoning not only guides what and how you think and act as a practitioner, but also your engagement as a citizen in society (Fleming, 1991).

In clinical practice, reasoning is occurring whenever an occupational therapy practitioner is thinking about or doing occupational therapy. Fleming (1994) writes that it is impossible to fully explain, as one must experience what an occupational therapy practitioner experiences and think how they think to understand their reasoning. It is "knowing more than we can tell" (p. 24). For example, reasoning is used to select one treatment technique over another, or deciding to postpone or terminate occupational therapy services. However, the value of this skill set is significant beyond the clinical world alone. The workforce today requires individuals who can work out problems on their own, and individuals who aren't afraid to develop and implement innovative solutions or take risks. Professionals are needed to think critically and creatively, share thoughts and opinions, use good judgment, and make decisions. In fact, according to the 2012 Critical Skills Survey by the American Management Association, critical thinking and problem solving skills were rated as priority competencies by 71.9% of participants (American Management Association, 2012).

Integrity and Honesty

It is hard to describe professional and ethical behavior without including integrity and honesty. Having integrity can be described as adhering to moral and ethical principles, and displaying a soundness of moral character ("Integrity," 2017). Therefore, it is not only important to do the right thing, but do the right thing the right way. Professionals never compromise their values (both personal and professional), and will do the right thing, even when it means taking a harder road. This ability to stick with something despite the task becoming tough is called tenacity, and is a very important element of being a professional. Martin Luther King, Jr., one of the most famous American civil rights activists, once said that "the time is always right to do what is right" (Electronic Oberlin Group, n.d.). For example, in the classroom, honesty is deeply connected to academic integrity, which guides students to refrain from cheating. In the clinic, honesty and integrity are required to appropriately bill for services or document real client results. As an administrator or manager, it is necessary to be honest when providing feedback to employees on their performance, or as a fieldwork educator accurately scoring the performance of a fieldwork student using the AOTA Fieldwork Performance Evaluation (FWPE) of the Level II Student.

Dependability and Reliability

Dependability is a characteristic that shows the reliability of a person to others ("Dependability," 2016). What makes you dependable or reliable to others is integrity and honesty; this is what allows others to trust what you say or do. For example, what are some of the qualities you look for when you need to hire someone to do a job? Many marketing materials or job descriptions list desired traits such as "dependable," "reliable," and "loyal." Dependability is the first step towards building trust and gaining respect as a professional. It is important to point out that being dependable is not just about being punctual (which will be discussed further as an extrinsic professional quality). It is a symbol of your commitment and trust that makes you an important asset to your profession. By being dependable, it not only causes those around you to trust you and respect you, but it teaches an individual that they can depend on and trust themselves! For example, in a student's educational training, one may have to collaborate with his or her peers on a group project. It is necessary to contribute and pull your weight so that your peers can depend on you to complete your part. In the clinic, if a staff member is going to be scheduled off for a day, it is helpful to create a caseload coverage plan for whomever may be treating that person's patients instead. These intrinsic qualities of professionalism have a direct effect on a professional's self-worth and self-efficacy by building self-confidence.

Generational and Cultural Sensitivity

Today's workforce is undeniably diverse in regards to gender, race, ethnicity, and age. It is essential for professionals to possess strengths in generational and cultural sensitivity—displaying the ability to build rapport with a diverse workforce in multicultural settings, which overall enhances one's moral core. Generational or intergenerational competence is the ability to understand, appreciate, and respond to the specific needs of individuals from generations different than your own (Friedman, 2011). A generation is defined as all of the people born and living at about the same time, regarded collectively ("Generation," n.d.). For the first time in society, there are four generations together in both higher education and the workforce. Other than within one's own family dynamic, the workplace is typically the only other context where you will regularly engage with individuals and groups from various generations. Having a strong skill set in interaction and working alongside each generation is critical for a professional (Taylor, 2008). Each generation has its own distinct set of values regarding family, career, work and life balance, gender roles, communication styles, work ethic, education, and so on that was developed from the social and historical factors they experienced during their formative years. The four generations most prominent in society today are: Silent/Traditionalists, Baby Boomers, Generation X and Generation Y. The newest generation is Generation Z, which will be college-bound in the next decade or so, and will also be briefly discussed. The specific date ranges of each generation may vary depending on the source.

Traditionalists (Silents)

Although many of these individuals may be retired, the Traditionalist generation, or the Silents, comprise the oldest generation in the workforce today. About 6.5% of the workforce consists of Traditionalists (Bureau of Labor Statistics, 2016). This generation includes individuals born before 1945. Individuals in this generation were strongly influenced by the Great Depression era and World War II. They were raised with strict regimen that taught them to value fiscal restraint, quality, respect, patriotism, and authority. The Traditionalists can be described as disciplined individuals who prefer social order including formality in the workforce such as a top-down hierarchy and chain of command. Authority is viewed by seniority and age as opposed to skill level and performance. Problem-solving and decision-making abilities are preferred with experience. They embrace a strong work ethic, and embody a sense of obligation and commitment towards teamwork and collaboration. Communication skills, particularly face-to-face, are highly regarded. They are often averse to risk and conflict, and keep work and family life separate. The Silents embrace a strong sense of morality and tend to do "what is right."

Baby Boomers

The Baby Boomer generation identifies people born between 1943 and 1965. It can be argued that this population has had the largest effect on American society due to its size—78 million roughly, according to the U.S. Census Bureau. The Baby Boomers are the highest population within the workforce at around 41%. This generation was influenced by the Vietnam War, the civil rights movement, the Kennedy and King assassinations, Woodstock, and the Watergate Scandal.

A trend of protest against power characterized these formative events, which propelled many of the individuals in this generation into leadership positions in their fields. The Baby Boomers started the workaholic trend, and are known for being competitive, risk-takers, and loyal towards their employers and colleagues (Karp, Fuller, & Sirias, 2002; Niemiec, 2000). Like their parents, who were Silents, Baby Boomers were raised to respect authority figures, yet wanted to be viewed as equals, and learned not to "trust anyone over 30" (Karp et al., 2002). They dislike authoritarianism and micromanage others (Francis-Smith, 2004). They equate work with self-worth, contribution, and personal fulfillment (Yang & Guy, 2006, p. 270). Some have described them as being more process-oriented than result-oriented (Zemke, Raines, & Filipczak, 2000), although they have also been characterized as being goal-oriented Baby Boomers value health and wellness as well as personal growth and gratification (Zemke et al., 2000), and seek job security (Rath, 1999).

Generation X

The U.S. Census Bureau defines this segment of the population as consisting of individuals born between 1968 and 1979. However, the upper limit of Generation X in some cases has been set as late as 1982. These are the children of the Baby Boomers and are characterized as being raised in the "dot-com era" and the age of entrepreneurship. Generation X accounts for about 29% to 30% of all people in the workforce. People from this generation grew up in a stagnant job market, full of corporate downsizing and limited wage mobility, and are referred to as the first generation to earn less than their parents did. These are the children of the workaholic Baby Boomers, and are often referred to as the "latchkey kids" or the Lost Generation. Some unique characteristics of Generation X is that they aspire more than previous generations to achieve a balance between work and life (American Management Association, 2007; Karp et al., 2002). Generation X'ers are more independent, autonomous, and self-reliant than previous generations (American Management Association, 2007; Zemke et al., 2000). They demonstrate strong technical skills, and value continuous learning and skill development (Bova & Kroth, 2001; Zemke et al., 2000). People from Generation X tend to be outcome-focused, and seek specific and constructive feedback on their performance and role.

This generation is likely to find a way to get things done smart, fast, and well, even if it means bending the rules. They tend to respond well to a coaching management style that provides prompt feedback, focuses upon results (Crampton & Hodge, 2006), and is "ruled by a sense of accomplishment and not the clock" (Joyner, 2000). X-ers naturally question authority figures and are not intimidated by them. They are adaptable to change (Zemke et al., 2000) and prefer flexible work schedules and environment (Joyner, 2000). They can tolerate work, as long as it is enjoyable (Karp et al., 2002). This generation approaches authority casually and are not afraid to ask questions. Although they are individualistic, Generation X'ers also like teamwork, collaborative work, and group decision making. (Corporate Leadership Council, 2002; Rath, 1999).

Generation Y

Generation Y, also known as the Millennials or Cyberkids, represent those that are born between 1980 and 1999. The lower limit for Generation Y may be as low as 1978, however, while the upper limit may be as high as 2002, depending on the source. This generation accounts for about 22% to 23% of all people within the workforce. This generation has been shaped by parental excesses, computers (Niemiec, 2000), and dramatic technological advances. One of the most frequently reported characteristics of this generation is their comfort with technology (Kersten, 2002). In general, Generation Y shares many of the characteristics of Xers, yet represent the most diverse generation of our time.

They are purported to value teamwork and collective action (Zemke et al., 2000), embrace diversity (The National Oceanographic and Atmospheric Office of Diversity, 2006), be optimistic (Kersten, 2002), and be adaptable to change (American Management Association, 2007). Furthermore, they seek flexibility (Martin, 2005), are independent, desire a more balanced life (Crampton & Hodge, 2006), are multi-taskers (The National Oceanographic and Atmospheric Office of Diversity, 2006), and are the most highly-educated generation in the workforce today. They are focused, but lack direction and initiative, which is why they often seek out rubrics and "samples" as guidelines in the classroom. They also value comprehensive training. They have been characterized as demanding and entitled (Martin, 2005), and as the most confident generation (Glass, 2007). Like Xers, Generation Y is also purported to be entrepreneurial, and as being less process-focused (Crampton & Hodge, 2006).

This generation will most likely have great influence in the occupational therapy academic world and the workforce. According to the most recent American Occupational Therapy Association Faculty Workforce Survey, the median age among occupational therapy faculty is 50, program directors is 52, and the average projected year for retirement is 2022 (AOTA, 2007b). This indicates a significant need for qualified and prepared occupational therapy educators in the near future. There is a perceived decline in work ethic among Generation Y, which is perhaps one of the major contributors of generational conflicts in the workplace today. For instance, Generation Y has been labeled the 'slacker' generation (American Management Association, 2007), and a common stereotype made by older generations such as Baby Boomers or Traditionalists is that "younger workers don't work as hard as the older do."

Another point of contention among generations is loyalty towards employers. While Traditionalists and Boomers have been characterized as being extremely loyal toward their employers, a lack of loyalty of younger workers, especially X-ers, has been noted. For instance, it has been postulated that X-ers may value their relationships with their co-workers above the relationship with their company, especially if a co-worker is a friend (Karp et al., 2002). As employees, Generation Y desires immediate feedback on performance, and need frequent validation on their role and performance. Generation Y is the most technically literate, educated, and ethnically diverse generation in history, as they were socialized in a digital world. Through their routine use of technology, they have mastered the art of multitasking, but they often lack interpersonal skills. Generation Y may also have difficulty relating to X-ers and Boomers. For instance, they may have hundreds of Facebook and Twitter "friends," but often few real personal connections.

While the Baby Boomer generation is known for their "live to work" attitude, Generation Y are known for a "work to live" attitude. For example, Generation Y's typically prefer more paid time off as opposed to an increase in salary or job promotion. Some companies are tackling the challenges of recruiting and retaining Generation Y employees by using innovative strategies tailored to the generation's characteristics. These techniques include providing on-site leadership academies, creating formal mentor programs to maximize access, and giving early chances to do meaningful work. To better reach Generation Y, some are streamlining the recruitment process, and providing longer vacations after shorter service. For similar reasons, some are building comprehensive intranet sites, allowing conversion of unused administrative leave into cash, and permitting conversion of health benefits into deferred compensation accounts (Southard & Lewis, 2004). Additionally, Generation Y responds well to the mentorship model, which will be discussed in Chapter 5, as an important strategy to develop professionalism.

In regards to the changing health care environment, Generation Y is the most recent cohort to enter the workforce. Far larger than the generation before it, much of Generation Y was raised in a time of economic expansion and prosperity. They exhibit a strong sense of morality and will fight for what is right. This generation values work-life balance, learning about their unique needs, and serving them accordingly.

Generation Z

Generation Z or the new Millennials, Always-on Generation, or the eGeneration, are those individuals born around 1995 and are most likely current college students. This generation is facing the toughest economics since Great Depression and is often described as very sheltered—the protected "baby on board" children—who were raised in the post-Columbine era and doused in antibacterial gels. They are very familiar with structure, in both school and their leisure, and were raised with a sense of 'special-ness', surrounded by many enrichment programs in the classroom and within extracurricular activities. Generation Z are confident, optimistic over-achievers, yet also embody this sense of entitlement which is observed in Generation Y.

Many Generation Z individuals believe they will be more successful than their parents, and may have grown up fantasizing about owning a million-dollar home right out of college. Due to a sense of over-achievement as a necessity, this generation admits to having many pressures and concerns, demonstrated by a higher prevalence of anxiety disorders and depression. According to the Anxiety and Depression Association of America (ADAA) (n.d.), anxiety disorders affect 1 in 8 children, and also commonly co-occurs with other disorders such as depression, eating disorders, and attention deficit disorders. Furthermore, anxiety disorders are one of the most common mental health problems on college campuses. Forty million U.S. adults suffer from an anxiety disorder, and 75% of them experience their first episode of anxiety by age 22. A study commissioned by the American Psychological Association (2012) reported that the millennials are the most stressed demographic. The study asked participants to rank their stress level on a scale of 1 ("little or no stress") to 10 ("a great deal of stress"). Millennials led the stress parade, with a 5.4 average. Boomers registered 4.7, and the group the study labeled the "Matures" gave themselves a 3.7. In addition, a 2009 Associated Press and mtvU survey of college students (Half of Us, 2009) found the following:

- 80% say they frequently or sometimes experience daily stress
- 34% have felt depressed at some point in the past three months
- 13% have been diagnosed with a mental health condition such as an anxiety disorder or depression
- 9% have seriously considered suicide in the past year

EFFECT OF MILLENNIALS AND GENERATION Z MINDSET ON OCCUPATIONAL THERAPY PRACTICE

By all accounts, Millennials are unlike preceding generations. They view the world differently and have redefined the meaning of success, personally and professionally. However, there is a consensus that professionalism is on the decline in America, especially among the younger generation. Differences between the generations in the workplace is not a new phenomenon, but there are clear illustrations in how Generation Y may be changing the professional work culture dramatically. By changing the way we educate, manage, and interact with Generation Y, we may facilitate greater intergenerational competence and ultimately have a more positive affect on professional practice in the occupational therapy workforce. The over-arching theme of this textbook is ... that professionalism needs to make a comeback!

Generation Z is extremely tech-savvy, which will benefit implementation of electronic health records and the continual emphasis on evidenced-based practice and telehealth. In later chapters, we will examine more closely the affect of these generational stereotypes on the occupational therapy student in the classroom, on fieldwork, and in clinical practice. While the personal and professional viewpoints presented in this chapter can be helpful to understand the various viewpoints of these generations, it is important to focus on each individual in his or her context and to avoid stereotypes.

Clearly, an inherent part of being an occupational therapy professional is influenced by an individual's internal set of values, beliefs, and mindset (Table 1-5). These intrinsic qualities are formed both by the individual's experience and the context in which his or her identity was formed. Sometimes positive use of these qualities may be more innate, and must simply be further developed to support professionalism. Other times, unfamiliar qualities must be consciously learned and practiced. Regardless of the origin, a large component of professionalism is rooted in and grows from within the individual occupational therapy practitioner

EXTRINSIC QUALITIES OF PROFESSIONALISM

"If you want to change attitudes, start with a change in behavior. In other words, begin to act the part, as well as you can, of the person you would rather be, the person you most want to become. Gradually, the old, fearful person will fade away."

—William Glasser, Psychiatrist

If intrinsic qualities refer to being a professional, extrinsic qualities refer to acting like a professional. These are contrasted with the idea of an extrinsic value, which depends on how much it generates intrinsic value, and is displayed outward such as such as one's behaviors, actions and contributions. Extrinsic qualities of professionalism refers to an individual's behavior, actions, and outward contributions to and affect on their profession and society. Therefore, displaying these extrinsic qualities demonstrates one's ability to apply their intrinsic professional values. Examples of extrinsic characteristics of professionalism include:

- Professional image, manners, and etiquette
- Time management, adaptability, and organizational skills
- Interpersonal skills and intelligence
- Teamwork
- Conflict management
- E-professionalism

Professional Image, Manners, and Etiquette

There is no way around the fact that people are assessed by their personal appearance. There, I said it! Appearances matter! In the academic and clinical environment, clean scrubs or attire, neat hair, clean shoes, and a well-groomed look makes the statement that you care about yourself as a person, and therefore you have the capacity to care about and for others. Practitioners who look sloppy or unkempt may be perceived by others as unorganized, lazy, and uncaring. If you do not care about yourself, how can you truly care for others? A little attention to how you look and portray yourself goes a long way to display your professionalism. In society today, consideration of the use of clothing, make-up, cologne, tattoos, and piercings are often part of the dialogue regarding professional image and professionalism. Although image is identified as an important aspect of professional behavior and conduct, everyone dreads having that awkward conversation or providing feedback to one of their peers, colleagues, or students about their dress, hygiene, and/or cleanliness.

Clothing

Why is what we wear, and how we wear it, important to being a professional? What does "business casual attire," "business attire," or "clinically-appropriate attire" mean?

The three main reasons for implementing a professional dress code or policy are:

- To ensure safety
- To present or create a professional or identifiable appearance to others
- To promote a positive working environment and limit distractions caused by provocative or inappropriate dress

Whether in the classroom, clinic, or workplace, professionals should avoid wearing clothing or displaying accessories that depict or allude to an obscenity, violence, or sex; advertises alcohol, tobacco, or illegal substances; or conveys political or religious opinions and other unsuitable slogans. As a professional, your clothing should be consistent with the culture of your environment. The dress code in a private-practice pediatric outpatient clinic will most likely be very different than for a practitioner who serves as a consultant to a high-powered large health care organization. For example, Steve Jobs, one of the most influential entrepreneurs and inventors from this century, was known for wearing his black turtleneck, Levi's jeans, and white shoes in each and every keynote and public appearance. Same with Mark Zuckerberg, creator and CEO of Facebook, who is notorious for his denim jeans and hoodie sweatshirts. Students and practitioners should follow the dress code policy established by their academic program or work place. However, here are a few general rules of thumb for professional dress:

- Clothing should be clean and pressed.
- Clothing should not to be worn in such a manner as to be inappropriately revealing or to expose undergarments. Avoid clothing that fits too tight, or reveals skin including cleavage, stomach, midriff, or low back.
- Shoes should be polished or clean and coordinate with your clothing.

TABLE 1-5
SUMMARY OF GENERATIONS

GENERATION	FORMATIVE EVENTS	SOCIALIZATION	VALUES	POSITIVE QUALITIES	
Generation Traditionalists 75 million born pre-1945; 6.5% of workforce	Great Depression World War II	Hardship; parent at home	Consistency, patriotism Conformity, discipline, and authority	Loyal, self-sacrificing, morals	
Baby Boomers 80 million born 1943-1965; 41% of workforce	Anti-war movement, Civil rights, Woodstock	Post-war prosperity, activism, increase in consumerism	Civil rights, reform, equality, optimism	Loyal, workaholic	
Generation X 46 million born 1968-1979; 30% of workforce	Globalization, dot.com boom	Latchkey kids, parents are workaholics	Balance between work and life	Independent, autonomous	
Generation Y 75 million born 1980-1999; 23% of workforce	Terrorism, violence	Trophy kids Structured life/live at home Child-centric era, helicopter parent Rewarded for for effort vs performance	Values innovation	Curious, energetic, civil, tech savvy, not afraid of change, multitasking	
Generation Z Always-On Year 2000 to present	Toughest economics since Great Depression; raised in the post-Columbine era	Very sheltered	Sense of entitlement	Confident, optimistic over-achievers	

TABLE 1-5 (CONTINUED)
SUMMARY OF GENERATIONS

AREAS OF NEED	WORK ETHIC	EDUCATIONAL VIEW	VIEW OF AUTHORITY	COMMUNICATION STYLE
Technology, adapting to change	Work is an obligation; tend to stay with company	A dream	Correlates seniority with age, respects experience, top-down hierarchy	Prefers face to face, formal
Wants it all, competitive, Micro-managers	Paid dues (comes in early, stays late), climbs ladder, adventurous	Hardworking	A birthright	Face to face
Lack loyalty Skeptical Reluctant to network	Job hop, outcome-focused	Value continuous learning and skill development	A way to get there	Like learning to be entertaining— "edutainment"— allow innovation and creativity
Expect to make decisions Need to achieve, demanding, lack direction/focus, interpersonal skills Tries to negotiate vs. earn	Entitlement and sense of validation, Desired immediate result Rely on external motivation vs. internal, lack maturity Lack self confidence and self-esteem	Incredible expense Micromanaged by parents so they expect it from educators and authority figures	Desire to have more control over their time, activities, and work culture Aren't' afraid to challenge authority, "what can you do for me?" attitude vs. "what I can do for you?"	Need a lot more coaching and modeling of interprofessional skills, Provide them a voice, assign work groups clarify big picture, mentor, work-life balance Informal i.e emoticons and texting lingo
Sense of over-achievement; admits to having many pressures and concerns, demonstrated by a higher prevalence of anxiety disorders and depression	Over-achievers	Sense of "special-ness' "surrounded by many enrichment programs in the classroom and within extra-curricular activities	Believe they will be more successful than parents	Informal

- If you have a moment's doubt about whether something is appropriate to wear in the workplace, don't wear it!

- You should always dress at least to the level of your direct authority. It is easier to "dress down" if you are over-dressed than it is to dress up if you are under-dressed.

- If you underdress, the affect is significant; if you overdress, the affect is minimal.

Jewelry, Piercings, and Tattoos

Tattoos, body art, and piercings are becoming more and more of a norm in today's society. According to a 2006 report in the Journal of the American Academy of Dermatology, 24% of Americans ages 18 to 50 reported having at least one tattoo, and one in seven reported at least one body piercing (Laumann & Derick, 2006). The study also revealed that tattooing was equally common in both sexes, but body piercing was more common among women. Notably, nearly one in ten respondents reported experiencing discrimination in the workplace related to body art. Many employers will have specific policies regarding concealing tattoos for their employees; in 2012, 60% of HR managers indicated on a survey that a tattoo could hinder a candidate's chance of being hired, an increase from 57% in 2011 (Polk-Lepson Research Group, 2012). Miller, McGlashan, Nicols, and Eure (2009) demonstrate both a trajectory of increasing prevalence of tattoos and piercings, as well as a continued stigma towards employees with them. Because of the increased prevalence of body art and tattoos and lack of change in opinions towards people with them, the regulation of their appearance in the classroom, health care environment, and the workplace has become more mainstream. While they can be viewed as a form of self-expression, they can also communicate an unprofessional, immature, and irresponsible message to our consumers, peers, and colleagues. Professionals in health care shall conceal all tattoos. In particular, tattoos containing words or images which depict or allude to the items referenced as inappropriate in the previous passage shall not be visible while engaged in work. It would be prudent for students and/or job candidates who have (or are considering getting) a visible tattoo to look into policies for tattoos held by potential future employers.

Jewelry and accessories worn in the workplace should be unassuming and complementary to the professional appearance. In most circumstances, discreet jewelry is acceptable. Discreet earrings are limited to no more than two ear piercings in each ear, and no large hoops or dangling earrings should be worn. Dangling earrings or necklaces in the health care environment may be hazardous during self-care or transfer training sessions, imposing a safety risk to both you and the patient. Body piercings other than in the ears shall not be visible while engaged in work.

Make-up, Perfume, and/or Cologne

Make-up, perfume and/or cologne should never be excessive or distracting. Whether you are a student or an educator, whether you work for a small non-profit organization, a large health care system, or something in between, chances are that you spend many hours a day in proximity to other people. Maintaining hygiene and a low-profile yet well-groomed professional appearance are essential. Here are a few recommendations:

- Keep hair style professional and modern.

- Use colognes, aftershave, and perfumes in moderation. (Avoid scents that may be overpowering, offensive, unpleasant, or distracting to others.)

- Choose subtle, natural, or neutral shades for make-up. (Avoid make-up that is flashy, glossy, and glittery.)

- Use light-colored nail polish, and keep nails manicured short. (Many health-care facilities strictly prohibit artificial nails and enforce a nail length of no more than ¼ inches due to hygiene reasons. Long nails are hard to maintain hygienically, and may cause injury to you or a potential patient.)

It appears that this advice may contradict the long-standing metaphor which states that you can't judge a book by its cover. However, being professional is all about your representation of what being professional means. Different people have different ways of being an effective professional, depending on context and personality. It is alright to develop your own representation of professionalism to reflect your individual professional identity. Demonstrating professionalism comes from a combination of displaying a professional image, having good manners and etiquette, and other behaviors.

Manners and Etiquette

"Your manners are always under examination, awarding or denying you high prizes when you least think of it."

—Ralph Waldo Emerson

Good manners and etiquette is essential for a professional. Etiquette is a "code of ethical behavior regarding professional practice or action among the members of a profession in their dealings with each other" ("Etiquette," 2017). The foundation of etiquette is basically behavior that is accepted as gracious and polite in social situations, as well as within cultural norms. Historically, good manners result from common sense and an individual's upbringing. Here is a short list of some common courtesies that should not be forgotten:

- Be polite! Say "please," "thank you," and "you're welcome"
- Address individuals by their surname—Mr. Smith, Mrs. Jones, Dr. Wells, etc.
- Wait to be asked to enter an office or room, or sit in a chair
- Don't interrupt when someone else is talking
- Give and receive compliments graciously
- Avoid put-downs or participating in "gossip"

More information regarding professional image, including visual examples, for the occupational therapy student in the classroom and on fieldwork will be discussed in Chapters 6 to 8.

Time Management, Adaptability, and Organizational Skills

Having a strong skill set in time management and organization is a must for a professional. This includes a combination of traits such as being punctual, adaptable, and flexible. In my childhood, I was taught a life lesson called Lombardi time, derived from the late, great, football coach Vince Lombardi. This phrase states "If you're early you're on time, if you're on time you're late, if you're late, don't bother showing" (Snarkville, 2009). A student who comes late to class or a colleague who arrives late to a meeting both send a clear message to those around them. This message most often includes negative connotations such as disrespect, immaturity, irresponsibility, and ultimately, unprofessionalism.

For instance, the employee that punches in on time, but then ever-so-comfortably takes time to "settle in" may have a morning that looks like this. First comes the stashing of personal items, then, the enjoyment of the requisite cup of coffee and breakfast pastry. Next up is a quick bathroom break—and don't forget the greetings that are necessary all around. By the time real work starts, a good 10 to 15 minutes have gone by. There are no specific statistics, but you can do the math. Multiply those few minutes by five days a week, times several—even tens—of employees, and you are talking about a hefty hunk of time and money. Benjamin Franklin once said that "time is money," and he was right! Being punctual strengthens and reveals your integrity. If you tell someone that you will meet them at a certain time, you have essentially made them a promise. If you say you'll be there at 8 o'clock, and yet arrive at 8:15, you have essentially broken that promise. Being on time shows others that you are a person of your word.

Being punctual also shows that you are dependable. A professional can always be found at his or her post, carrying out the duties that are needed for that time. People know that they can rely on a professional—that if he or she says they will be there, they will be there. But if an individual is not punctual, others cannot depend on them; they do not know where he or she will be when they need them. Their associates will begin to feel he or she cannot organize his or her own time, and these doubts will seep into matters beyond the clock, as it naturally raises the question: "If this person is careless about time, what else are they careless about?"

The occupational therapy profession has written extensively about adaptability. Occupational therapy practitioners are trained to assist individuals, organizations and populations to modify, or adapt their occupations and/or environment to ensure independent, success, and/or fulfillment. However, as professionals, it is important that we demonstrate a skill of being adaptable, which is the ability to adjust to new conditions or change. How you deal with expected or unexpected change is a true marker for professionalism. Former Prime Minister Winston Churchill once said "to improve is to change."

Due to changes in higher education, health care, technology, and the workforce, perhaps at no other time in recent history has the trait of adaptability been more important than it is now. The ability to demonstrate positive emotions and energy, be open to new ideas, and handle unexpected demands is a crucial requirement of a professional. Hercalitus, a Greek philosopher, once proclaimed the only thing that is constant is change ("Heraclitus," 2015). The health care environment is dynamic, complex, and requires health care professionals to be adaptable and flexible. Flexibility is a very important component of time management, and ultimately professionalism. Being flexible indicates that one is receptive to modification or adaptation. Employers appreciate workers that are both versatile and resourceful. Therefore, being a professional requires that an individual be flexible in both his or her thinking and his or her actions, which reflect emotional maturity and adjustment.

Organizing is all about keeping things in proper order. For any business, organization plays a significant role in helping an individual to achieve their goals. A study by Kerr and Zigmond (1986) identified that 67 percent of high school teachers viewed organizational skills as a crucial component necessary for student success. Practicing effective organizational skills will help you personally and professionally, and your good organization skills will be reflected in the completion of all of your everyday responsibilities. Organization also gives you a sense of control and allows for increased productivity (Table 1-6). People with strong organizational skills often achieve success in their personal and professional lives, as they use their time more efficiently and are more productive.

Interpersonal Skills and Intelligence

As you may have noticed, various skills are important to being professional, but two undeniably key aspects are interpersonal skills and interpersonal intelligence. Interpersonal skills can also be referred to as "people skills," "communication skills," or "social skills." Interacting with others appropriately and respectfully, communicating clearly and directly, and having the ability to relate to and feel comfortable with people at different levels are essential to being professional. In his book *Frames of Mind: The Theory of Multiple Intelligences*, Howard Gardner (1993) describes interpersonal intelligence as the ability to work cooperatively with others in a group, as well as the ability to communicate verbally and nonverbally with other people. According to Gardner, characteristics of Interpersonal Intelligence include:

- Good at communicating verbally
- Skilled at nonverbal communication

TABLE 1-6 STRATEGIES TO STAY ORGANIZED	
ROLE	**STRATEGY**
Student	Keep a planner or schedule book, and update frequently with upcoming meetings, deadlines, and due dates
Clinician	Use a checklist to organize patient caseload, or a calendar to schedule important meetings or due dates, e.g. when to acknowledge your time-card, submit reimbursement forms, or send productivity records to your administrator
Manager/Fieldwork Educator	Keep a calendar or checklist of dates of performance reviews, upcoming competencies, or midterm and final evaluations of students

- See situations from different perspectives
- Create positive relationships with others
- Good at resolving conflict in groups

In addition to exhibiting respect, interactions with other individuals should also be equal—meaning how you treat the receptionist, is the same as to how you treat the CEO, is how you treat the housekeeper, is the same as how you treat the surgeon, and so on and so forth. Communication is simply the act of transferring information from one place to another. Information can be conveyed via different methods, including written communication, verbal or oral communication, nonverbal communication, and listening skills.

Professionalism in written communication involves the ability to write clearly, concisely, legibly (if handwritten), use appropriate terminology, and attend to required formatting (regardless if it is a research paper that needs to be in APA formatting or preparing an abstract for dissemination of a research project or manuscript for a professional conference). Demonstration of acceptable spelling and grammar is also a must. Another important aspect of strong written communication is knowing your audience. For instance, in a medical setting, it may be necessary to use approved abbreviations during documentation. The use of text messages and emails is a modern form of written communication. Be cautious of certain features such as "reply all" and blind cc'ing, which have the potential to send written communication to unknown users.

Professional verbal or oral communication is more than just what you say, but how and when you say it. It includes word choice, clarity, tone of voice, affect, and volume. Professionals should be polite and respectful when they communicate verbally. Knowing your audience is also an important of verbal communication. For example, how you communicate with a patient will most likely be different than how you communicate with a colleague, and how you communicate with an administrator will also be different.

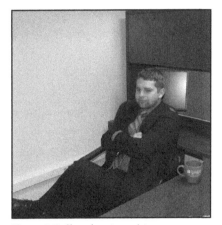

Figure 1-3. Closed posture picture.

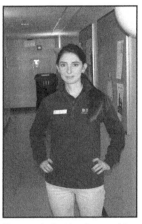

Figure 1-4. Hands on hips shows dominance.

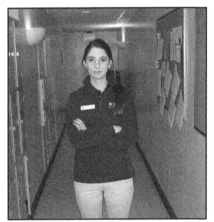

Figure 1-5. Crossed arms shows defensiveness and resistance.

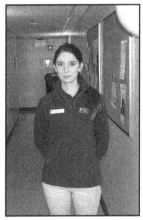

Figure 1-6. Arms around back shows passiveness and nervousness.

Nonverbal communication refers to what and how we communicate without the use of words. According to Mehrabian (1972), nonverbal communication accounts for 55% of how we communicate as human beings, whereas your actual "words" are only 7%. This includes:

- Body movements
- Eye contact
- Facial expression
- Use of touch
- Proxemics (personal space)

Body movements include gestures, postures and head, hand, or whole body movements. Open and closed postures may reflect an individual's degree of confidence, status or receptivity to another person. Someone seated in a closed position might have his or her arms folded, legs crossed, or be positioned at a slight angle from the person with whom they are interacting (Figures 1-3 to 1-5). This can give the impression of boredom, hostility, or detachment (Figure 1-6).

In an open posture, you might expect to see someone directly facing you with hands apart on the arms of the chair (Figure 1-7).

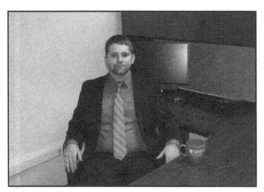

Figure 1-7. Open posture.

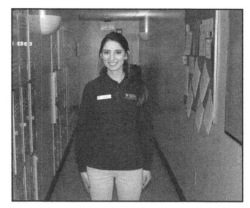

Figure 1-8. Open posture and good body language.

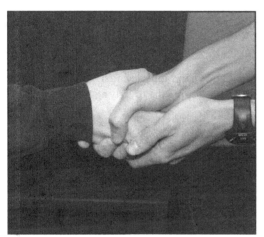

Figure 1-9. Hand hug handshake.

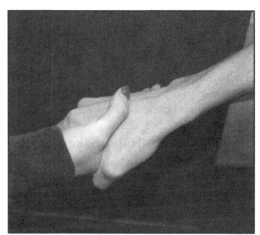

Figure 1-10. Dominator handshake.

An open posture can be used to communicate openness or interest in someone and a readiness to listen (Figure 1-8), whereas the closed posture might imply discomfort or disinterest. Open posture portrays friendliness (Mehrabian, 1972).

Hand movements, such as a handshake, communicate a lot about one's personality; this can demonstrate characteristics of one's professionalism and assist in developing rapport.

Unprofessional Handshakes

Hand Hug Handshake

This type of handshake is when one individual wraps both hands around the others hand. While it can be perceived as a warm, friendly gesture, it can also be misinterpreted as an invasion of intimacy, or unprofessional (Figure 1-9).

Dominator Handshake

This handshake is when one individual forcibly displays their palm downward, which can be interpreted as a sign of authority or domination (Figure 1-10).

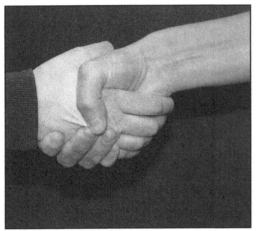

Figure 1-11. Bone crusher handshake.

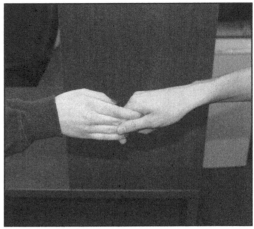

Figure 1-12. Queen fingertips handshake.

Bone Crusher Handshake

This handshake may make your knuckles white, and your hand muscles hurt. This handshake may appear to demonstrate confidence, however, it can be interpreted as overly aggressive, intimidating, and authoritative (Figure 1-11).

Queen Fingertips Handshake

This handshake occurs when an individual outstretches his or her hand from a distance, only allowing the other person to barely grasp two or three fingers, without a good grip of the hand. It causes an awkward embrace (Figure 1-12) (The Guardian Jobs, 2007; Sol, n.d.).

Professional Handshake

To demonstrate a good handshake, you should:

- Keep the fingers together with the thumb up and open (Figure 1-13)
- Slide your hand into the other person's, so that each person's web of skin between thumb and forefingers touches the other's (Figure 1-14)
- Squeeze firmly (Figure 1-15)

A proper handshake should last from 3 to 6 seconds, be equally balanced (meaning each person's hand is vertically side by side), thumbs locked around each other's upper hand, and fingers in a firm grip. Always reciprocate the same amount of pressure you are receiving from the other person's hand, and release after the shake. A good handshake includes eye contact with the person.

One of the most important nonverbal communication skills is eye contact. Eye contact helps you capture attention, shows that you have genuine interest and respect, exhibits honesty/sincerity, shows confidence, and your eyes strengthen your message when you have passion and enthusiasm. In fact, physiologically, there is some truth to the familiar analogy of having that "twinkle" or "sparkle" in your eye. When a person is authentically interested in a conversation, there is a chemical released, the hormone oxytocin, and their eyes dilate (Leknes et al., 2013). This sparkle inspires the listener, letting them know that your adrenaline is up and that you are interested and engaged. Making and maintaining eye contact is not only important, it is an essential part of professionalism.

Eye contact refers to the act of looking directly into another's eyes, or a meeting of eyes of two persons, regarded as a meaningful, nonverbal form of communication. It does not mean staring into someone's eyes without taking a break. Not enough eye contact and people can deem you

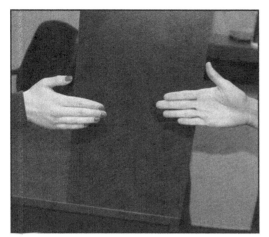

Figure 1-13. Professional handshake 1.

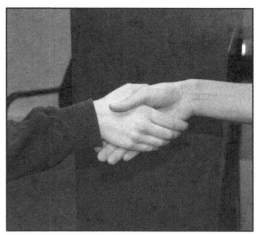

Figure 1-14. Professional handshake 2.

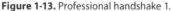

Figure 1-15. Professional handshake 3.

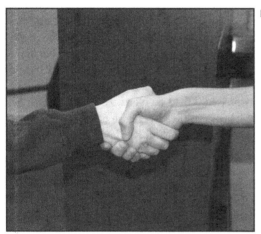

untrustworthy or disinterested, and excessive eye contact may be misconstrued to be inappropriate. According to Toastmasters International (2011), appropriate eye contact includes 3 to 5 seconds of constant engagement of a listener before you look away. It is important to note that how and when you make eye contact may depend on the customs of where you are, and who you are with. For example, some cultures consider making direct eye contact aggressive, rude, or a show of disrespect. While direct and prolonged eye contact is seen as a sign of respect and trustworthiness in Western culture, it may seem like a sign of disrespect if you look directly at a superior in Eastern cultures. Eye contact is a very important nonverbal communication skill to master use of.

An individual's facial expressions can communicate a lot to the external world. Your face is the primary source for communicating your emotions. During oral communication, our facial expressions change continually and are constantly observed and interpreted by the listener. Examples can include a smile, frown, raised eyebrow, eye-rolling, grimace, or sneer. These expressions either enhance, emphasize, or disagree with the spoken statement. I believe that the age-old adage that smiles are contagious is true! Try it out. Turn to your partner and say the following statement without smiling: "Today will be a great day." Now, repeat the same statement, but do it with a big smile on your face! What did you notice? Did the tone of the message change?

Haptic communication refers to the ways in which people and other animals communicate and interact through the sense of touch (Straker, n.d.). Touch is extremely important for humans,

Figure 1-16. Schematic of proxemics.

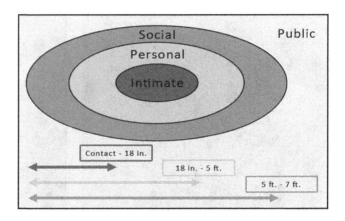

and is vital in conveying emotion, appreciation, inclusion, support, affection, attention-seeking, personal interaction, and task-orientation. The use of touch can include a handshake, or a tap on the shoulder. Professionals should know the effectiveness of touch while communicating, but need to be cautious and understand how touch can be understood. A hand on the shoulder could be interpreted as a supportive gesture, or could potentially mean an inappropriate advance to another person. When working with others, you need to be aware of each person's touch tolerance.

Proxemics, or the use of personal space, is an often overlooked component of nonverbal communication skills (Sheppard, 1996). The four main distances that can be described as the norm in Western Society and they are intimate distance, personal distance, social distance and public distance. Each of these proxemics has a close and far phase (Skills You Need, 2016).

Intimate Distance: Ranges from close contact (touching) to the 'far' phase of 15 cm to 45 cm. In British society, this tends to be seen as an inappropriate distance for public behavior and, as mentioned above, entering the intimate space of another person with whom you do not have a close relationship can be extremely disturbing.

Personal Distance: The 'far' phase of personal distance is considered to be the most appropriate for people holding a conversation. At this distance, it is easy to see the other person's expressions and eye movements, as well as their overall body language. Handshaking can occur within the bounds of personal distance (Figure 1-16).

Social Distance: This is the normal distance for impersonal business, for example working together in the same room, or during social gatherings. Seating is also important; communication is far more likely to be considered as a formal relationship if the interaction is carried out across a desk. In addition, if the seating arrangements are such that one person appears to look down on another, an effect of domination may be created. At a social distance, speech needs to be louder and eye contact remains essential to communication; otherwise, feedback will be reduced and the interaction may end.

Public Distance: Educators and public speakers address groups at a public distance. At this distance, exaggerated nonverbal communication is necessary for communication to be effective. Subtle facial expressions are lost at this distance, so clear hand gestures are often used as a substitute. Larger head movements are also typical of an experienced public speaker who is aware of changes in the way body language is perceived at longer distance.

Listening

Contrary to popular belief, there is a difference between hearing and listening. Hearing is a passive occurrence where the physical manifestation of sound waves are transmitted to the ear, into the brain, and are processed into audible information. Simply put, hearing is the act of perceiving sound by the ear. Listening, on the other hand, requires an active, conscious choice to involve the processes of concentration and learning. The art of listening is another component of communication skills that is often overlooked. Active listening is an interactive process that involves all senses, comprehension and mindfulness to assess verbal and nonverbal communication (Clark, 2003). Good listening skills in a health care provider's interactions are one of the behaviors most highly correlated with client satisfaction, as is the behavior of a provider who does not interrupt when the client is speaking (Wanzer, Booth-Butterfield, & Gruber, 2004). To be truly professional, we must listen actively to those around us, whether they are our peer, supervisor, client, or the family of our client; we must listen to all of them with equal respect and mindfulness.

The ability to communicate information accurately, clearly, and as intended is a vital life skill whose importance should not be disregarded. Studies show that the communication skills of health care professionals do not necessarily improve over time or with clinical experience (Fallowfield et al., 2002). Therefore, there is a need to specifically focus on improving communication skills with formal educational training. This will mainly begin in the classroom, and continue on in fieldwork education as well as in clinical practice. Specific to health care, patients' perceptions of the quality of the health care they received are highly dependent on the quality of their interactions with their health care clinician and team (Institute for Healthcare Communication, 2011). This desired rapport between an occupational therapy practitioner and a client in occupational therapy literature is defined as therapeutic use of self. Mosey (1986) discusses therapeutic use of self as "the use of oneself in such a way that one becomes an effective tool in the evaluation and intervention process" (p. 199).

Teamwork

Teamwork has been described as the combined action of a group of people, especially when effective and efficient ("Teamwork," 2016). The importance of a team-based approach in health care is not new, and has in fact evolved over time. Teamwork has to be more than just a group of clinicians who happen to work with the same patient or in the same facility. Being a professional team player involves the skill of working constructively with others, while also having a keen sense of personal responsibility. Part of being a professional in health care is figuring out how each of our individual contributions and actions affect the actions and work of others and the patient. Communication skills are an important aspect of teamwork, but just one part of a wider skill set that includes networking, building relationships, and creating a culture that supports both the exchange of thought processes and allows feedback to happen organically and regularly. More information regarding team-based approaches and interprofessional professionalism will be discussed in Chapter 3.

Conflict Management

Conflict arises in every person's personal and professional life at some point in time. Conflict arises from differences. It occurs whenever people disagree in their values, motivations, perceptions, ideas, or desires. Sometimes these differences appear to be trivial, but when a conflict triggers strong feelings, a deep personal and relational need is at the core of the problem—a need to feel safe and secure, a need to feel respected and valued, or a need for greater closeness and intimacy. The key to resolving conflict is to maintain professionalism. Regardless of the type of conflict that presents itself, maintaining an environment of respect in spite of differences is vital to sustaining a professional work environment. Colleagues who listen attentively and respectfully to one another's viewpoints, however different they may be, are better positioned to work through troubling issues and reach a consensus. Professionals learn to disagree without being disagreeable.

Compromise is a professional, effective way to resolve conflict in the workplace. A compromise essentially involves a give and take between disagreeing parties, often overseen by a mediator ("Compromise," 2016). A compromise settlement allows conflicted colleagues the opportunity to maintain their professional position on a matter while creating an equitable and respectful agreement; for example, if an adolescent desires to stay out with friends until midnight, but the parents request that their child be home by 10 o'clock. If both parties were to agree to an 11 o'clock curfew, that would be a compromise. In a clinical setting, a department manager and staff members may have opposing viewpoints in scheduling staff during legal holidays. The department manager believes that this should be a random, lottery-like process, while the staff members believe it should be completed based upon seniority (date of hire). A compromise would be when the legal holidays are divided up into two groups, and half of the holidays are determined by lottery, and the other half by seniority.

In no instance should professional individuals resort to name calling, threats, or undermining work efforts when conflicts arise. Professionals should treat others with respect, and use their critical thinking skills to attempt to handle the conflict on their own, but be knowledgeable about following the proper chain of command when necessary. For example, in the classroom setting, if a student has a concern within a particular course, the student should first go to the course instructor to try to resolve the issue, not the Dean of the school or the Chancellor of the University. During a fieldwork experience, if a fieldwork student has an issue with their fieldwork educator, they should first attempt to communicate and resolve the issue with the fieldwork educator, under support of the Academic Fieldwork Coordinator, prior to involving the facility director or department head. In closing, professionals should strive to learn from mistakes, always trying to improve, refrain from holding grudges, and move past difficulties.

E-PROFESSIONALISM

Within the past 20 years, technology and cyberspace advances have brought many new and exciting concepts to our culture: email, video conferencing, webinars, text messaging, blogs, social media networking sites, smart devices, apps, to name just a few. These innovations have changed the way we communicate with our colleagues, patients, selves, and society. They have provided us, as well as consumers, immediate access to information. They allow us to meet new people without leaving the comfort of our own home, school, or job. They allow us to quickly search for evidence to support and/or justify clinical intervention. They allow individuals who live in rural areas of the country to engage in telehealth and receive access to various health care and therapeutic services. However, with these pleasures and advantages also come disadvantages and potential professional pitfalls. It is just as important to instruct future health care professionals about how to act, dress, and portray themselves in cyberspace as it is person.

According to the third edition of the *Occupational Therapy Practice Framework: Domain and Process*, the virtual environment or context refers to interaction which occurs in "simulated, real-time or near-real-time situations, absent of physical contact" (AOTA, 2014, p. S28). As an occupational therapy student, fieldwork educator, or clinician, there are various occupations that take place in a virtual context, such as communication and documentation. In recent literature, the term *e-professionalism* has been used to describe the etiquette of using technology, social media, and navigating cyberspace that reflect traditional professionalism paradigms (Kaczmarczyk et al., 2013). These attitudes and behaviors of e-professionalism are no different than the intrinsic and extrinsic qualities of professionalism that have already been discussed in this chapter. The American Medical Association has made strong statements surrounding this concept, including a part of medical curricula (American Medical Association, 2011). Other health care professional academic programs are making clear policies to guide student behavior in classroom, as well as model expectations in the real world (Ventola, 2014). Clinical sites and employers are also creating social media or technology policies to govern their employee and student use. For example, many health care facilities now have social media guidelines and policies for employees to ensure that their social networking activity does not interfere with the workplace, as well as federal legislation such as Health Insurance Portability and Accountability Act.

| TABLE 1-7 |
| CLINICAL USES OF TECHNOLOGY |

USES	POSITIVES	POTENTIAL PROBLEMS
Billing	Storage	Privacy/security concerns
Apps for treatment	Mobility	Loss or theft of device
Voice-activated interfaces	Speed	Poor bandwidth/speed of connection or application
Narration	Efficiency	
Telemedicine; consultation or treatment tool between client and remote therapist		Distractors, pop ups, notifications

It could be argued in some sense that the 24/7 access to technology, especially for individuals within Generations Y and Z, is eroding certain long-standing principles of professionalism. Text-based communication is growing at a rapid pace. Research indicates that the use of hand-held mobile devices, such as tablets and smartphones, has increased significantly in recent years (Berolo, Wells, & Amick, 2011). Although 83% of adults between the ages of 18 and 29 own a smartphone, mobile device ownership among college students is even higher; according to a 2014 EDUCAUSE report, 86% of undergraduates owned a smartphone, and nearly half (47%) owned a tablet (Dahlstrom & Bichsel, 2014).

There is a growing body of evidence that suggests that texting and emailing has fostered poorer spelling and grammar during written communication (Barker, 2007; Crystal, 2008). Text lingo or textism is the language used in text messages, characterized by the use of single letters and symbols (such as emojis) and abbreviations, which can include BTW (by the way), BRB (be right back), tho (though) or IIRC (if I remember correctly). The concern arises when this text lingo makes its way into more professional scenarios such as school assignments, clinical documentation, or work memos.

Smart Device Use

The use of mobile devices such as smartphones and tablets is rapidly increasing in both social and work-based contexts (Madden & Smith, 2010; Sadeh, 2011; Solove, 2007). Let's be honest … smart devices have almost become an additional appendage to our bodies. It is almost like a Pavlovian response to check your device when you hear it ding, vibrate, or ring (Pavlov, 1960). However, it is necessary for professionals to be aware of appropriate and inappropriate scenarios to use smart devices and technology. Here are some basic guidelines providing certainty around the use of smart devices in clinical practice and the professional world (Table 1-7).

In the academic setting, it can be beneficial to use smart devices. Many academic programs require their students to use some type of smart device in the classroom. For example, a smart device can be used to access a web-based platform such as Blackboard or Moodle to communicate with peers and faculty, to access course materials, to access library materials, or to perform evidenced-based literature searches. Quick response (QR) codes are a type of mobile-readable bar code that can also be used by smart devices. By using the camera feature, QR codes can be scanned and then automatically provide linkage to websites or resources. For example, an occupational therapy classroom would have QR codes listed around the room for the AOTA website. However, there are some negative implications to smart device presence. The use of technology and smart devices in the classroom can be a distraction. As an instructor, how do you ensure that your students are using their laptop to take notes and follow along with the PowerPoint lecture? Are they using their device to enhance their classroom experience, or are they online shopping, using a personal social media network, or doing unrelated work?

Social Media

The use of social media and social networking sites and/or apps has evolved quickly over the course of recent decades. In an individual's personal life, social media can be an easy way to communicate with friends and family, and to share life events. In the professional world, it can provide a platform to disseminate evidence or scholarly work, and foster collegiality and camaraderie within the profession through networking. Similar to the use of smart devices, the accessibility and routine use of social media can present professional pitfalls. Several important issues are:

- Privacy and confidentiality
- Professional boundaries
- Professional image

Privacy and Confidentiality

Regardless of how you have set-up your privacy settings, social media is a public forum. Through the use of various features such as "likes," "share," and "hashtags" (#), information that you initially intended for one audience has the possibility of being shared with a much wider and unintended audience. For example, let's imagine an occupational therapy student whose profile has strict privacy settings; this person posts a blurb about something that occurred during fieldwork. The student's mother, who is in their social media network, "likes" the page. Anyone who is now in the mother's network now has the possibility of viewing this information. More recently, there are new networking sites that have time-released features, where a post or picture will appear for a short-time frame and then supposedly be deleted. Health Insurance Portability and Accountability Act violations can be both intentional and unintentional; therefore, even a light-hearted post or an innocent picture regarding a patient, health care institution, or workplace scenario has potential civil and legal consequences. Professionals have a responsibility to remain ethical and abide by all privacy and confidentiality policies and legislation at all times.

Professional Boundaries

Social media promotes networking. In the professional setting, it can create blurring of professional boundaries between student and faculty, and between patient and health care provider. This must be avoided consciously at all costs. Maintaining appropriate boundaries within the therapeutic relationship is not only suggested by the literature, but also specifically upheld at the professional level; this can be seen in the Occupational Therapy Code of Ethics (AOTA, 2015) under Principle 4, Justice.

Professional Image

Social media profile pages can be viewed by your educators, colleagues, prospective employers, and anyone else who wishes to search your name and 'see what you are about'. Yes, there are privacy settings, and if you are technology-savvy, you may have yours set so that only the people you want can see your page. However, what if you are not so good with technology? Or better yet, can you be entirely sure that the fieldwork educator and/or instructor you're complaining about isn't the relative or neighbor of one of your friends? Perceptions may be based on any of the information featured in a social media profile, such as photos, nicknames, posts, and comments liked or shared, as well as the friends, causes, organizations, games, and media that a person follows. With that in mind, it is essential to remain professional and adhere to our code of ethics at all times when we are posting things that nearly anyone can read. Your opinion is your opinion, but you

Box 1-3

- Be knowledgeable about your privacy settings
- Never post or comment anything about a patient or a health care setting
- Clean up your "virtual image": delete inappropriate photos, comments, or pages your profile may be linked with
- Do not be afraid to untag yourself from something inappropriate
- Above all, be a responsible and ethical Internet user!

never know who you will offend with your words. If you have to think twice about a post you are about to send, chances are you probably shouldn't send it. Bottom line: you never know who might be looking (Box 1-3)!

Summary of Extrinsic Factors

The extrinsic qualities discussed in this chapter enable the principles of professionalism to be enacted and observed by those around you. Awareness and portrayal of these extrinsic factors is crucial to becoming and being a professional. Both intrinsic and extrinsic attributes of professionalism as discussed in this chapter will be referred to throughout this text, specifically within various contexts such as the classroom, fieldwork, and the clinic.

SUMMARY

This chapter introduced you to the general concepts and terminologies associated with professionalism. You learned that professionalism and the associated words discussed in this chapter have a wide range of uses and interpretations, and that it all tends to raise many questions. Now that you have a better understanding of what constitutes professionalism, you can ask yourself: are you demonstrating these characteristics to the people around you? As an occupational therapy student, it is likely that you are already exhibiting some of these internal and external characteristics, but you may find yourself lacking in some areas, or potentially unaware of the importance of others. This text will challenge you to build your own sense of professionalism and a professional identity as an occupational therapy practitioner.

Professionalism is one of those concepts that is so familiar to all associated with it, yet so complex that each of those people could each have a different understanding of its meaning. However, it is undeniable that professionalism is a trait that is highly valued, not only in the occupational therapy profession, but within society as a whole. As stated previously, there is currently no formal definition of professionalism within the occupational therapy profession. For the purpose of this text, the following definition should be used.

> Professionalism in occupational therapy clinical practice is a dynamic sophistication exemplified by a combination of an individual's personal skill set, knowledge, behaviors, and attitudes, and the adoption of the moral and ethical values of the profession and society.

Promoting this multifaceted definition of professionalism, and more importantly, establishing a recognized body of individuals who possess these internal and external characteristics, will have a number of tangible benefits that will accrue to the individual, client, occupational therapy profession, and society as a whole. Appearances and conduct are important, but these are underpinned by senses of internal values, attitudes, and behavior that are displayed by a person's approach to work and the way they relate to, work with, and communicate with others. The development of professionalism in not unlike human development, which "flows along a continuum that is not linear but bumpy, at times convoluted and unpredictable, and certainly only partially planned. Many choose to go with the flow, content to make the best of what befalls them" (Robertson & Savio, 2003).

LEARNING ACTIVITIES

1. Using the information gathered in this chapter, as a foundation, how would you define professionalism?

2. Provide examples of professional and unprofessional behavior in your personal and professional life.

3. Think of a person you consider to be a professional. What attributes does this person possess? How does this person interact with others? How does this person react to stress or conflict? Describe what makes this person a professional.

4. Identify a person in your life from each of the five generations discussed in this chapter. Compare and contrast qualities and viewpoints in their personal and professional lives.

REFERENCES

American Management Association. (2007). Leading the four generations at work. Retrieved from http://www.ama-net.org/training/articles/leading-the-four-generations-at-work.aspx

American Management Association. (2012). American Management Association 2012 critical skills survey. Retrieved from http://playbook.amanet.org/wp-content/uploads/2013/03 /2012-Critical-Skills-Survey-pdf.pdf

American Medical Association. (2011). Professionalism in the use of social media. In *AMA code of medical ethics (Section 9)*. Retrieved from http://www.ama-assn.org/ama/pub/ physician-resources/medical-ethics/code-medical-ethics/opinion9124.page

American Occupational Therapy Association. (1993). Occupational therapy roles. *American Journal of Occupational Therapy, 47*(12), 1087-1099.

American Occupational Therapy Association. (1999). Guide for supervision of occupational therapy personnel in the delivery of occupational therapy services. *American Journal of Occupational Therapy, 53*, 592-594.

American Occupational Therapy Association. (2007a). AOTA's American Centennial Vision and executive summary. *American Journal of Occupational Therapy, 61*(6), 613-614.

American Occupational Therapy Association. (2007b). *2007 Faculty workforce survey*. Bethesda, MD: AOTA Press.

American Occupational Therapy Association. (2014). Occupational therapy practice framework: Domain and process (3rd ed.). *American Journal of Occupational Therapy, 68*(Suppl. 1), S1-S48.

American Occupational Therapy Association. (2015). Occupational therapy code of ethics. Retrieved from http://www.aota.org/-/media/corporate/files/practice/ethics/code-of-ethics.pdf

American Physical Therapy Association. (2010). APTA guide for professional conduct. Retrieved from http://www.apta.org/uploadedFiles/APTAorg/Practice_and_Patient_Care/Ethics/ GuideforProfessionalConduct.pdf

American Physical Therapy Association. (2013). Code of ethics for the physical therapist. Retrieved from http://www.apta.org/uploadedFiles/APTAorg/About_Us/Policies/Ethics/CodeofEthics.pdf#search=%22code%20of%20 ethics%22

American Psychological Association. (2012). Stress by generation. *Stress in America 2012* (section 6). Retrieved from http://www.apa.org/news/press/releases/stress/2012/ generations.aspx

American Speech-Language-Hearing Association. (2016). Code of ethics. Retrieved from http://www.asha.org/uploadedFiles/ET2010-00309.pdf

Anxiety and Depression Association of America. (n.d.) Children and teens. Retrieved from http://www.adaa.org/living-with-anxiety/children

Bannigan, K. (2000). Passion is our greatest asset in marketing occupational therapy. *British Journal of Occupational Therapy, 63*(10), 463.

Barker, I. (2007, February 2). Txts r gr8 but not in exams. *Times Educational Supplement.* Retrieved from https://www.tes.com/article.aspx?storycode=2341958

Beauchamp, T. L., & Childress, J. F. (2012). *Principles of biomedical ethics,* (7th ed.). New York, NY: Oxford University Press.

Behavior. (2016, January 26). In Merriam-Webster dictionary. Retrieved from http://www.merriam-webster.com/dictionary/behavior

Benner, P. (1984). *From novice to expert: Excellence and power in clinical nursing practice.* Menlo Park, CA: Addison-Wesley.

Benner, P. A. (2004). Using the Dreyfus model of skill acquisition to describe and interpret skill acquisition and clinical judgment in nursing practice and education. *Bulletin of Science, Technology, & Society, 24*(3), 188-199.

Berolo, S., Wells, R. P., & Amick, B. C. (2011). Musculoskeletal symptoms among mobile hand-held users and their relationship to device use: A preliminary study in a Canadian university population. *Applied Ergonomics, 42*(2), 371-378.

Bierema, L. (2011). Reflections on the profession and professionalization of adult education. *PAACE Journal of Lifelong Learning, 20,* 21-36.

Boutin-Lester, P., & Gibson, R. W. (2002). Patients' perceptions of home health occupational therapy. *Australian Occupational Therapy Journal, 49*(3), 146–154.

Bova, B., & Kroth, M. (2001). Workplace learning and generation X. *Journal of Workplace Learning, 13*(2), 57-65.

Brayman, S. J., Clark, G. F., DeLany, J. V., Garza, E. R., Radomski, M. V., Ramsey, R., ... & Liberman, D. (2009). Guidelines for supervision, roles, and responsibilities during the delivery of occupational therapy services. *American Journal of Occupational Therapy, 63*(6), 797-803.

Brykcznski, K. A. (2010). Benner's philosophy in nursing practice. In M. R. Alligood (Ed.), *Nursing theory: Utilization and application* (4th ed., pp. 137-159). Maryland Heights, MO: Mosby Elsevier.

Bureau of Labor Statistics. (2016). Labor force statistics from the current population survey. Retrieved from http://www.bls.gov/cps/

Clark, P. A. (2003). Medical practices' sensitivity to patients' needs: Opportunities and practices for improvement. *Journal of Ambulatory Care Management, 26*(2), 110-123.

Competence. (2016, January 1). In Dictionary.com. Retrieved from http://dictionary.reference.com/browse/competence

Compromise. (2016, January 1). In Dictionary.com. Retrieved from http://dictionary.reference.com/browse/compromise

Cooper, J. E. (2012). Reflections on the professionalization of occupational therapy: Time to put down the looking glass. *Canadian Journal of Occupational Therapy, 79*(4), 199-209.

Corporate Leadership Council. (2002). *Building the high-performance workforce: A quantitative analysis of the effectiveness of performance management strategies.* Washington, DC: Corporate Executive Board.

Crampton, S. M., & Hodge, J. W. (2006). The supervisor and generational differences. *Proceedings of the Academy of Organizational Culture, Communications and Conflict, 11,* 19-22.

Crystal, D. (2008). *Txting: The gr8 db8.* Oxford, United Kingdom: Oxford University Press.

Dahlstrom, E., & Bichsel, J. (2014). ECAR study of undergraduate students and informationtechnology, 2014. Retrieved from https://net.educause.edu/ir/library/pdf/ss14/ers1406.pdf

Dependability. (2016, January 1). In Your Dictionary. Retrieved from http://www.yourdictionary.com/dependability

Dickinson, R. (2003). Occupational therapy: A hidden treasure. *Canadian Journal of Occupational Therapy, 70*(3), 133-135.

Dreyfus, H., & Dreyfus, S. (1980). *A five-stage model of mental activities involved in directed skill acquisition.* Berkeley, CA: Operations Research Center, University of California.

Driscoll, J. W. (2002). Paradigms for assessment: Women's knowledge and skill attainment. *American Journal of Maternal/Child Nursing, 27*(5), 288-293.

Electronic Oberlin Group. (n.d.). The Reverend Dr. Martin Luther King, Jr. at Oberlin. Retrieved from http://www.oberlin.edu/external/EOG/BlackHistoryMonth/MLK/MLKmainpage.html.

Emotional Intelligence. (2017). In Dictionary.com. Retrieved from http://www.dictionary.com/browse/emotional-intelligence?s=t

Employee. (2017). In Dictionary.com. Retrieved from http://www.dictionary.com/browse/employee?s=t

Epstein, R. M., & Hundert, E. M. (2002). Defining and assessing professional competence. *Journal of the American Medical Association, 287,* 226-235.

Etiquette. (2017). In Dictionary.com. Retrieved from http://www.dictionary.com/browse/etiquette

Fallowfield, L., Jenkins, V., Farewell, V., Saul, J., Duffy, A., & Eves, F. (2002). Efficacy of a cancer research UK communication skills training model for oncologists: A randomized control trial. *The Lancet, 359,* 650-656.

Fisher, A. (1998). Utilizing practice and theory in an occupational framework. *American Journal of Occupational Therapy, 52*(7), 509-521.

Fleming, M. H. (1991). The therapist with the three-track mind. *American Journal of Occupational Therapy, 45*(11), 1007-1014.

Fleming, M. H. (1994). The search for tacit knowledge. In C. Mattingly & M. H. Fleming (Eds.), *Clinical reasoning: Forms of inquiry in a therapeutic practice* (pp. 22-33). Philadelphia, PA: F. A. Davis.

Friedman, M. B. (2011, Spring). "Generational competence": A conceptual framework for an aging America. Retrieved from http://www.michaelbfriedman.com/mbf/images/stories/GENERATIONAL_COMPETENCE.pdf

Francis-Smith, J. (2004, August 26). Surviving and thriving in the multigenerational workplace. Retrieved from https://www.questia.com/newspaper/1P2-2120458/ surviving-and-thriving-in-the-multigenerational-workplace

Gardner, H. (1993). *Frames of mind: The theory of multiple intelligences.* New York, NY: Basic Books.

Generation. (2016, February 5). In Merriam-Webster dictionary. Retrieved from http://www.merriam-webster.com/dictionary/generation

Glass, A. (2007). Understanding generational differences for competitive success. *Industrial and Commercial Training, 39*(2), 98-103.

Gripper, P. (2008). Letter to the editor: The image of occupational therapy in mental health. *British Journal of Occupational Therapy, 71*(1), 40-41.

The Guardian Jobs. (2007). The top 10 handshakes. Retrieved from https://jobs.theguardian.com/article/the-top-10-handshakes/

Half of Us. (2009). mtvU AP 2009 economy, college stress and mental health poll. Retrieved from http://www.halfofus.com/wp-content/uploads/2013/10/mtvU-AP-2009-Economy-College-Stress-and-Mental-Health-Poll-Executive-Summary-May-2009.pdf

Heraclitus. (2015, October 25). In Wikiquote. Retrieved from https://en.wikiquote.org/wiki/Heraclitus

Hill, W. T., Jr. (2000). White paper on pharmacy student professionalism. *Journal of the American Pharmaceutical Association, 40*(1), 96-102.

Institute for Healthcare Communication. (2011, July). Impact of communication in healthcare. Retrieved from http://healthcarecomm.org/about-us/impact-of-communication-in-healthcare/

Integrity. (2017). In Dictionary.com. Retrieved from http://www.dictionary.com/browse/integrity?s=t

Joyner, T. (2000, May 1). Gen X-ers focus on life outside the job fulfillment. Retrieved from http://findarticles.com/p/articles/mi_qa5352/is_200005/ ai_n21455443

Kaczmarczyk, J. M., Chuang, A., Dugoff, L., Abbott, J. F., Cullimore, A. J., Dalrymple, J. … & Casey, P. M. (2013). e-Professionalism: A new frontier in medical education. *Teaching and Learning in Medicine, 25*(2), 165-170.

Karp, H., Fuller, C., & Sirias, D. (2002). *Bridging the boomer-Xer gap. Creating authentic teams for high performance at work.* Palo Alto, CA: Davies Black Publishing.

Kerr, M. M., & Zigmond, N. (1986). What do high school teachers want? A study of expectations and standards. *Education & Treatment of Children, 9*(3), 239–249.

Kersten, D. (2002, November 15). Today's generations face new communication gaps. Retrieved from http://usatoday30.usatoday.com/money/jobcenter/workplace/communication/2002-11-15-communication-gap_x.htm

Lamb, A. J., & Metzler, C. A. (2014). Defining the value of occupational therapy: A health policy lens on research and practice. *American Journal of Occupational Therapy, 68*(1), 9-14.

Lamb, A. J. & Robosan-Burt, S. (n.d.) Documenting the distinct value of occupational therapy. Retrieved from http://files.abstractsonline.com/CTRL/26/6/C1A/3EC/5A8/4CF/D95/0DE/2BD/2E3/227/3D/a1828_1.pdf.

Laumann, A. E., & Derick, A. J. (2006). Tattoos and body piercings in the United States: A national data set. *Journal of the American Academy of Dermatology, 55*(3), 413-421.

Leach, D. C. (2002). Building and assessing competence: The potential for evidence-based graduate medical education. *Quality Management in Healthcare, 11*(1), 39-44.

Leknes, S., Wessberg, J., Ellingsen, D., Chelnokova, O., Olausson, H., & Laeng, B. (2013). Oxytocin enhances pupil dilation and sensitivity to hidden emotional expression. *Social Cognitive and Affective Neuroscience, 8*(7), 741-749.

Low, J. F. (1992). The reconstructive aides. *American Journal of Occupational Therapy, 46*(1), 38-43.

Madden, M., & Smith, A. (2010, May 26). Reputation management and social media. Retrieved from http://www.pewinternet.org/Reports/2010/Reputation-Management.aspx

Martin, C. (2005). From high maintenance to high productivity: What managers need to know about Generation Y. *Industrial and Commercial Training, 37*(1), 39-44.

Mehrabian, A. (1972). *Nonverbal communication.* Chicago, IL: Aldine-Atherton.

Miller, B. K., McGlashan Nicols, K., & Eure, J. (2009). Boday art in the workplace: Piercing the Prejudice? *Personnel Review, 38*, 621-640. doi: 10.1180/00483480910992247

Mootz, R. D., Coulter, I., & Schultz, G. D. (2005). Professionalism and ethics in chiropractic. In S. Haldeman (Ed.), *Principles and practice of chiropractic* (3rd ed., pp. 201 205). Columbus, OH: McGraw-Hill.

Mosey, A. (1986). *Psychosocial components of occupational therapy.* New York, NY: Raven Press.

The Myers & Briggs Foundation. (n.d.). The 16 MBTI types. Retrieved from http://www.myersbriggs.org/my-mbti-personality-type/mbti-basics/the-16-mbti-ypes.htm

The National Oceanographic and Atmospheric Association Office of Diversity. (2006). Tips to improve the interaction among the generations: Traditionalists, boomers, X'ers and nexters. Retrieved from http://honolulu.hawaii.edu/intranet/committees/FacDevCom/guidebk/teachtip/intergencomm.htm

Newkirk, G. (1982, Spring). The home economics professional and professionalism. *Distaff of Kappa Omicron Phi, 48*(2), 1, 4, 8.

Niemiec, S. (2000). Finding common ground for all ages. *Security Distributing & Marketing, 30*(3), 81-84.

Occupation. (2017). In Dictionary.com. Retrieved from http://www.dictionary.com/browse/occupation?s=t

Ozar, D. (2004). Profession and professional ethics. In *Encyclopedia of Bioethics* (3rd ed., vol 3, pp. 2158-2169). New York, NY: Macmillan.

Pattison, M. (2006). OT—Outstanding talent: An entrepreneurial approach to practice. *Australian Occupational Therapy Journal, 53*(3), 166-172.

Pavlov, I. P. (1960). *Conditional reflexes.* New York, NY: Dover.

Peloquin, S. M. (2005). Embracing our ethos, reclaiming our heart. *American Journal of Occupational Therapy, 59*(6), 611-625.

Polk-Lepson Research Group. (2012). 2012 professionalism in the workplace study. Retrieved from http://www.ycp.edu/media/york-website/cpe/2012-Professionalism-in-the-Workplace-Study.pdf

Practitioner. (2017). In Dictionary.com. Retrieved from http://www.dictionary.com/browse/practitioner?s=t

Profession. (2017). In Dictionary.com. Retrieved from http://www.dictionary.com/browse/profession?s=t

Professional. (2017). In Dictionary.com. Retrieved from http://www.dictionary.com/browse/professional?s=t

Professionalism. (2016). In Merriam-Webster dictionary. Retrieved from http://www.merriamwebster.com/dictionary/professionalism

Professionalization. (2016). In Wikipedia. Retrieved from https://en.wikipedia.org/wiki/Professionalization

Quiroga, V. A. (1995). *Occupational therapy: The first 30 years, 1900-1930.* Bethesda, MD: American Occupational Therapy Association.

Rath, D. (1999). Bridging the generation gap. *InfoWorld, 21*(45), 84.

Responsibility. (2016). In Merriam-Webster dictionary. Retrieved from http://www.merriam-webster.com/dictionary/responsibility

Robertson, S. C., & Savio, M. G. (2003). Mentoring as professional development. *OT Practice, 8*, 20-27.

Robinson, A. J., Tanchuck, C. J., & Sullivan, T. M. (2012). Professionalism and occupational therapy: An exploration of faculty and student perspectives. *Canadian Journal of Occupational Therapy, 79*(5), 275-284.

Sadeh, N. (2011). Smartphone privacy & security: What should we teach our users? Retrieved from EDUCAUSE website http://www.educause.edu /Resources/SmartphonePrivacySecurityWhatS/227595

Sauter-Davis, D. (2014). Local to global resources for the occupational therapy professional. In K. Jacobs, N. MacRae, & K. Sladyk (Eds.), *Occupational therapy essentials for clinical competence* (2nd ed., pp. 647-662). Thorofare, NJ: SLACK Incorporated.

Sheppard, M. (1996). Proxemics. Retrieved from http://www.cs.unm.edu/~sheppard/proxemics.htm

Skills You Need. (2016). Non-verbal communication. Retrieved from http://www.skillsyouneed.com/ips/nonverbal-communication.html#ixzz3ArVWWXTx

Snarkville, L. (2009). Time according to Vince Lombardi. Retrieved from http://bleacherreport.com/articles/300787-time-according-to-vince-Lombardi

Sol, M. (n.d.). Body language: Hand shakes. Retrieved from http://lonerwolf.com/body-language-handshakes/

Solove, D. J. (2007). *The future of reputation: Gossip, rumor, and privacy on the internet.* New Haven, CT: Yale University Press.

Southard, G., & Lewis, J. (2004). Building a workplace that recognizes generational diversity. *PM.Public Management, 86*(3), 8-12.

Straker, D. (n.d.). Haptic communication. Retrieved from http://changingminds.org/explanations/behaviors/body_language/ haptic_touch.htm

Taylor, R. R. (2008). *The intentional relationship: Occupational therapy and use of self.* Philadelphia, PA: F. A. Davis.

Teamwork. (2016). In Oxford Dictionaries. Retrieved from http://www.oxforddictionaries.com/us/definition/american_english/teamwork

Toastmasters International. (2011). Gestures: Your body speaks. Retrieved from http://www.toastmasters.org/~/media/E202D7AA84E24A758D1BAAE8A77FD496.ashx

Ventola, C. L. (2014). Social media and health care professionals: Benefits, risks, and best practices. *Pharmacy and Therapeutics, 39*(7), 491-499, 520.

Wanzer, M. B., Booth-Butterfield, M., & Gruber, K. (2004). Perceptions of health care providers' communication: Relationships between patient-centered communication and satisfaction. *Health Care Communication, 16*(3), 363-384.

Wilding, C., & Whiteford, G. (2008). Language, identity and representation: Occupation and occupational therapy in acute settings. *Australian Occupational Therapy Journal, 55*(3), 180-187.

Wilensky, H. L. (1964). The professionalization of everyone? *American Journal of Sociology, 70*(2), 137-158.

Withers, S., & Shann, S. (2008). Embracing opportunities: Stepping out of the box. *British Journal of Occupational Therapy, 71*(3), 122-124.

World Health Organization. (2010). *Framework for action on interprofessional education and collaborative practice.* Geneva, Switzerland: WHO Press.

Yang, S. M., & Guy, M. E. (2006). GenXers versus boomers: Work motivators and management implications. *Public Performance & Management Review, 29*(3), 267-284.

Yusoff, M. S. B. (2009). Professional behaviour: What does it mean? *Education in Medicine Journal, 1*(1), 1-5.

Zemke, R., Raines, C., & Filipczak, B. (2000). *Generations at work: Managing the clash of veterans, boomers, Xers, and nexters in your workplace.* New York, NY: AMACOM.

Zimmerman, M. J. (2014, December 24). Intrinsic vs. extrinsic value. Retrieved from http://plato.stanford.edu/entries/value-intrinsic-extrinsic/

2

The Evolution of Professionalism

Elizabeth D. DeIuliis, OTD, OTR/L

INTRODUCTION

Over the course of the evolution of the concept which is now described as professionalism, there have been many factors influencing its development. Ranging from ancient, internally-imposed codes of ethics in the Hippocratic Oath, to federal legislation such as the Health Insurance Portability and Accountability Act of 1996, there are historical, societal, and humanistic influences which have shaped the way that we conceptualize what it means to be a professional.

KEY WORDS

Health Insurance Portability and Accountability Act: Passed in 1996; legislation which protects the health insurance and private health information of health care consumers

Health Maintenance Organizations: Organizations with a business model that provide contract-based health insurance to consumers

Patient Protection and Affordable Care Act: Also referred to as ObamaCare; health care reform legislation passed in 2010 focused on improving quality of care, increasing access to care, and decreasing costs of care

Telehealth: An emerging area in the profession of occupational therapy, which allows for services to be provided at a distance through means of technology

DeIuliis, E.D.
Professionalism Across Occupational Therapy Practice (pp 43-50).
© 2017 Taylor & Francis Group.

OBJECTIVES

By the end of reading this chapter and completing the learning activities, the reader should be able to:

1. Understand the historical origination of the basic principles of professionalism

2. Identify past and current societal influences on professionalism

3. Examine critical issues related to expectations and demands placed on professionals by societal and practice contexts

PAST INFLUENCES ON PROFESSIONALISM

The notion of ethics and morality has been written about as early as the third century, when Hippocrates, a Greek physician often called the father of medicine, created the Hippocratic Oath and ultimately established medicine as a profession. In the mid-to-late 1990s, the concept of professionalism began to have a stronger emergence in the realm of health care and medical education (Shrank, Reed, & Jernstedt, 2004). For example, in 1990, the American Board of Internal Medicine established a task group to enhance the evaluation of professionalism as a component of clinical competence in internal medicine. Furthermore, it was during this time that significant changes began to occur within the health care system—such as within health maintenance organizations, where the provision of health care came to be treated more like a business and adversely affected certain aspects of professionalism. Therefore, maintaining and improving standards of service and care became central to reinforcing professionalism and ethical principles in health care. More recently, due to new changes in health care, educational standards, and societal influence, professionalism has been under greater scrutiny across health and social care professions. Here is a quick analysis of past societal influences on professionalism and the effect they had on the occupational therapy profession.

Ancient Philosophers

Hippocrates, often referred to as the "father of medicine," was an ancient Greek physician who promoted outstanding moral values and ethical practice, and has served as a vision and foundation for many health care professions' codes of conduct and ethics. Hippocrates is also responsible for creating the Hippocratic Oath, which is a rite of passage as well as one of the most quoted documents of the medical field. There is a classic as well as modern version of the Hippocratic Oath, yet both echo the ethical and moral elements calling those who take it to use only beneficial treatments, to refrain from causing harm, to preserve patient privacy, and to live an exemplary personal and professional life (Tyson, 2001). Furthermore, Plato, a Greek philosopher, teaches us in *The Republic* that the ideal leader (or professional) is someone who commits themselves and is trained for a life of service and devotion to their fellow citizen (Waterfield, 1994). In other words, leadership (or professionalism) requires competence. Plato was influential in setting standards for just and virtuous conduct. Both of these ancient philosophers were fundamental in creating a foundation for the principles of ethics and morality in society today, which are, ultimately, the pillars of the occupational therapy profession.

Professionalization of Other Health Care Professions

Many health care practitioners identify themselves as professionals. Although we are approaching our centennial birthday, the professionalization of occupational therapy is undoubtedly influenced by the professionalization of other health care professions. Chapter 3 will provide an in-depth discussion on the origination, scope of practice, beliefs, and values regarding professionalism of six other health care disciplines.

Federal Legislation

There have been several laws passed by the federal government that have had a significant effect on professionalism in health care. Two specifically that will be discussed are the American with Disabilities Act and the Health Insurance Portability and Accountability Act.

The Americans with Disabilities Act is a civil law passed in 1990 that prohibits discrimination against individuals with disabilities in all areas of public life, including employment, education, transportation and all public and private places that are open to the general public. It is this law which mandates that employers must provide reasonable accommodations to qualified employees and applicants, as well as make accommodations in public spaces, such as restaurants and shopping centers. Health care professionals who are employers and/or administrators have a legal obligation to obey by this law. This law promotes equality and sensitivity, which are critical elements of being an ethical professional (Americans With Disabilities Act, 1990).

The Health Insurance Portability and Accountability Act that was passed by Congress in 1996 is deeply connected to long-standing principles of ethics and professionalism. The purpose of HIPAA is twofold. One was to ensure that individuals would be able to maintain their health insurance between jobs. This is the Health Insurance Portability part of the Act. It is relatively straightforward, and has been successfully implemented. The second part of the Act is the "Accountability" portion. This section is designed to ensure the security and confidentiality of patient information and data. In addition, it mandates uniform standards for electronic transmission of administrative and financial data relating to patient health information. HIPAA has created industry-wide standards regarding protection, privacy, security, and confidentiality of protected health information. The Privacy Rule states that the following identifiers are protected health information and must be protected:

- Names
- Contact information such as addresses, telephone numbers, and email addresses
- Dates, such as birth, admission, discharge, and death dates
- Social security numbers
- Medical record numbers
- Health plan beneficiary numbers
- Account numbers
- Certificate/License numbers
- Vehicle identifiers and serial numbers (including license plate)
- Device identifiers and serial numbers
- Web Universal Resource Locators
- Internet Protocol addresses
- Biometric identifiers, including finger and voice prints
- Full face photographic images and any comparable images
- Any other unique identifying number, characteristic, or code such as past, present, or future physical or mental health condition or treatment provided to a patient

Health information can exist in any form or medium, including paper, electronic, and oral communications. As a health care professional, protected health information is part of

Box 2-1
Health care professional students are required to complete HIPAA training. Did you know that the training you receive is the same training that practitioners receive? Therefore, students are held to the same standards as practitioners, as well as the same consequences under HIPAA law.

everything you do. It exists in verbal and written communication, interactions with technology (i.e. faxing, electronic health records), and activities related to the privacy rules. For example, we come in contact with a patient's health information when we speak to a colleague about a patient's treatment, review a patient's medical record or bill, and when we access information using a computer. A HIPAA violation can occur with both an intentional and unintentional breach. As a health care professional, our consumers entrust us with their health information; therefore, we must protect it. The consequences of not complying with HIPAA can include both federal and civil penalties such as demotion, dismissal from academic program or place of employment, monetary fine, and imprisonment. Compliance with HIPAA is required of all health care professionals, providers, and students in training, regardless of your career stage (Box 2-1). As discussed in Chapter 1, an essential part of being a professional is professional responsibility, which involves abiding by laws and regulations (see Box 2-1).

CURRENT INFLUENCES ON PROFESSIONALISM AND THEIR EFFECT ON OCCUPATIONAL THERAPY

While the concept of professionalism has been evolving in health care professions for many decades, there has been a stronger emphasis as of late on this issue due to changes in society as a whole.

The Effect of Health Care Reform

The Patient Protection and Affordable Care Act (2010), also referred to as ObamaCare, is a United States health reform law aimed to:

- Increase the rate of health insurance coverage for Americans
- Reduce the overall cost of health care
- Improve health care outcomes
- Streamline the delivery of health care services

Furthermore, the Patient Protection and Affordable Care Act contains nine titles, each addressing an essential component of reform:

1. Quality, affordable health care for all Americans
2. The role of public programs
3. Improving the quality and efficiency of health care
4. Prevention of chronic disease and improving public health
5. Health care workforce
6. Transparency and program integrity

7. Improving access to innovative medical therapies

8. Community living assistance services and supports

9. Revenue provisions

This legislation is often referred to as the triple aim, as it has three main focal points: care, health, and cost. The current environment of health care and health care reform, including the triple aim, creates an ethical dilemma for many health care providers, such as occupational therapy practitioners. Providers are challenged to maintain their level of clinical care, increase collaboration with the larger health care team, and yet also increase productivity and decrease costs. Furthermore, economic influences, such as health care reform, have resulted in increased expectations of health care consumers. The involvement of the consumer body (patients) in their health care has certainly evolved. Current consumers and members of society as a whole are more sophisticated, educated, technology-savvy, and socially-connected (Bachman, n.d.). Some literature labels these individuals as "empowered health care consumers" as opposed to patients. These factors and others have contributed to the increased global focus on professionalism, specifically competency and behavior, in health care professionals.

Health care reform has also created a paradigm shift from the notion of quantity of care or life to quality of care or life for consumers. The overall push of wellness and prevention due to health care reform has increased the number of individuals that have access to health care due to no pre-existing medical conditions. Health care has been evolving and moving away from a "disease-centered model" and toward a "patient-centered" or "concierge model," aimed to bring health care services to the patient, focusing on how to make things more convenient and satisfying for the consumer body. Therefore, intrinsic and extrinsic factors of professionalism (discussed in Chapter 1) such as communication skills, generational and cultural sensitivity, and more are skills that are in high demand today.

Health care reform presents many opportunities for the occupational therapy profession. The American Occupational Therapy Association (AOTA) believes that occupational therapy practitioners are well-prepared to contribute to interprofessional care teams addressing the primary care needs of individuals across the lifespan, particularly those with or at risk for one or more chronic conditions. Occupational therapy practitioners' knowledge of how habits and routines significantly affect individuals' health and wellness will make their contribution to primary care distinct. In the official position paper titled "The Role of Occupational Therapy In Primary Care," authors Roberts, Farmer, Lamb, Muir, and Siebert (2014) showcased how occupational therapy practitioners are "distinctly qualified" to be a player in the dynamic health care environment, which requires a coordinated and team-based approach to promote collaborative care and shared decision-making. Unfortunately, despite many advocacy and legislative efforts by the occupational therapy profession, occupational therapy is not listed as a primary care provider by the Affordable Care Act. This begs the question: will increasing our profession's overall definition and language surrounding professionalism benefit this situation?

Telehealth

The use of technology in health care, specifically telehealth, has been growing and is labeled as an emerging niche in the occupational therapy profession. The AOTA (2013) "defines telehealth as the application of evaluative, consultative, preventative, and therapeutic services delivered through telecommunication and information technologies" (p. S69). Telehealth is a service-delivery model that allows increased access to services by providing "services at a location that is physically distant from the client, thereby allowing for services to occur where the client lives, works, and plays, if that is needed or desired" (AOTA, 2013, p. S69). Specific competencies related to telehealth include appropriate, effective, proficient, and safe use of telehealth technologies. An understanding of

Box 2-2
(POTENTIAL) SHIFTS IN ENTRY-LEVEL DEGREES
Due to these changes caused by health care reform, in addition to the impending transition of other health care disciplines to an entry-level doctorate degree, the occupational therapy profession has been having a profession-wide dialogue and debate about the shift in the entry to occupational therapy education for some time.

technology is needed, as well as an expertise in the knowledge, skills, and clinical reasoning necessary due to the factor of distance. Enhanced communication skills are an integral part of using this medium to deliver health care.

As telehealth provides access to consumers in more diverse geographical areas, a strong skill set in generational and cultural sensitivity is required. Telehealth practitioners are required to adhere to the same standards of quality, patient privacy, security of patient-protected information, and confidentiality as established in the traditional face-to-face clinical settings and governed by law (AOTA, 2013). Similar to any new treatment intervention or approach, it is recommended that practitioners interested in using telehealth seek out training and education to gain and demonstrate service competency prior to using this medium in clinical practice. Clearly, the service delivery model of telehealth requires a specific professional skill set.

The Buzzword of Interprofessional

Did you know if you google the word interprofessional, nearly a million results are returned? The recent focus on interprofessional education, collaboration, practice and professionalism has been rapidly accelerating in health and social care professions over the past decade. Research indicates that interprofessional practice, collaboration, and communication improves care and outcomes while reducing costs. However, a unique skill set and knowledge are needed to effectively display interprofessional professionalism. Chapter 3 will provide an in-depth overview of the unique skills and knowledge required to be an interprofessional professional.

Occupational Therapy Education

As of August 2015, the Accreditation Council for Occupational Therapy Education has determined that the entry-level-degree requirement for the occupational therapy practitioner will remain at both the master's and the doctorate degree. The council's decision is based on a comprehensive review of available literature, specific reports, and extensive commentary from stakeholders (AOTA, 2015). The overarching justifications for the Council's decision are: limited outcomes differentiate master and doctorate graduates; the academic infrastructure of many institutions is not sufficient to meet the occupational therapy doctorate standards, especially with respect to faculty resources and institutional support; the readiness and capability of institutions to deliver quality fieldwork and experiential components of the program is constrained; and retaining two entry levels allows for flexibility of the profession to assess and address the changing health care needs of individuals and populations (Box 2-2).

Occupational Therapy Assistant Education

The Accreditation Council for Occupational Therapy Education has determined that the entry-level-degree for the occupational therapy assistant will be offered at both the associate and bachelor's degree. A motion to move to the single entry-level baccalaureate was defeated, but the motion to move to a dual entry-level for the occupational therapy assistant was approved.

The Council's decision is based on a number of findings, which were informed in significant part by information and commentary from stakeholders, including: the ability to better prepare individuals for further academic advancement and leadership positions; the expansion of opportunities within the current scope of practice; and two entry levels permits additional flexibility to assess and address the changing health care needs of individuals and populations (Kalahar, 2014).

Like occupational therapy clinical practice, the concept of professionalism is continually changing in light of changes in societal and workforce demands, as well as generational differences and constraints imposed by the educational and health care delivery systems. One cannot deny that society has had an influence on occupational therapy practice and the expectations of its practitioners and students. Not only does our clinical practice evolve with research, but the expectations of practitioners changes as well. Evolution of the occupational therapy profession, including elevating the educational requirements for occupational therapy programs, is not something that we can currently predict with certainty. Will it have an effect on the autonomy of the profession, and the development of occupational therapy students' professionalism to better prepare them for the current and future health care arena? Howard (1991) stated that occupational therapy practitioners "need to understand who they are as occupational therapists" (p. 880). Does the profession agree as a whole upon what one needs to be successful in the current and future health care environment? More discussion regarding professionalism and occupational education will be provided in Chapters 5 and 6.

Generation Z

The next generation of occupational therapy practitioners is on the horizon, and currently holds the greatest potential for initiating change. As discussed in Chapter 1, the rise of Generation Z into higher education settings and the workforce may present many professional challenges. These individuals are very dependent on organizational structure, strive toward over-achievement at their baseline, and often struggle with anxiety and other emotional difficulties when faced with adversity. Therefore, it would be prudent for the current leaders in the occupational therapy profession to be well-educated and knowledgeable about the values and needs of Generation Z, and incorporate these values as they shape and model the future of the profession.

SUMMARY

In conclusion, there have been numerous past and current organizational, environmental, and societal factors which have shaped the evolution of professionalism. Containing costs, promoting high quality care, and sustaining professionalism have been ongoing goals in health care as a whole. The history of professionalism and its evolution is long, and will continue to be written as society and technology continue to progress. It is our duty as occupational therapy professionals to be aware not only of the historical influences which have shaped the past of our conduct, but those of the future which may be forthcoming and to which we must adapt.

LEARNING ACTIVITIES

1. The Hippocratic Oath was written more than 2,000 years ago. If you were to write a new oath for health care practitioners today, how might this document look? What values would you want to keep, and what may change?

2. Read the Hippocratic Oath and compare its tenets to the Occupational Therapy Code of Ethics (2015) document. What occupational therapy ethical principles are discussed in the Oath?

3. As both society and the workforce grow and change, the meaning of professionalism will continue to evolve along with new norms and policies. Is there anything that you have observed around you influencing the direction of professionalism at present, or for the near future?

REFERENCES

American Occupational Therapy Association. (2013). Telehealth. *American Journal of Occupational Therapy, 67*(6), S69-S90.

American Occupational Therapy Association. (2015). Occupational therapy entry-level survey. Retrieved from http://www.aota.org/-/media/Corporate/Files/EducationCareers/Accredit/ 7OTEntryLevelSurvey.pdf

Americans With Disabilities Act of 1990, Pub. L. No. 101-336, 104 Stat. 328 (1990).

Bachman, R. E. (n.d.). The future of healthcare consumerism: Empowering consumers through new medical delivery models. Retrieved from http://www.theihcc.com/en/communities/health_access_alternatives/the-future-of-health-care-consumerism--empowering-_htln3omt.html

Howard, B. (1991). How high do we jump? The effect of reimbursement on occupationaltherapy. *American Journal of Occupational Therapy, (45)*10, 875-881.

Kalahar, J. (2014). American Occupational Therapy Association Ad Hoc Committee to OTA Entry-Level-Degree Requirements: Final report to the Representative Assembly. Retrieved from http://www.aota.org/-/media/Corporate/Files/EducationCareers/ Accredit/2OTAEntryLevelDegreeADHoc.pdf

Patient Protection and Affordable Care Act, Pub. L. No. 111-148, §2702, 124 Stat. 119, 318-319 (2010).

Roberts, P., Farmer, M. E., Lamb, A. J., Muir, S., & Siebert, C. (2014). The role of occupational therapy in primary care. *American Journal of Occupational Therapy, 68*(Suppl. 3), S25-S33.

Shrank, W. H., Reed, V. A., & Jernstedt, G. C. (2004). Fostering professionalism in medical education: A call for improved assessment and meaningful incentives. *Journal of General Internal Medicine, 19*(8), 887-892.

Tyson, P. (2001, March 27). The Hippocratic Oath today. Retrieved from http://www.pbs.org/wgbh/nova/body/hippocratic-oath-today.html

Waterfield, R. (1994). *Plato: Republic: Translated, with notes and an introduction.* Oxford, United Kingdom: Oxford University Press.

3

Interprofessional Professionalism

Sarah E. Wallace, PhD, CCC-SLP; Elizabeth D. DeIuliis, OTD, OTR/L; and Leesa M. DiBartola, EdD, DPT, PT, MCHES

INTRODUCTION

Becoming an occupational therapy professional requires learning outside of the occupational therapy profession. In addition to being knowledgeable of the roles, responsibilities and expectations of other disciplines in which we work with, professionals are expected to have a distinguished skill set that allows them to communicate, collaborate, and mutually respect one another. Interprofessionalism is working together within interprofessional teams to best meet the needs of the patient and family. Professional interaction among members of the interprofessional team leads to improved practice, safety, and client outcomes. To be an effective member of a team, a practitioner must understand the roles and responsibilities of the other interprofessional team members. Practicing interprofessional professionalism is a key aspect of being an occupational therapy professional. This chapter will explore the professionalization, scope of practice, and key discipline-specific information of six allied health professions. Current educational and health care terminology, such as interprofessional education (IPE), interprofessional collaboration (IPC), and interprofessional professionalism (IPP), will also be discussed.

KEY WORDS

Accreditation Body: Typically a third party that oversees and ensures the quality of organizations or processes that provide certification(s)

- Example: The Joint Commission is an independent agency that sets performance standards for health care organizations in the United States such as hospitals (The Joint Commission, 2015)

- Accreditation Council for Occupational Therapy Education is an accrediting body that sets the minimum educational and administrative requirements for occupational therapy educational programs

DeIuliis, E.D.
Professionalism Across Occupational Therapy Practice (pp 51-87).
© 2017 Taylor & Francis Group.

Code of Conduct: Outward looking, governs relationship between members and society as a whole

- Example: "In your professional role you shall have regard for the public health, safety, and environment"

Code of Ethics: A set of published guidelines developed by an organization or institution describing appropriate behaviors

Code of Practice: Inward looking, governs how to practice the profession

- Example: "Every statement in the code must be executed at least once during testing."

Interprofessional Collaboration: "When multiple health workers from different professional backgrounds work together with patient, families, and communities to deliver the highest quality care"; elements of collaboration include respect, trust, shared decision making, and partnerships (World Health Organization, 2010, p. 7)

Interprofessional Education: Occurs when two or more professions learn with, from, and about each other to improve collaboration and the quality of care (Center for Advancement of Interprofessional Education, 2008)

Interprofessional Professionalism: "Consistent demonstration of core values evidenced by professionals working together, aspiring to and wisely applying principles ... to achieve health and wellness in individuals and communities" (Arnold & Stern, 2006, p. 19)

Intraprofessional Collaboration: Collaboration among colleagues from the same profession who share a common professional education, values, socialization, identity, and experience

- Example: registered occupational therapists and certified occupational therapy assistants or physical therapists and physical therapist assistants

Professional Organization: Also called a professional body or professional society; is usually a nonprofit organization seeking to further a particular profession, the interests of individuals engaged in that profession, and the public interest

- Example: American Occupational Therapy Association, American Society for Hand Therapists

OBJECTIVES

By the end of reading this chapter and completing the learning activities, the reader should be able to:

1. Identify how professionalism is described within multiple allied health care professions
2. Understand the basic professional traits of multiple allied health care professions
3. Explain the importance of interprofessional professionalism in the current health care environment

PROFESSIONALISM IN OTHER HEALTH CARE PROVIDERS

Professions emerged in the Middle Ages when specialized practitioners began to develop and provide an array of significant, unstandardized personal services that were central to human values.

These services, such as health, education, religion, and welfare, were adapted to meet the needs of individuals and required knowledge and skills that the typical person did not possess. Health care providers are often held to higher standards of professional behavior than other professional groups. Historically, society expects health care professionals "to be of high moral standing" (Horowitz, 2002, p. 5). Health care providers use human relations when dealing with patients and coworkers. Therefore, personal traits like character, values, morals, ethics, integrity, and trustworthiness are vital in the health care environment. The health care industry works on behalf of individuals and families, and therefore, unethical or unprofessional behavior is not acceptable. One approach to understanding the purpose of professions in society is to examine the unique service needs and how an organized body of professions meet those needs. Professionals, through a representative body of peers, are often sanctioned by a state or national organization, are given the unusual authority to determine who may be permitted to practice and under what conditions. This chapter will provide a general overview of the core values, ethics, and professionalism associated with the allied health professions of medicine, nursing, pharmacy, physical therapy, physician assistant, and speech-language pathology. Professionalism in these fields implies commitment, training, and competence in the practice of the discipline. In each of these professions, the essence of professionalism begins with ethics, competence, and responsibility. Concepts and terminology associated with interprofessional professionalism will be discussed later in this chapter.

To effectively work together and collaborate, health care practitioners must have a basic understanding of each other's professions' qualifications, core values and philosophy, expertise, terminology, professional body/organization(s), and possible contributions to the team. Additionally, it is important to consider the common characteristics across the professions such as the following.

Characteristics common to many professions:

- Substantial education and training required
- The members of the profession decide the nature of the training and control entry to the profession
- The profession is organized into one or more professional bodies or organizations
- Typical functions developed by professional bodies:
  - Setting standards of education and experience that must be met by its members
  - Accreditation of university courses or curriculum that are judged to meet these standards to facilitate entry into the profession
  - Establishing a code of conduct to regulate how members behave in their professional lives.

Professional bodies have codes of conduct and/or practice that their members must obey (Bullock & Trombley, 1999). The purpose of a code of conduct is to define standards of behavior and expected performance of its members.

To display interprofessional professionalism, individuals must understand the roles, responsibilities, and scope of practice of the colleague's profession. Let's investigate the value of professionalism across six other allied health professions: medicine, nursing, pharmacy, physical therapy, physician assistant, and speech-language pathology.

MEDICINE

History of Professionalization

In England around the 17th century, medical practice included three professions: physicians, surgeons, and apothecaries. These professions were distinguished at the time based on area of practice and education. For example, physicians typically had a degree from a university.

Surgeons were trained through an apprenticeship at a hospital and served as barbers and surgeons. Apothecaries also completed apprenticeships to learn how to prescribe, as well as make and sell medicines. Although the medical profession in the United States can be traced back to the early 1600s, these distinctions did not exist in the colonies. Early on, physicians were expected to also perform surgery and prescribe medications.

The first organization of medical professions in the United States, the New Jersey Medical Society, was chartered in July 1766. Its purpose was to regulate medical practice, develop educational standards, monitor fee schedules, and maintain a code of ethics. The first medical college, the Medical Society of the County of New York, was founded in March 1807. Later, in 1846 a national convention was held to determine standards for medical education. Then, shortly after this national convention, the first meeting of the American Medical Association (AMA) was held in 1847, bringing together 40 medical societies and 28 colleges from 22 states. Many changes in standards for medical education followed including the development of a residency program.

Medical education changed dramatically in 1910 with the Flexner Report and later, in 1984, with the General Professional Education of the Physician Report, both aimed at advancing the professionalization of medicine. The Flexner Report resulted in standardization of medical education in the basic sciences and clinical expectations. The General Professional Education of the Physician Report resulted in a focus on the art of medicine and aspects of professionalism that appeared lacking.

In 1930, most medical schools required a liberal arts degree for admission which was followed by 3 to 4 years of curriculum in medicine and surgery. Around the 19th century, physicians in the United States began to specialize in aspects of medicine. These specialties were recognized in the 1930s through work of the AMA and the Advisory Board of Medical Specialties (later named the American Board of Medical Specialties) (U.S. National Library of Medicine, 2013).

Professional Organizations

Founded in 1847 by Nathan Smith Davis, the AMA serves to promote scientific advancement, improve public health, and support the doctor and patient relationship. The mission is stated as "To promote the art and science of medicine and the betterment of public health." Within the seven AMA councils, the Council of Ethical and Judicial Affairs is responsible for ethical and professionalism issues. This council serves to maintain and update the AMA Code of Medical Ethics (AMA, n.d.a; AMA, n.d.c).

Brief Description of Scope of Practice

Physicians diagnose, treat, and counsel patients in an effort to address issues related to any human disease, ailment, injury, infirmity, deformity, and pain. They can also prescribe medications. Physicians can work in private practices, group practices, hospitals, teaching facilities, and public health organizations.

Accrediting Agency for Education

The Association of American Medical Colleges (AAMC) is the agency that serves and leads the academic community to improve the lives of all (Association of American Medical Colleges, 2017).

Minimum Entry-Level Professional Education/Current Education Trends

After completing a bachelor degree that includes the required prerequisite courses, students can attend an allopathic or osteopathic medical school as a path to become a physician.

Allopathic medicine results in a degree in medicine with the distinction of MD (medical doctor) and osteopathic medicine results in a degree of DO (osteopathic doctor). Typically, MDs practice the classical or traditional form of medicine with an emphasis on diagnosis and treatment of human diseases. In contrast, DOs practice medicine with an emphasis on a holistic view of treating or diagnosing the whole person rather than treating only symptoms. Most physicians continue their education by completing residencies in one of the variety of specialties available such as internal medicine, family practice, pediatrics, surgery, psychiatry, dermatology, and many others.

Required Educational Content

Physician education includes undergraduate education, medical school, a residency program, and an optional fellowship. An undergraduate degree can be either a bachelor of science or bachelor of arts degree and will typically include a strong emphasis in basic sciences such as biology, chemistry, and physics. Medical education is considered a graduate-level training, and will include four years of preclinical and clinical course work at one of the accredited United States medical schools. After completion of medical school, a student earns a doctor of medicine degree, but is not able to independently practice until he or she has completed additional training. Instead of an MD, some students earn a doctor of osteopathic medicine degree (DO) from a college of osteopathic medicine. Graduate medical education includes a residency program that students are assigned to through a national matching program. Physician residents are expected to master core competencies that include patient care, medical knowledge, practice-based learning and improvement, systems-based practice, professionalism, and interpersonal skills and communication. Residency programs typically last three to seven years and are completed under the supervision of senior physician educators. Some students will elect to complete a fellowship that includes an additional one to three years of subspecialty to become highly specialized in a particular area.

Regulatory Body/Practice Credentials (National/State)

Upon completion of graduate medical education, physicians must earn a state license to practice medicine. This typically involves a series of exams before the physician can apply for a permanent license. Physicians in some states are required to earn a certain number of continuing medical education (CME) credits per year, although these vary by state and professional organizations.

The United States Medical Licensing Examination is a three-step examination for medical licensure in the United States. It is sponsored by the Federation of State Medical Boards and the National Board of Medical Examiners. The United States Medical Licensing Examination was designed to assess a physician's ability to apply knowledge, concepts, and principles as well as demonstrate fundamental patient-centered skills. Most states require at least a one-year residency program and the passage of a board certification in whatever medical specialty a student has chosen.

Intraprofessional Roles

Physicians provide ongoing supervision to physician assistants (PAs), whose role will be discussed later in this chapter. The regulations regarding supervision responsibilities of physicians over PAs vary by state. The definition of supervision should convey the idea that direction of the medical practice of the PA is provided and assured by supervising physicians, but this does not necessarily require the physical presence of a supervising physician at the place where services are rendered. It is imperative, however, that the PA and a supervising physician are or can be in contact with each other by telecommunication. Supervising physician should be defined as an allopathic or osteopathic physician (MD or DO) licensed to practice in the state, who accepts responsibility for the supervision of services provided by PAs (American Academy of Physician Assistants [AAPA], 2011).

Box 3-1

THE PROFESSIONALISM REQUIREMENTS OF THE ACCREDITATION COUNCIL FOR GRADUATE MEDICAL EDUCATION

Residents must demonstrate a commitment to carrying out professional responsibilities, adherence to ethical principles, and sensitivity to a diverse patient population. Residents are expected to:

- Demonstrate respect, compassion, and integrity; a responsiveness to the needs of patients and society that supersedes self-interest; accountability to patients, society, and the profession; and a commitment to excellence and ongoing professional development

- Demonstrate a commitment to ethical principles pertaining to provision or withholding of clinical care, confidentiality of patient information, informed consent, and business practices

- Demonstrate sensitivity and responsiveness to patients' culture, age, sex, and disabilities

---

Specializations or Advanced Practice Areas

Most physicians choose to become board certified, although this process is optional. Physicians can be certified in 36 general medical specialties and an additional 88 subspecialty fields. These specialty certifications must be renewed every 6 to 10 years. The most frequently entered specialties include emergency medicine, family practice, internal medicine, obstetrics-gynecology, orthopedic surgeon, pediatrics, psychiatry, and surgery (National Resident Match Program, 2015). Most specialty areas have a specialty medical board. For example, the American College of Emergency Physicians oversees the specialization of emergency medicine physicians.

Definitions and Terminology for Professionalism

Although the field of medicine does not have an endorsed definition of professionalism, in 1999, the Accreditation Council for Graduate Medical Education implemented general competencies, applicable to every specialty, that need to be imparted during residency or fellowship training. One of these six competencies is professionalism (Box 3-1).

Official Documents Related to Professionalism

The AMA's Code of Ethics focuses on benefiting the patient. It states that physicians must recognize responsibility to patients first and to society and other health professions. Nine guiding principles describe the conduct that defines the essentials of behavior expected for the physician. The principles are as follows: A physician shall

1. Be dedicated to providing competent medical care, with compassion and respect for human dignity and rights.

2. Uphold the standards of professionalism, be honest in all professional interactions, and strive to report physicians deficient in character or competence, or engaging in fraud or deception, to appropriate entities.

3. Respect the law and recognize a responsibility to seek changes in those requirements which are contrary to the best interests of the patient.

4. Respect the rights of patients, colleagues, and other health professionals and safeguard patient confidences and privacy within the constraints of the law.

5. Continue to study, apply, and advance scientific knowledge; maintain a commitment to medical education; make relevant information available to patients, colleagues, and the public; obtain consultation; and use the talents of other health professionals when indicated.

6. In the provision of appropriate patient care, except in emergencies, be free to choose whom to serve, with whom to associate, and the environment in which to provide medical care.

7. Recognize a responsibility to participate in activities contributing to the improvement of community and the betterment of public health.

8. While caring for a patient, regard responsibility to the patient as paramount.

9. Support access to medical care of all people.

The AMA developed multiple policies or statements to guide physicians' decision-making and action. AMA Policies include those established by the AMA House of Delegates, the Code of Medical Ethics, and AMA's Constitutions and Bylaws. The AMA website provides a policy finder program that allows individuals to reference particular policies. Policies put forward by the AMA House of Delegates typically elaborate on issues discussed in the code of ethics such as gifts to physicians and end of life care.

The AMA Code of Medical Ethics is composed of 10 sections. The first section introduces important terminology. The remaining nine sections provide opinions on particular issues including social policy issues; interprofessional relations; hospital relations; confidentiality, advertising, and communications media relations; fees and charges; physician records; practice matters; professional rights and responsibilities; and patient-physician relationship. This Code of Ethics was developed over 160 years ago and is updated every couple of decades, and most recently in 2001. The Council of Ethical and Judicial Affairs and other groups convened by AMA's Institute for Ethics frequently publishes rules related to important ethical topics. For example, The AMA's House of Delegates reaffirmed its policy in 2009 that physicians "must oppose and must not participate in torture for any reason." The Code of Medical Ethics is also available in a pocket-sized guide (AMA, n.d.b).

Nursing

History of Professionalization

After an influx of nurses were needed during the Civil War, three nurse educational programs began in 1873 and were referred to as Nightingale Schools because they were greatly influenced by the work of Florence Nightingale. In the 1890s, nurses formed two major professional organizations: the American Society of Superintendents of Training Schools for Nurses and the Associated Alumnae which later became the American Nurses Association. Later, nurse registration acts passed resulting in nurses acquiring the title of registered professional nurses (RN) (Whelan, n.d.).

Professional Organizations

The primary professional organization for nursing is the American Nurses Association (ANA). The ANA represents 3.1 million registered nurses in the United States and has three subsidiary organizations: the American Academy of Nursing, the American Nurses Foundation, and the American Nurses Credentialing Center. American Nurse Association's mission is "Nurses advancing our profession to improve health for all" (ANA, n.d.a).

Brief Description of Scope of Practice

The ANA describes nursing as "the protection, promotion, and optimization of health and abilities, prevention of illness and injury, alleviation of suffering through the diagnosis and treatment of human response, and advocacy in the care of individuals, families, communities, and populations" (ANA, 2016).

Accrediting Agency for Education

The American Association for Colleges of Nursing provides accreditation for nursing educational programs. Students cannot take the licensing exam (i.e., National Licensing Exam: Practical Nurse [NCLEX-PN] or Registered Nurse) unless they have earned a degree from an accredited school (American Association of Colleges of Nursing, 2015).

Minimum Entry-Level Professional Education/Current Education Trends

Nurses can enter into the profession as a registered nurse through many educational paths:

- Diploma Program: the length of time can vary, but most diploma programs are shorter than three years, from which students earn a diploma versus a degree. In many instances these are programs run out of a hospital or health system. Diploma graduates can take the same state licensing exam for RNs as students that graduate with an associate or baccalaureate degrees.

- Associate Program: 2-year community college program from which students earn an associate degree.

- Bachelor of Science in Nursing (BSN): 4-year program at an accredited college or university

Once completing one of the above programs, students can take the NCLEX-RN. Upon successful completion of the examination, the student is then licensed to practice as a registered nurse (RN). Students who earned a diploma or associate degree can then attend an RN to BSN program. A Licensed Practical Nurse (LPN) earns a degree from a 2-year technical school program and then takes the National Licensing Exam: Practical Nurse. Licensed Practical Nurses are supervised by RNs and have a limited scope of practice.

Required Educational Content

All of the paths to becoming a nurse include core nursing courses such as fundamentals of nursing, nutrition, pathophysiology, adult medical surgical nursing, gerontology, obstetrics, community, behavioral health, and pediatrics. These courses also incorporate a theoretical component. Additionally, all paths include clinical practicums to provide clinical experience working with a variety of patient populations in a variety of practice settings. Typically, the clinical practicums correlate to the clinical theory courses.

> Baccalaureate nursing programs encompass all of the course work taught in associate degree and diploma programs plus a more in-depth treatment of the physical and social sciences, nursing research, public and community health, nursing management, and the humanities. The additional course work enhances the student's professional development, prepares the new nurse for a broader scope of practice, and provides the nurse with a better understanding of the cultural, political, economic, and social issues that affect patients and influence health care delivery. (American Association of Colleges of Nursing, 2015)

Regulatory Body/Practice Credentials (National/State)

Nurses are certified by the American Nurses Credentialing Center, a subsidiary of the ANA, and are typically licensed by the State Board of Nursing. Some states provide licensure to nurses who pass the NCLEX-RN examination. Continuing education units are required every two years.

Intraprofessional Roles

Certified Nursing Assistants (CNAs) are supervised by RNs or LPNs to address patients' health care needs. Sometimes CNAs are referred to as Nursing Assistant, Patient Care Assistant, or State Tested Nurse Aid. CNAs can gather patient data and administer basic care as well as tend to patients' hygiene needs.

> An LPN may initiate and maintain IV therapy only under the direction and supervision of a licensed professional nurse or health care provider authorized to issue orders for medical therapeutic or corrective measures (such as a certified registered nurse practitioner, physician, physician assistant, podiatrist or dentist). (The Pennsylvania Code, 2012)

Specializations or Advanced Practice Areas

After earning a BSN, nurses can take additional course work, typically as part of a master's degree or doctorate degree, to pursue an advanced practice degree and become a certified registered nurse anesthetist, certified nurse practitioner, clinical nurse specialist, or certified nurse-midwife. During continued practice, many nurses obtain additional certification for a variety of specialty areas such as medical-surgical nursing, intravenous therapy nursing, wound, ostomy and continence nursing, critical care nursing, as well as many others. These are all referred to as advanced practice registered nurses and require a minimum of a master's degree. Individual states determine advanced practice registered nurses' scope of practice, recognized roles and responsibilities, and the certification examinations accepted (American Association of Nurse Practitioners [AANP], n.d.).

Definition and Terminology for Professionalism

The American Nurses Association (2014) provides a position statement to guide professionalism in the nursing profession (Box 3-2):

> The public has a right to expect registered nurses to demonstrate professional competence throughout their careers. American Nurse Association believes the registered nurse is individually responsible and accountable for maintaining professional competence. The American Nurse Association further believes that it is the nursing profession's responsibility to shape and guide any process for assuring nurse competence. Regulatory agencies define minimal standards for regulation of practice to protect the public. The employer is responsible and accountable to provide an environment conducive to competent practice. Assurance of competence is the shared responsibility of the profession, individual nurses, professional organizations, credentialing and certification entities, regulatory agencies, employers, and other key stakeholders.

Box 3-2

OFFICIAL NURSING DOCUMENTS RELATED TO PROFESSIONALISM

- Policy Statement: The ANA Code for Nurses (see text).

- Code of Ethics. The code is a 76-page document with interpretative statements to assist with interpretation of each statement. The code contains nine provisions; the first three reiterate nurses' values and commitments, the second three describe the boundaries of duty and loyalty, and the final three describe nurses' responsibilities beyond patient care. Similarly, the ANA website features a list of ethics resources on topics such as ethics during health care reform as well as spiritual and religious issues (ANA, n.d.c).

- ANA principles for Nursing Practice. Reports with guidelines and principles for various issues such as community paramedics, principles of collaborative relationships, documentation, and environmental health (ANA, n.d.b).

- Nursing: Scope and Standards of practice 2nd edition. This document, published in September 2010, Contains 15 national standards of practice and performance.

- ANA position statements on ethics and human rights provide additional information about important current issues in the nursing industry. Topics covered in these documents include do not resuscitate orders and capital punishment.

PHARMACY

History of Professionalization

The field of pharmacy has existed for centuries. Globally, pharmacists have been referred to as apothecaries, chemists, or druggists. Pharmacy is the field of health sciences focusing on safe and effective medication use ("Pharmacy," 2015).

Professional Organizations

American Pharmacists Association

Founded as the American Pharmaceutical Association (AphA) on October 6, 1852, APhA currently represents more than 62,000 practicing pharmacists, pharmaceutical scientists, student pharmacists, pharmacy technicians, and others interested in advancing the profession. It was the first-established professional society of pharmacists within the United States. There are many specialized pharmacy organizations, which are briefly discussed below, and nearly all of them trace their roots to the APhA.

American College of Clinical Pharmacy

The American College of Clinical Pharmacy is a professional and scientific society that provides leadership, education, advocacy, and resources enabling clinical pharmacists to achieve excellence in practice and research. American College of Clinical Pharmacy's membership is composed of practitioners, scientists, educators, administrators, students, residents, fellows, and others committed to excellence in clinical pharmacy and patient pharmacotherapy. Over the years a number of specialized organizations have evolved in clinical pharmacy, focusing on practice location (e.g., American Society of Hospital [now Health-System] Pharmacists), professional specialization (e.g., American Society for Pharmacy Law), or category of patients served (e.g., American College of Veterinary Pharmacists). For a full list of these additional professional organizations see: https://www.accp.com/stunet/compass/organizations.aspx.

American Association of Colleges in Pharmacy

Founded in 1900, the American Association of Colleges of Pharmacy is the national organization representing pharmacy education in the United States. Their mission is to lead and partner with members in advancing pharmacy education, research, scholarship, practice, and service to improve societal health.

Brief Description of Scope of Practice

Pharmacy is the science and technique of preparing and dispensing drugs. It is a health profession that links health sciences with chemical sciences and aims to ensure the safe and effective use of pharmaceutical drugs. The scope of pharmacy practice includes traditional roles such as compounding and dispensing medications. Additionally, pharmacy practice includes modern services related to health care, such as clinical services, reviewing medications for safety and efficacy, and providing drug information. Pharmacists, therefore, are the experts on drug therapy and are the primary health professionals who optimize use of medication for the benefit of the patients. Pharmacists practice in a variety of settings including retail (e.g., drugstore or supermarket), hospitals, nursing homes, drug industry, and regulatory agencies.

Accrediting Agency for Education

The Accreditation Council for Pharmacy Education is the national agency for the accreditation of professional degree programs in pharmacy and providers of continuing pharmacy education. The Accreditation Council for Pharmacy Education was established in 1932 for the accreditation of pre-service education, and in 1975, its scope of activity was broadened to include accreditation of providers of continuing pharmacy education. The Accreditation Council for Pharmacy Education expanded its activities to include evaluation and certification of professional degree programs internationally in 2011 and entered into a collaboration with the American Society of Health-System Pharmacists to accredit pharmacy technician education and training programs beginning in 2014 (Accreditation Council for Pharmacy Education, n.d.).

Minimum Entry-Level Professional Education/Current Education Trends

Doctor of Pharmacy

The following didactic content areas and associated learning expectations are viewed as central to a contemporary, high-quality pharmacy education and are incorporated at an appropriate breadth and depth in the required didactic Doctor of Pharmacy curriculum:

- Biomedical Sciences (such as biochemistry and microbiology)
- Pharmaceutical Sciences (such as biopharmaceutics and compounding)
- Social/Administrative/Behavioral Sciences (such as ethics, cultural awareness, and professional development)
- Clinical Sciences (such as health informatics and public health)

In addition to didactic training, clinical training is a requirement curriculum component for pharmacy education. The Accreditation Council for Pharmacy Education requires 1440 hours of

Advanced Pharmacy Practice Experience in the following four settings: community, ambulatory patient care, hospital/health system, and inpatient general medicine patient care

- (Optional) Postgraduate Training
  - ○ Residency is an option for post-graduates that is typically 1 to 2 years long. A residency gives licensed pharmacists decades of clinical experience in an extremely condensed time frame of only a few short years. For new graduates to remain competitive, employers generally favor residency-trained applicants for clinical positions.
  - ○ Graduates from a PharmD program may also elect to do a fellowship that is geared toward research. Fellowships can vary in length but typically last 1 to 3 years depending on the program and usually require 1 year of residency at minimum.

Estimated timeline for Pharmacist: 4 years undergraduate + 4 years doctorate + 1 to 2 years residency + 1 to 3 years fellowship = 8 to 13 years

Education Trends

- Increase in number of graduates entering post-graduate training (residency/fellowship)
- Board certification for clinical pharmacists
- Disease state management certification programs
- Interprofessional education/collaboration/practice

Required Educational Content

The Accreditation Council for Pharmacy Education requires the programs it accredits to meet the expectations of all 30 standards of Accreditation Council for Pharmacy Education's accreditation standards. There are a handful of accreditation standards that directly relate to professionalism. Here are a few:

- Standard 3: Approach to care (problem solving, cultural sensitivity and communication)
- Standard 4: personal and professional development.

Standard 4 imparts to the graduate the knowledge, skills, abilities, behaviors, and attitudes necessary to demonstrate self-awareness, leadership, innovation and entrepreneurship, and professionalism as described in the key elements listed below.

- **4.1. Self-awareness:** The graduate is able to examine and reflect on personal knowledge, skills, abilities, beliefs, biases, motivation, and emotions that could enhance or limit personal and professional growth.
- **4.2. Leadership:** The graduate is able to demonstrate responsibility for creating and achieving shared goals, regardless of position.
- **4.3. Innovation and entrepreneurship:** The graduate is able to engage in innovative activities by using creative thinking to envision better ways of accomplishing professional goals.
- **4.4. Professionalism:** The graduate is able to exhibit behaviors and values that are consistent with the trust given to the profession by patients, other health care providers, and society
- **4.5. Professional attitudes and behaviors development:** The curriculum inculcates professional attitudes and behaviors leading to personal and professional maturity consistent with the Oath of the Pharmacist.

Regulatory Body/Practice Credentials (National/State)

Pharmacy practice is regulated by several agencies and regulatory bodies:

- National Association for Boards of Pharmacy

- ○ The National Association of Boards of Pharmacy is an impartial professional organization that supports the state boards of pharmacy in protecting public health
- North American Pharmacist Licensure Examination
- National clinical exam used for every state
- Multistate Pharmacy Jurisprudence Examination
- Individual state law exam
- Continuing Education units: 30 hours every 2 years (by September 30 on even years)
- Continuing Education (must be accredited by Accreditation Council for Pharmacy Education)
- 2 hours of patient safety
- 2 hours of child abuse
- Some states require live credits
- Immunization License (within 2 years of APhA certificate program)
- 2 hours of Continuing Education (required every 2 years regarding vaccinations/biologics)

Once licensed, the pharmacist, like other health care practitioners, has a professional, ethical, and legal obligation to maintain competence to practice.

Intraprofessional Roles

Assistant pharmacists fall into two categories: assistants, who provide mostly clerical support to pharmacists; and technicians, who deal more with medications and the technical aspects of the pharmacy. Both of these professionals work alongside licensed pharmacists in a variety of settings. Assistants (sometimes called clerks or aides) are considered the more junior of these two roles. They primarily fulfill administrative functions such as typing medical labels, stocking shelves, and keeping the pharmacy clean. The typical minimum requirement for this role is a high school diploma and on-the-job training from either pharmacists or certified pharmacy technicians. Although pharmacy technicians can perform clerical tasks, they also can help the pharmacist in a variety of other pharmacy-related functions, including dispensing prescription drugs and other medical devices to patients and instructing on their use. They may also perform advanced administrative duties in pharmaceutical practice, such as reviewing prescription requests with physicians' offices and insurance companies to ensure correct medications are provided and payment is received. Although they may perform, under supervision, most dispensing, compounding, and other tasks, they are not generally allowed to perform the role of counseling patients on the proper use of their medications. Some states require formal training program or certification.

Specializations or Advanced Practice Areas

Pharmacists in the United States can become certified in recognized specialty practice areas by passing an examination administered by one of several credentialing boards. Outside of clinical pharmacy, pharmacists can participate in specialized or advanced practice areas such as:

- Academic Pharmacy
- Ambulatory Care Pharmacist
- Community Pharmacy
- Consultant Pharmacy
- Federal Pharmacy: Armed Services
- Federal Pharmacy: Public Health
- Hospital and Institutional Pharmacy

- Informatics
- Managed Care Pharmacy
- Pain and Palliative Care
- Poison Control
- Pharmaceutical Sciences/Industry

In the United States, specializations in pharmacy practice recognized by the Board of Pharmaceutical Specialties include cardiovascular, infectious disease, oncology, pharmacotherapy, nuclear, nutrition, and psychiatry. For instance, The Commission for Certification in Geriatric Pharmacy certifies pharmacists in geriatric pharmacy practice. The American Board of Applied Toxicology certifies pharmacists and other medical professionals in applied toxicology.

Definitions and Terminology for Professionalism

Chalmers provides the following definition to guide professionalism in the pharmacy profession:

Professionalism is displayed in the way pharmacists conduct themselves in professional situations. This definition implies a demeanor that is created through a combination of behaviors, including courtesy and politeness when dealing with patients, peers, and other health care professionals. Pharmacists should consistently display respect for others and maintain appropriate boundaries of privacy and discretion. (1997, p. 10)

Official Documents Related to Professionalism

- Pharmacist Code of Ethics and Oath Code:

These principles, based on moral obligations and virtues, are established to guide pharmacists in relationships with patients, health professionals, and society (APhA, 1994).

- Pharmacy Pledge and Sworn Statement
- Pharmacy-Specific Resources on Professionalism (American Association of Colleges of Pharmacy, 2012).
- APhA-ASP: Professionalism Toolkit for Students and Faculty(http://www.aacp.org/resources/studentaffairspersonnel/studentaffairspolicies/Documents/Version_2%200_Pharmacy_Professionalism_Toolkit_for_Students_and_Faculty.pdf)
- APhA Pharmaceutical Care Guidelines Advisory Committee (1995): Principles of Practice for Pharmaceutical Care (https://www.pharmacist.com/principles-practice-pharmaceutical-care)
- Quality Standards and Practice Principles for Senior Care Pharmacists: Standard 9: Professionalism (https://www.ascp.com/articles/quality-standards-and-practice-principles-seniorcare-pharmacists)
- Tenets of Professionalism for Pharmacy Students (www.accp.com/docs/positions/commentaries/TenetsProfessionlsmFinal.pdf)
- American Association of Colleges of Pharmacy Professionalism Task Force

The Task Force was specifically charged to examine the current status of the various initiatives. These initiatives aimed to build and assess professional attitudes and behaviors in student pharmacists, as well as help raise awareness to lead action on the issue of professionalism among student pharmacists. Their focus includes:

- Leadership
- Interprofessional professionalism
- Honesty, ethics, and e-professionalism
- Admissions implications

Box 3-3

The 10 traits of a student pharmacist professional displayed in the "White Paper on Pharmacy Student Professionalism" are:

1. Knowledge of skills of a profession
2. Commitment to self-improvement of skills and knowledge
3. Service-orientation
4. Pride in the profession
5. Covenantal relationship with the client
6. Creativity and innovation
7. Conscience and trustworthiness
8. Accountability for his/her work
9. Ethical and sound decision making
10. Leadership

Adapted from Popovich, N. G., Hammer, D. P., Hansen, D. J., Spies, A. R., Whalen, K. P., Beardsley, R. S., ... & Athay, J. L. (2011). Report of the AACP professional task force. *American Journal of Pharmaceutical Education, 75*(10), 1-4; American Society of Health-System Pharmacists. (2008). American Society of Health-System Pharmacists statement on professionalism. *American Journal of Health-Systems Pharmacists, 65*, 172-174.

A branch of this committee also focused specifically on student professionalism. This committee convened in 2011 and was charged to examine the status of various initiatives, which aim to build and assess professional attitudes and behaviors in student pharmacists, using the same four concepts outlined above.

This group also created a white paper on professionalism in student pharmacists that outlines the essential attitudes and behaviors that signify professionalism and that should be developed and practiced by all students (Box 3-3) (American College of Clinical Pharmacy, 2009).

- Altruism
- Honesty and integrity
- Respect for others
- Professional presence
- Professional stewardship
- Dedication and commitment to excellence Tenets of Professionalism for Pharmacy Students

PHYSICAL THERAPY

History of Professionalization

The development of the physical therapy profession in the United States was a response to the polio epidemic in the late 1800s to early 1900s that rendered many children in need of physical therapy services. During World War I, the Surgeon General sent a group of physicians to Europe to learn physical therapy specific to the care of wounded soldiers. This lead to the Division of Special Hospitals and Physical Reconstruction in 1917. The charge was to train "reconstructive aides" who provided physical reconstruction to injured soldiers. After the war, reconstructive aides moved into the workforce and provided care to civilians. The need for physical therapy expanded again after World War II. To meet these demands, eight emergency 6-month courses were authorized among 15 approved full-length programs in physical therapy. The U.S. Army recognized the importance of physical therapy and established the Women's Medical Specialists Core in 1947. This included physical therapists, occupational therapist practitioners, and dieticians. Monumental professional growth occurred in the 30-year period of the 1960s through the 1980s. Physical therapists and physical therapist assistants were recognized as professionals and educational programs were developed to meet the growing demand for these professionals. The educational development evolved from a certificate program, to a bachelor degree, and today most programs offer a doctorate of physical therapy. The goal for year 2020 is to have all education programs offer the doctorate of physical therapy as the entry-level degree for physical therapists (American Physical Therapy Association [APTA], 2013b).

Professional Organizations

The APTA is the professional association for physical therapists and physical therapist assistants. The mission is to further the profession's role in the prevention, diagnosis, and treatment of movement dysfunctions and the enhancement of the physical health and functional abilities of members of the public. Each state has a state chapter in APTA as well as district sections. The APTA has specialty sections that include acute care, aquatic physical therapy, cardiovascular and pulmonary, clinical electrophysiology, education, geriatrics, hand rehabilitation, health policy and administration, home health, neurology, oncology, orthopedics, pediatrics, private practice, research, sports physical therapy, federal physical therapy, and women's health (APTA, 2015).

Brief Description of Scope of Practice

The primary role of the physical therapist (PT) involves direct patient care (APTA, 2014). In addition to the provision of patient care, PTs may serve in other professional roles such as administration, education, and research. The Standards of Practice for Physical Therapy is the foremost document approved by APTA, which identifies conditions and performances that are essential for provision of high quality physical therapy (APTA, 2013a). The physical therapy profession's commitment to society is to promote optimal health and function in individuals by pursuing excellence in practice. The Standards include statements related to ethical/legal considerations, administration of physical therapy service, patient/client management, education, research, and community responsibility.

Accrediting Agency for Education

The Commission on Accreditation in Physical Therapy Education (CAPTE) is the unit of APTA responsible for accrediting professional entry-level physical therapist and physical therapist assistant education programs. Commission on Accreditation in Physical Therapy Education is responsible for the development of criteria in which educational institutions are bound to uphold. Each educational institution is reviewed and deemed appropriate for accreditation as determined by Commission on Accreditation in Physical Therapy Education. Students must graduate from an accredited institution to be eligible to take the physical therapy licensing examination (APTA, 2013b; Commission on Accreditation of Physical Therapy Education [CAPTE], 2015).

Minimum Entry-Level Professional Education/Current Education Trends

The entry-level degree for physical therapists is a master's of physical therapy; however, beginning in 2020 all programs must offer a doctorate of physical therapy to replace the master's degree.

Educational Trends

- Adoption of professional core values
- Online course series offered through APTA
- Interprofessional Education

Required Educational Content

- Courses in biology, chemistry, physics, and biostatistics provide foundational knowledge. Specific physical therapy courses typically cover topics such as anatomy, physiology, histology, biomechanics, orthopedics, ergonomics, pharmacology, neurologic conditions, and principles of research. Three years of graduate level education

- 4 years + 3 years (Bachelor degree before entry to the doctorate of physical therapy program)

- 3 years + 3 years (three years of pre-professional/undergraduate education followed by three years of graduate level education). The curriculum must be approved by CAPTE. In addition to these academic courses and labs, students must complete a minimum of 30 weeks of clinical education with most programs offering between 32 and 52 weeks of clinical education (CAPTE, 2015).

Regulatory Body/Practice Credentials (National/State)

All physical therapists must pass the national licensing examination administered by the Federation of State Boards of Physical Therapy. Additionally, physical therapists need to apply for state licensure to practice. After two years of practice, physical therapists practicing in a private practice setting are eligible to apply for a Direct Access License. Direct access means the removal of the physician referral mandated by state law to access physical therapists' services for evaluation and treatment. However, in many jurisdictions, such treatment is limited by arbitrary restrictions in state law (APTA, 2013b).

Intraprofessional Roles

Physical therapist assistants provide physical therapy services under the direction and supervision of a licensed physical therapist. The physical therapist must perform the evaluation and reassessment of the patient (APTA, 2014). Physical therapist assistants work in a variety of settings including hospitals, private practices, outpatient clinics, home health, nursing homes, schools, and sports facilities. Physical therapist assistants may also measure changes in the patient's performance as a result of the physical therapy provided. To work as a physical therapist assistant, an individual must graduate with an associate degree (two years, usually five semesters) from an accredited physical therapist assistant program at a technical or community college, college, or university. Graduates must pass the national examination for licensing/certification/regulation in most states to be eligible to work.

Specializations or Advanced Practice Areas

Specialization is the process by which a physical therapist builds on a broad base of professional education and practice to develop greater depth of knowledge and skills related to a particular area of practice. Clinical specialization in physical therapy responds to a specific area of patient need and requires knowledge, skill, and experience which exceeds that of the entry-level physical therapist and which is unique to the specialized area of practice. The approved specialty areas via the American Board of Physical Therapy Specialties are:

- Cardiovascular and Pulmonary Physical Therapy
- Clinical Electrophysiologic Physical Therapy
- Geriatric Physical Therapy
- Neurologic Physical Therapy
- Orthopedic Physical Therapy
- Pediatric Physical Therapy
- Sports Physical Therapy
- Women's Health Physical Therapy

(American Board of Physical Therapy Specialists, 2014).

Definitions and Terminology for Professionalism

According to the APTA website, the definition of professionalism is when "physical therapists consistently demonstrate core values by aspiring to and wisely applying principles of altruism, excellence, caring, ethics, respect, communication and accountability, and by working together with other professionals to achieve optimal health and wellness in individuals and communities" (Arnold & Stern, 2006).

Official Documents Related to Professionalism

In 2000, the American Physical Therapy Association House of Delegates adopted Vision 2020 and the Strategic Plan for Transitioning to a Doctoring Profession. The plan includes six elements: doctorate of physical therapy, evidence-based practice, autonomous practice, direct access, practitioner of choice, and professionalism. It describes how these elements relate to and interface with the vision of a doctoring profession. One of the initiatives describes the concept of professionalism by explicitly articulating what the graduate of a physical therapist program will demonstrate with respect to professionalism. Professionalism was integrated into a Normative Model of Physical Therapist Professional Education in 2004 to include core values of the profession, indicators consistent with the core values, and a professional education matrix that includes educational outcomes, terminal behavioral objectives, and instructional objectives for the classroom and clinical practice. In 2003, Professionalism in Physical Therapy: Core Values was reviewed by the APTA Board of Directors and adopted as a core document on professionalism in physical therapy practice, education, and research. The core values are:

- **Accountability:** The active acceptance of responsibility for the diverse roles, obligations, and actions of the physical therapist including self-regulation and other behaviors that positively influence patient/client outcomes, the profession, and the health needs of society.
- **Altruism:** The primary regard for devotion to the interest of patients/clients, thus assuming the fiduciary responsibility of placing the needs of the patients/clients ahead of the physical therapist's self-interest.

- **Compassion/Caring:** The desire to identify with or sense something of another's experience: a precursor of caring. The concern, empathy, and consideration for the needs and values of others.

- **Excellence:** Physical therapy practice that consistently uses current knowledge and theory while understanding personal limits, integrates judgment and the patient/client perspective, challenges mediocrity, and works toward development of new knowledge.

- **Integrity:** Steadfast adherence to high ethical principles or professional standards; truthfulness, fairness, doing what you say you will do, and speaking forth about why you do what you do.

- **Professional Duty:** Commitment to meeting one's obligations to provide effective physical therapy services to individual patients/clients, to serve the profession, and to positively influence the health of society.

- **Social Responsibility:** Promotion of a mutual trust between the profession and the larger public that necessitates responding to societal needs for health and wellness (APTA, 2014).

Furthermore, the APTA has offers online educational modules focused on various principles of professionalism for the physical therapy student, clinical instructor, and practitioner.

Physician Assistant

History of Professionalization

Various nations have been training non-physicians to provide health care services in remote or dangerous locations for centuries. In 1942, physician shortages and an uneven distribution of primary care physicians were creating a stain on the nation's health care delivery system. Dr. Eugene Stead developed a fast-track 3-year curriculum for education of physicians in military service during World War II at Emory University. This became the model for the medical curriculum used in 1965 to educate four former military corpsmen as physician assistants (PA) at Duke University. By 1969, the American Hospital Association and the Joint Commission on Accreditation of Hospitals release a report on the Utilization of Physician's Assistants in the Hospital (Physician Assistant History Society, n.d.).

Professional Organizations

Founded in 1968, the American Academy of Physician Assistants (AAPA) is the national professional society for PAs. It represents a profession of more than 100,000 certified PAs across all medical and surgical specialties in all 50 states, the District of Columbia, the majority of the U.S. territories and the uniformed services. American Academy of Physician Assistants advocates and educates on behalf of the profession and the patients whom PAs serve. The AAPA works to ensure the professional growth, personal excellence, and recognition of physician assistants.

Brief Description of Scope of Practice

PAs practice medicine as part of a physician-PA team. They can take medical histories, perform physical examinations, make diagnoses, prescribe medications, develop comprehensive treatment plans, assist in surgery, counsel patients, and perform minor medical procedures. Scope of practice may vary slightly based on the supervising physician and state law.

Accrediting Agency for Education

The Accreditation Review Commission on Education for the Physician Assistant is the accrediting agency that protects the interests of the public and physician assistant profession by defining the standards for physician assistant education and evaluating physician assistant educational programs within the territorial United States to ensure their compliance with those standards.

Minimum Entry-Level Professional Education/Current Education Trends

The entry-level degree for PAs is a master's degree.

Required Educational Content

The model described here is typical for an entry-level masters programs; however, a significant number of programs are post-bachelorette across the United States. Physician assistant students complete foundational courses covering topics such as biology, anatomy, physiology, pathophysiology, biostatistics, and social/behavioral sciences and humanities. The following topics are examined comprehensively during undergraduate studies: medical history and physical exam, medical procedures, pharmacology, diagnostic modalities, and disease management. Graduate studies include continued academic coursework and clinical practice. Academic coursework allows students to apply their basic medical knowledge to pediatric, adolescent, adult, obstetric, and geriatric patient populations. Physician assistants are required to complete a total of more than 2,000 hours of clinical rotations with documented experience in all of the following areas:

- Family medicine
- Internal medicine
- Obstetrics and gynecology
- Pediatrics
- General surgery
- Emergency medicine
- Psychiatry

Regulatory Body/Practice Credentials (National/State)

Upon graduation from a master's program, graduates must successfully pass the Physician Assistant National Certification Exam (PANCE). The National Commission on Certification for Physician Assistants (NCCPA) is the governing body responsible for PANCE development and delivery. Physician Assistants must earn CME credits that are evaluated by the NCCPA. One hundred CME credits must be earned every 2 years to maintain certified status. Every 10 years, PAs must successfully pass the Physician Assistant Recertification Exam, which is also developed by the NCCPA. All states require that PAs graduate from an accredited PA program and pass the PANCE; however, additional state licensure requirements may vary.

Intraprofessional Roles

Physician assistants are provided ongoing supervision by physicians relative to patient care. Physician assistants should consult with the supervising physician whenever it will safeguard or advance the welfare of the patient. This includes seeking assistance with a conflict situation with a patient or another health care professional.

Specializations or Advanced Practice Areas

Physician assistants can opt to specialize or advance their clinical practice in the following areas:

- Surgery
- Allergy and immunology medicine
- Cardiology
- Dermatology
- Emergency medicine
- Gastroenterology and hepatology
- Geriatrics
- Nephrology
- Neurosurgery
- Obstetrics and gynecology
- Occupational medicine: promoting employee health
- Oncology
- Orthopedic surgery
- Otolaryngology
- Palliative care
- Pediatrics
- Plastic surgery
- Primary care
- Psychiatry
- Rheumatology
- Urology

(American Academy of Physician Assistants, n.d.).

Definitions and Terminology for Professionalism

The PA profession's four national organizations (AAPA, NCCPA, Physician Assistant Education Association [PAEA], and Accreditation Review Commission on Education for the Physician Assistant [ARC-PA]) have adopted the Competencies for the Physician Assistant Profession (CPAP), which defines professionalism as "the expression of positive values and ideals as care is delivered" (NCCPA, ARC-PA, AAPA, & PAEA, 2012).

Official Documents Related to Professionalism

The AAPA published the Guidelines for Ethical Conduct for the Physician Assistant Profession which outlines principles of the profession and provides descriptions to assist with applying these principles to professional situations. Four primary bioethical principles were used in the development of these guidelines: autonomy, beneficence, nonmaleficence, and justice. First adopted in 2000, this document has been amended to meet the changing needs in the profession and was reaffirmed in 2013. The 12-page document includes a statement of foundational values for the profession with 11 individual statements. Then, the guidelines are listed from within five categories: the PA and the patient, the PA and individual professionalism, the PA and other health professionals, the PA and the health care system, and the PA and society. Guidelines within these categories include, for example, statements about team practice, the PA-physician relationship, and community well-being (AAPA, 2013).

A second document, Competencies for the Physician Assistant Profession, was developed by NCCPA, ARC-PA, AAPA, and PAEA. The document was adopted in 2005 and revised in 2012. The purpose of this document is to support the development and maintenance of professional competencies among physician assistants. The competencies are grouped into the following six major areas: medical knowledge, interpersonal and communication skills, patient care, professionalism, practice-based learning and improvement, and systems-based practice (NCCPA, ARC-PA, AAPA, & PAEA, 2012).

As outlined in the AAPA Judicial Affairs Procedures Manual, if after due notice and a hearing, the AAPA finds any member or organization recognized by the House of Delegates Academy in violation of bylaws, rules, or ethical guidelines, appropriate disciplinary action will be taken (AAPA, 2009).

SPEECH-LANGUAGE PATHOLOGY

History of Professionalization

The first speech-language pathologists were experts in other areas (e.g., medicine, education, elocution) who developed an interest in people with communication impairments. Frequently they were referred to as speech correctionists and most often treated people who stuttered and people with voice disorders. In the early 1900s, the professionals identifying themselves as speech correctionists in the United States began to form special interest groups. One group included speech correctionists who were originally schoolteachers. While attending the meetings of the National Education Association, they formed an affiliated subgroup led by Walter Babcock Swift, an academic at Western Reserve University in Cleveland. This subgroup named itself the National Society for the Study and Correction of Speech Disorders and continued under the leadership of Swift from 1918 to 1939.

A group of physicians, scholars, and public school administrators from the National Association of Teachers of Speech formed a second subgroup in 1925 called the American Academy of Speech Correction. The original group had 25 members (15 women and 10 men). In 1952, this group (renamed the American Speech and Hearing Association) initiated the development of national standards for audiologists and speech-language pathologists and providing certification. After several name changes, this group eventually became the American Speech-Language-Hearing Association (ASHA) in 1978 (ASHA, 2015a; Duchan, 2002; Duchan, 2011).

Professional Organizations

ASHA is the professional organization for speech-language pathologists, audiologists, and speech, language, and hearing scientists. It has more than 186,000 members and affiliates. American Speech-Language-Hearing Association's mission is "to empower and support audiologists, speech-language pathologists, and speech, language and hearing scientists through advancing science, settings standards, fostering excellence in professional practice, and advocating for members and those they serve" (ASHA, 2017).

American Speech-Language-Hearing Association's Board of Ethics is a semi-autonomous body that formulates and if needed, amends the Code of Ethics. Additionally, this board develops educational programs and materials on ethics, formulates and publishes procedures for processing alleged Code of Ethics violations, and determines sanctions for such violations (ASHA, 2013b).

Brief Description of Scope of Practice

Speech-language pathologists serve individuals, families, and groups from diverse linguistic and cultural backgrounds. Speech-language pathologists address typical and atypical communication and swallowing in multiple areas including speech sound production, resonance, voice, fluency, language, cognition, as well as feeding and swallowing.

Accrediting Agency for Education

The Council on Academic Accreditation in Audiology and Speech-Language Pathology of ASHA oversees accreditation of institutions of higher learning that offer graduate degree program in audiology and/or speech-language pathology. The Council on Academic Accreditation in Audiology and Speech-Language Pathology formulates standards for accreditation of graduate education programs in speech-language pathology and audiology and evaluates programs that voluntarily apply for accreditation.

Minimum Entry-Level Professional Education/Current Education Trends

The entry level degree for speech language pathologists is a masters degree. Recently a clinical doctorate degree has been introduced by some institutions; however, currently no guidelines are available for such degrees and they are not widely offered.

Required Educational Content

In addition to courses in biology, physiology, statistics, and social/behavioral sciences and humanities, the following topics are examined more in-depth during undergraduate studies: normal language and speech development, language disorders and phonology, linguistics, anatomy of hearing and speech mechanisms, and introduction to audiology.

Graduate studies include academic coursework and clinical practice. Academic coursework provides students with an in-depth knowledge on the various disorders and populations seen within the field (e.g., aphasia, speech-sound disorders, fluency disorders, voice disorders). Students are required to complete a minimum of 375 hours of direct client contact with specific guidelines designating a number of clinical hours for diagnostics and treatment across various specialties of the field. Students work with a variety of patient populations and in varied practice settings while also taking required coursework.

Regulatory Body/Practice Credentials (National/State)

The Council for Clinical Certification in Audiology and Speech-Language Pathology through ASHA defines the standards for clinical certification and applies those standards in the certification of individuals. This council may also develop and administer a credentialing program for speech-language pathology assistants.

Upon graduation from an accredited master's degree program, graduates must complete a Clinical Fellowship Year under the supervision of an ASHA certified speech-language pathologist to earn Clinical Competence. Additionally, candidates for certification must pass the Praxis Examination in Speech-Language Pathology. National Certification from ASHA is referred to as the Certificate of Clinical Competence in the field of Speech-Language Pathology.

State licensure requirements vary by state, but are frequently required to practice. Teacher certification requirements are often required by the state Department of Education to practice in school settings.

Certified speech-language pathologists must complete 30 Continuing Education Units (1 CEU = 10 contact hours) every three years to maintain their certification (e.g., Certificate of Clinical Competence in the field of Speech-Language Pathology).

Intraprofessional Roles

Speech-language pathology assistants are support personnel who perform tasks prescribed, directed, and supervised by ASHA-certified speech-language pathologists. Speech-language pathology assistants must complete relevant academic coursework, fieldwork, and on-the-job training. The terminology for speech-language pathology assistants may vary by state (e.g., communication aides, paraprofessionals, service extenders). Despite recent increased attention, speech-language assistants have been used and regulated by many states since the 1970s. The increase in the use of assistants is likely due to the need to expand services while containing costs. In 2000, ASHA began development of an approval process for associate degree speech-language pathology assistant training programs and a registration process for speech-language pathology assistants. In 2011, ASHA began processing applications for the Associate Affiliation Membership Category. In 2013, ASHA published a Speech-Language Pathology Assistant Scope of Practice document.

The supervision of speech-language pathology assistants must adhere to guidelines established by ASHA. First, appropriate training and supervision of speech-language pathology assistants is to be provided by speech-language pathologists who hold ASHA's Certificate of Clinical Competence (CCC) in Speech-Language Pathology. Additionally, a speech-language pathologist should not supervise or be listed as a supervisor for more than two full-time speech-language pathology assistants simultaneously. All activities conducted by the speech-language pathology assistant must be directed by the supervising speech-language pathologist, and should fall within the Scope of Practice for speech-language pathology assistants. Speech-language pathology assistants should not be used to increase or reduce the speech-language pathologists caseload size, but rather to manage existing caseloads. Speech-language pathology assistants should not have full responsibilities for a caseload or function autonomously (ASHA, 2013b).

Specializations or Advanced Practice Areas

The Clinical Specialty Certification is a voluntary program that enables an audiologist or a speech-language pathologist with advanced knowledge, skills, and experience beyond the CCC to be recognized as a board-certified specialist in a specific area of clinical practice. As of August 2015, the current specialty area of practice recognized by the Council on Academic Accreditation in Audiology and Speech-Language Pathology includes child language and language disorders, fluency and fluency disorders, swallowing and swallowing disorders, and intraoperative monitoring. Each specialty certification is also overseen by a specific specialty certification board that is semi-autonomous (e.g., American Board of Swallowing and Swallowing Disorders).

Definitions and Terminology for Professionalism

There is no single endorsed definition; however, ASHA (2000) stated that students should develop the following professionalism skills:

1. Planning and priority setting
2. Organization and time management
3. Managing diversity
4. Team building
5. Interpersonal savvy and peer relationships

6. Organizational agility

7. Conflict management

8. Problem solving, perspective and creativity

9. Dealing with paradox and learning "on the fly"

Official Documents Related to Professionalism

ASHA and the Council of Academic Programs in Communication Sciences and Disorders indicate that professional conduct can be achieved by following these documents:

1. Code of Ethics, which contains four principles of ethics, each with several rules. In summary, the principles indicate the speech-language pathologists should hold the welfare of the individuals they serve paramount, should achieve and maintain the highest level of professional competence, should provide accurate information to the public about the professions, and should honor the responsibilities to colleagues, students and other professionals. All members, non-members who are certified, and individuals seeking to fulfill standards for certification must follow this code of ethics.

2. Preferred Practice Patterns was approved by the ASHA Legislative Council in November 2004. It contains seven fundamental components and guiding principles applied to 47 areas of service provision for speech-language pathologists.

3. Technical Reports and Position Statements. These reports outline the roles and responsibilities of speech-language pathologists in specific areas of practice.

4. Consumer Bill of Rights. This guiding document was developed by ASHA and approved in 1993. It represents the 12 rights afforded to individuals needing services from speech-language pathologists. One such example is the right to be treated with dignity and respect (ASHA, 2015b).

Discipline-Specific Professional Development Tools and Measures

All students must meet the Knowledge and Skills Assessment competencies established by ASHA as a requirement for earning the CCC (ASHA, 2013a). These competencies are minimums for entry into the practice of speech-language pathology and include both academic knowledge and clinical skills. Academic programs must insure that students have the opportunity to learn and then demonstrate that they have acquired all the knowledge and skill competencies required for earning the CCC.

Three knowledge and skills assessment standards indicate student learning outcomes related to professionalism—Knowledge and skills assessment Standard IV-G—Interaction and personal qualities

1. Communicate effectively, recognizing the needs, values, preferred mode of communication, and cultural/linguistic background of the client/patient, family, caregivers, and relevant others.

2. Collaborate with other professionals in case management.

3. Adhere to the ASHA Code of Ethics and behave professionally

Summary

Across these various disciplines, professionalism is viewed as a combination of taught knowledge and skills, as well as learning gained through experience, such as experiential knowledge and the way to behave with particular people in specific situations. A review of the scholarly literature reveals that there are several shared characteristics and expectations among the different health care professions. You may refer to Table 3-1 to view this comparison. Although professionalism is a core competency for many professions, each profession articulates its own standards in professional-silos that list the attributes, behaviors, and values that professionals should exemplify. Gaining an understanding of the roles, responsibilities and expertise of other service providers is essential to work with and alongside them. Collaboration and team-based care are critical to effective patient care; therefore, higher education programs are currently examining at the best approaches and initiating new educational activities. These programs realize the importance of establishing a shared language among professionals and emphasizing the relationship between professionalism and interprofessional practice.

Interprofessional Professionalism

Human beings have worked in teams since ancient times. Whether hunting and gathering food centuries ago or providing sophisticated health care in the 21st century, teams are more effective than a group of individuals each working in isolation. Similarly, occupational therapy practitioners have engaged with other health care professionals since the beginning of our field. Occupational therapy practitioners are often part of a team of individuals involved in providing services to a client, group, or population. Teams frequently found in the delivery of health care services may be referred to as multidisciplinary teams, transdisciplinary teams, or interdisciplinary teams (Choi & Pak, 2006; Falk-Kessler, 2014). Team-based practice can be articulated in a number of ways, and often these terms are mistakenly used interchangeably. Let's briefly review the definition of each of these philosophies of team-based care.

A multidisciplinary team approach to service delivery (also called multi-professional practice) means that people from several disciplines are involved in the delivery of services. The approach, however, is discipline-oriented with each team member responsible only for the activities related to his or her own discipline (Melvin, 1989; Rothberg, 1981). Each team member will conduct separate assessments, planning, and provision of services with varying degrees of coordination. The team members, directly or indirectly, share information regarding the patient and discuss future directions for patient care, and consequently rely on a good communication system (e.g., team meetings, case conferences). As part of a multidisciplinary team, health professionals communicate regularly and share information with each other, but act autonomously. One team member is affected very little by the efforts of the other team members. This approach may be the easiest way to deliver services, because communication among team members may be less formal and may occur less frequently than with other approaches (Vanderhoff, 2010). However, it is not always in the best interest of the patient. Often team members feel responsible only for the clinical work of their discipline and need not share a sense of responsibility for program function and team effectiveness (Zeiss & Steffner, 1996). For example, an individual who sustained an acute cerebrovascular accident is currently in the hospital and receiving physical therapy, occupational therapy, and speech-language pathology services. Each of these disciplines evaluates the patient independently using his or her expertise and develops and implements an intervention program separate from the other services. In this scenario, the occupational therapy practitioner may not have a comprehensive

TABLE 3-1
SUMMARY OF HEALTH CARE PROFESSIONS

DISCIPLINE	DEFINITION OF PROFESSIONALISM	PROFESSIONALISM IN EDUCATION CURRICULAR STANDARDS	INTERPROFESSIONALISM IN EDUCATION CURRICULAR STANDARDS	PROFESSIONALISM IN CLINICAL EDUCATION EXPECTATIONS
Medicine	Yes	Yes	Yes	Yes Medical Student Performance Evaluation - MSPE Appendix C. Comparative Performance in Professional Attributes All students are evaluated in the area of Professionalism on each of their clinical clerkships. On the following attributes: ability to treat patients with compassion; honesty and ethical behavior; initiative and motivation; respect for patient autonomy and beliefs; communication skills; and ability to demonstrate effective and respectful working relationships with team members, peers, and physician colleagues. Other attributes such as: ability to treat patients with compassion; honesty and integrity; respect for others; ability to act as an advocate for patients; communication skills; and commitment to putting the needs of others before one's own needs are also evaluated (AAMC, 2002).

continued

TABLE 3-1 (CONTINUED)

SUMMARY OF HEALTH CARE PROFESSIONS

DISCIPLINE	DEFINITION OF PROFESSIONALISM	PROFESSIONALISM IN EDUCATION CURRICULAR STANDARDS	INTERPROFESSIONALISM IN EDUCATION CURRICULAR STANDARDS	PROFESSIONALISM IN CLINICAL EDUCATION EXPECTATIONS
Nursing	Yes	Yes	Yes	N/A Nursing does not have a national standard-ized evaluation tool for clinical education
Occupational Therapy	Not formally endorsed by profession	Yes	Yes	Yes American Occupational Therapy Association Fieldwork Performance Evaluation (FWPE) (AOTA, 2002)
Pharmacy	Yes	Yes	Yes	N/A Pharmacy does not have a national standard-ized evaluation tool for clinical education
Physical Therapy	Yes	Yes	Yes (new standards)	Yes APTA Physical Therapist Clinical Performance Instrument for Students Item 2 of Professional Practice is Professional Behavior, which includes 13 professional behaviors (APTA, 2015) *continued*

TABLE 3-1 (CONTINUED)
SUMMARY OF HEALTH CARE PROFESSIONS

DISCIPLINE	DEFINITION OF PROFESSIONALISM	PROFESSIONALISM IN EDUCATION CURRICULAR STANDARDS	INTERPROFESSIONALISM IN EDUCATION CURRICULAR STANDARDS	PROFESSIONALISM IN CLINICAL EDUCATION EXPECTATIONS
Physician Assistant	Yes	Yes	Yes	No Physical Assistant Studies does not have a national standardized evaluation tool for clinical education
Speech-Language Pathology	Not formally endorsed by profession	Yes	Yes	Yes While there is not a formal clinical education evaluation tool, The American Speech-Language-Hearing Association (ASHA) mandates that all graduate students abide by the principles of the ASHA Code of Ethics and that they demonstrate the Knowledge and Skills Acquisition consistent with the standards for ASHA certification (Standard IV and Standard V)

Figure 3-1. Multidisciplinary approach.

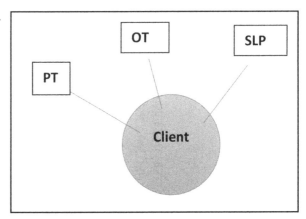

Figure 3-2. Transdisciplinary approach.

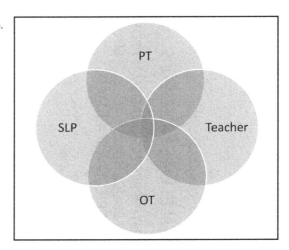

understanding of the client's needs, and the provision of services being implemented by the other service providers (Figure 3-1). A transdisciplinary approach is based on the premise that one person can perform multiple professionals' roles by providing services to the patient under the supervision of the individuals from the other disciplines involved. Representatives of various disciplines work together in the initial evaluation and care plan, but only one or two members directly provide the services. The transdisciplinary team model values the knowledge and skill of team members (Bruder, 1994). Transdisciplinary teamwork involves a certain amount of boundary blurring between disciplines and implies cross-training and flexibility in accomplishing tasks. Transdisciplinary practice becomes especially relevant in the remote and rural context, where health care professionals need to be more flexible about their roles and responsibilities. For example, a speech-language pathologist may provide guidance to a school-based occupational therapy practitioner who is providing direct services to an elementary-age student using an augmentative and alternative communication device to direct his or her personal care in the classroom setting. However, in a rural area, the speech-language pathologist in this situation may have very limited direct contact with the student and would instead meet regularly with the occupational therapy practitioner. Within this approach, two health care professionals (occupational therapy and speech-language pathology) bring their individually developed ideas to formulate a collective intervention plan to address the student's and family's needs in the school setting (Figure 3-2).

An interdisciplinary approach to service delivery presupposes interaction among the disciplines. Not only are individuals from several disciplines working toward a common goal, but also the team members have the additional responsibility of the group effort (Rothberg, 1981).

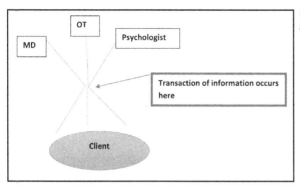

Figure 3-3. Interprofessional (interdisciplinary) approach.

This approach necessitates effective communication among the various individuals involved in the patient's rehabilitation (Melvin, 1989). Members contribute expertise from their specific profession and collaborate to interpret findings and develop a care plan. Team members negotiate priorities and reach agreement by consensus. The team includes not only the professionals, but also the patient, his or her family members, and his or her significant others. Recently, interdisciplinary practice has been referred to as interprofessional practice (Atwal & Caldwell, 2006).

While the concept of team-based care is not new, it is perhaps an understatement in current society to say that teamwork and collaboration are labeled as critical requirements for efficiency, cost effectiveness, and safe delivery of care within the current health care environment. In light of many changes in health care reform including an increased focus on outcomes, it has become necessary to integrate and coordinate the work of the various professions in the clinic. As such, there is an increased need to integrate opportunities for interprofessional education in the classroom to adequately prepare future professionals to participate in interprofessional practice.

Interprofessional education is defined as an educational experience during which two or more health professionals are learning interactively (WHO, 2010). The fundamental premise of IPE asserts that if health professional students learn interprofessional collaboration during their professional training, they will be better prepared to deliver an integrated model of collaborative clinical care after entering practice. Interprofessional education encourages learning to occur in a shared environment, versus in isolation or discipline-specific silos (Margalit et al., 2009). Training for interprofessional practice requires that members of the health care team know their discipline-specific roles, as well as the roles of other team members. Collaboration within interprofessional teams can promote sustainable and empowering patient-centered practice, health literacy, cultural sensitivity, increased critical thinking skills, and decision-making. Interprofessional collaborative practice is defined as multiple health care workers with various professional backgrounds working together with patients, families, caregivers, and communities to provide the highest quality of care and to provide the best outcomes (WHO, 2010). For example, an individual who sustained a work-related injury is referred to an outpatient chronic pain clinic. Using an interdisciplinary or interprofessional approach, service providers such as occupational therapist practitioners, psychologists, and physicians who specialize in pain management can work together to develop and implement a joint plan of care that encompasses physical and psychological deficits. Interventions such as pain management, body mechanics, joint protection, cognitive-behavioral strategies, and education on coping techniques may often overlap between the providers to support and increase intervention effectiveness for the client to eventually return to work (Figure 3-3).

Traditionally, health care professionals have been responsible for the education and training of students in their professions. Occupational therapy students primarily are taught by and learn from occupational therapy faculty (practitioners); medical students are primarily taught by and learn from physicians and so on and so forth. However, in actual patient care situations, health care professionals are expected to communicate with other health care disciplines to work

---

Box 3-4

FIVE ACCREDITATION COUNCIL FOR OCCUPATIONAL THERAPY EDUCATION STANDARDS FOR COLLABORATIVE PRACTICE

- B.5.20. Effectively interact through written, oral, and nonverbal communication with the client, family, significant others, communities, colleagues, other health providers, and the public in a professionally acceptable manner.

- B.5.21. Effectively communicate, coordinate, and work interprofessionally with those who provide services to individuals, organizations, and/or populations to clarify each member's responsibility in executing components of an intervention plan.

- B.5.22. Refer to specialists (both internal and external to the profession) for consultation and intervention.

- B.5.25. Identify and demonstrate techniques in skills of supervision and collaboration with occupational therapy assistants and other professionals on therapeutic interventions.

- B.5.31. Terminate occupational therapy services when stated outcomes have been achieved or it has been determined that they cannot be achieved. This process includes developing a summary of occupational therapy outcomes, appropriate recommendations, and referrals and discussion of post-discharge needs with the client and with appropriate others (ACOTE, 2011, pp. 26-27).

---

effectively and efficiently to provide the best patient care possible (Reeves, Perrier, Goldman, Freeth, and Zwarenstein, 2013). As a result, there is a pressing need to redesign health professions education (Box 3-4). "Changing the way we educate health professionals is key to achieving system change and to ensuring that health providers have the necessary knowledge and training to work effectively in interprofessional teams within the evolving health care system" (Thistlethwaite & Nisbet, 2007, p. 68). Academic institutions are considering methods to provide interprofessional education opportunities that prepare students to implement collaborative clinical practice due to new, common curricular mandates among medical and allied-health professions.

Preparing future professionals to work in this environment will require the culture of health care professional education to change. The AOTA supports interprofessional education to provide a higher level of patient-centered care and to better prepare the future of the profession (American Occupational Therapy Association, 2015; Moyers, & Metzler, 2014). Furthermore, for the first time, these changes have been supported through the Accreditation Council for Occupational Therapy Education (ACOTE), which has mandated clear educational standards regarding interprofessional practice. For example, ACOTE Standard B.5.21 states that the occupational therapy practitioner student must "effectively communicate and work interprofessionally with those who provide services to individuals, organizations, and/or populations to clarify each member's responsibility in executing an intervention plan" (2011, p. 26). Furthermore, within the current ACOTE Standards (2011), there are five other standards that relate to various components of collaborative practice. As discussed in Chapter 2, the high-performing team is now widely recognized as an essential tool for constructing a more patient-centered, coordinated, and effective health care delivery system (Mitchell, Parker, & Giles, 2011).

In 2011, the Interprofessional Education Collaborative (IPEC) developed the Core Competencies for Interprofessional Collaborative Practice (2011), which summarizes its efforts to facilitate a vision of IPC practice as a key to safe, high quality, accessible, patient-centered care. In February 2016, IPEC welcomed 9 new institutional members, expanding the professional representation

Box 3-5

Professionalism speaks to the values and expectations inculcated in the individual. Interprofessional professionalism considers the reciprocal collaborative elements at work in a holistic patient-centered model of care, where not only each health care provider must execute his or her particular role, but also all involved need to function as a comprehensive unit.

from 6 to 15, which now includes the AOTA. Its premise is continuous development of interprofessional competencies for health care students that will carry over as they enter the workforce, thus preparing them to practice a team approach to patient care. The four competency domains include (1) values/ethics for interprofessional practice, (2) roles and responsibilities of health professionals, (3) interprofessional communication, and (4) teams and teamwork. More specifically, each of these domains includes additional competency statements and objectives that further define the domain area (IPEC Expert Panel, 2011; IPEC, 2016). Although many of the competencies directly or indirectly relate to professionalism, a few are particularly related and warrant discussion within this chapter. The overarching objective of the values/ethics for interprofessional practice domain, for example, is to "work with individuals of other professions to maintain a climate of mutual respect and shared values" (p. 19). Within this domain are 10 competencies. These specific competencies relate to respecting, valuing, and developing trusting relationships with other health care professionals. Additionally, practitioners and future practitioners are expected to manage ethical dilemmas within the interprofessional team. Similarly, the eight competencies within the interprofessional communication domain also highlight professional behavior such as using respective language during difficult conversations or conflicts.

Although many similarities exist in how each of the health care professions conceptualize professionalism, "standards for professionalism have often been defined by individual program rather than across professions" (Hammer et al., 2012, p. e49). In 2006, representatives from seven national professional and educational groups in the United States convened to develop a concept of professionalism that could transcend and bridge the health care professions. This group, the Interprofessional Professionalism Collaborative, provides the most current definition of ineterprofessional professionalism (IPP).

Interprofessional professionalism is defined as "consistent demonstration of core values evidenced by professionals working together, aspiring to and wisely applying principles...to achieve health and wellness in individuals and communities" (Arnold & Stern, 2006, p. 19). Interprofessional professionalism focuses on the competencies, values, and norms that multiple professions have identified as critical to effective interactions in the provision of care (Box 3-5). Examples of IPP behaviors include altruism, caring, excellence, ethics, respect, communication, and accountability (Arnold & Stern, 2006). A high-performing, professional team is now widely recognized as an essential tool for constructing a patient-centered, holistic, coordinated, and effective health care delivery system (Mitchell et al., 2011). To effectively work together and collaborate, health care practitioners must have a basic understanding of each other's professions' qualifications, core values and philosophy, expertise, terminology, professional body/organization(s), and possible contributions to the team to foster interprofessional practice, collaboration, and professionalism. This chapter has identified many parallel, overlapping efforts as well as unique areas specific to individual disciplines related to professionalism within health care professions. Although professionalism is a core competency for many professions, each profession articulates its own standards in professional silos that list the attributes, behaviors, and values that professionals should exemplify, such as accountability, altruism, non-maleficence, respect, sensitivity to diversity, and so forth. Themes in the literature on interprofessional teams and leadership center on collaboration and communication. For example,

Lingard et al. (2012) state that "the growing body of literature on interprofessional care emphasizes the essential nature of collaboration and contains a strong discourse of partnership, shared leadership, and team interactions that are horizontal, relational, and situational" (p. 1762).

SUMMARY

Historically, health care professions have been exhibiting a silo mentality; each has articulated individual professional interests, values, and advocacy (Holtman, Frost, Hammer, McGuinn, & Nunez, 2011). The professional approach of the team including communication, collaboration, and a mutual respect for one another's role on the health care team is critical. In the contemporary context, professionalism contributes to safe, high-quality care primarily by supporting and fostering effective interprofessional care (Gilbert, Yan, & Hoffman, 2010). Elements of professionalism play a central role in service delivery. Understanding how the roles and responsibilities of the various team members complement each other is critical to team performance. The Institute of Medicine (IOM) highlights this point in stating "it is clear that how care is delivered is important as what care is delivered" (IOM, 2001). In other words, being a professional makes you a better practitioner and allows you to provide better care! The formation of a professional identity in occupational therapy is paramount in the journey to becoming an occupational therapy practitioner. As occupational therapy educators, the challenge lies within fostering a balance between the development of students' professional identity as an occupational therapy practitioner and identity as a member of the health care team. Although there are well-defined official documents regarding the differentiation of technical knowledge of the occupational therapy field, the distinction of professionalism and professional behaviors for occupational therapy practitioners is limited. The professionalism of the occupational therapy field will be discussed in Chapter 5.

LEARNING ACTIVITIES

1. Compare and contrast different approaches to team-based care (multidisciplinary, transdisciplinary, and interprofessional). What are the pros and cons to each?

2. Think back to previous courses completed as part of your degree program. Identify examples of interprofessional education.

3. Interview a health care professional outside of your discipline. Use the IPEC Core Competencies (2011) and explore similarities and differences between the two disciplines.

4. Observe a health care team meeting. What observations can you make regarding the communication among team members?

REFERENCES

Accreditation Council for Occupational Therapy Education. (2011). 2011 Accreditation Council for Occupational Therapy Education (ACOTE) standards and interpretive guide. Retrieved from https://www.aota.org/-/media/Corporate/Files/EducationCareers/Accredit/Standards/2011-Standards-and-Interpretive-Guide.pdf

Accreditation Council for Pharmacy Education. (n.d.) Retrieved from https://www.acpe-accredit.org/about/default.asp

American Academy of Physician Assistants. (n.d.). Issue briefs. Retrieved from https://www.aapa.org/advocacy/issue-briefs/

American Academy of Physician Assistants. (2009). Judicial affairs procedures manual 1: Complaints involving a potential judicial affairs committee (JAC) hearing. Retrieved from https://www.aapa.org/WorkArea/DownloadAsset.aspx?id=956

American Academy of Physician Assistants. (2011). Guidelines for state regulation of physician assistants. Retrieved from https://www.aapa.org/Workarea/DownloadAsset.aspx?id=795

American Academy of Physician Assistants. (2013). Guidelines for ethical conduct for the physician assistant profession. Retrieved from https://www.aapa.org/WorkArea/DownloadAsset.aspx?id=815

American Association of Colleges of Nursing. (2015). The Impact of Education on Nursing Practice. Retrieved from www.aacn.nche.edu/media-relations/fact-sheets/impact-of-education

American Association of Colleges of Pharmacy. (2012). Professionalism. Retrieved from http://www.aacp.org/resources/studentaffairspersonnel/studentaffairspolicies/Pages/professionalism.aspx

American Association of Nurse Practitioners. (n.d.). What's an NP? Retrieved from http://www.aanp.org/all-about-nps/what-is-an-np

American Board of Physical Therapy Specialists. (2014). ABPTS mission & responsibilities. Retrieved from http://www.abpts.org/About/Mission/

American College of Clinical Pharmacology. (2009). Tenets of professionalism for pharmacy students. *Pharmacotherapy, 29*(6), 757-759.

American Medical Association. (n.d.a). AMA councils. Retrieved from http://www.ama-assn.org/ama/pub/about-ama/our-people/ama-councils.page.

American Medical Association. (n.d.b). Developing AMA policies. Retrieved from http://www.ama-assn.org/ama/pub/about-ama/our-people/house-delegates/developing-ama-policies.page?

American Medical Association. (n.d.c). Our history. Retrieved from http://www.ama-assn.org/ama/pub/about-ama/our-history.page

American Nurses Association. (n.d.a). About ANA. Retrieved from http://nursingworld.org/aboutana

American Nurses Association. (n.d.b). ANA principles. Retrieved from http://www.nursingworld.org/principles

American Nurses Association. (n.d.c) Code of ethics for nurses with interpretivestatements. Retrieved from http://www.nursingworld.org/MainMenuCategories/EthicsStandards/CodeofEthicsforNurses/Code-of-Ethics-For-Nurses.html

American Nurses Association. (2014). Professional Role Competence. Retrieved from http://www.nursingworld.org/MainMenuCategories/ThePracticeofProfessionalNursing/NursingStandards/Professional-Role-Competence.html

American Nurses Association. (2016). What is nursing? Retrieved from www.nursingworld.org/EspeciallyForYou/What-is-Nursing

American Occupational Therapy Association. (2002). *Fieldwork performance evaluation for the occupational therapy student.* Bethesda, MD: American Occupational Therapy Association.

American Occupational Therapy Association. (2015). Importance of interprofessional education in occupational therapy curricula. *American Journal of Occupational Therapy, 69*(Suppl. 3).

American Pharmacists Association. (1994). Code of ethics. Retrieved from http://www.pharmacist.com/code-ethics.

American Pharmacists Association Pharmaceutical Care Guidelines Advisory Committee. (1995). Principles of Practice for Pharmaceutical Care. Retrieved from https://www.pharmacist.com/principles-practice-pharmaceutical-care

American Physical Therapy Association. (2013a). Standards of Practice. Retrieved from https://www.apta.org/uploadedFiles/APTAorg/About_Us/Policies/Practice/StandardsPractice.pdf

American Physical Therapy Association. (2013b). Vision statement for the physical therapy profession. Retrieved from http://www.apta.org/Vision/

American Physical Therapy Association. (2014). Guide to physical therapist practice 3.0. Retrieved from http://guidetoptpractice.apta.org/

American Physical Therapy Association. (2015). Physical therapist clinical performance instrument. Retrieved from http://www.apta.org/PTCPI/

American Society of Health-System Pharmacists. (2008). American Society of Health-System Pharmacists statement on professionalism. *American Journal of Health Systems Pharmacists, 65,* 172-174.

American Speech-Language Hearing Association. (2000). Responding to the changing needs of speech-language pathology and audiology students in the 21st century: A briefing paper for academicians, practitioners, employers, and students. Retrieved from http://www.asha.org/academic/reports/changing/

American Speech-Language-Hearing Association. (2013a). 2014 standards and implementation procedures for the certificate of clinical competence in speech-language pathology. Retrieved from http://www.asha.org/Certification/2014-Speech-Language-Pathology-Certification-Standards/

American Speech-Language-Hearing Association. (2013b). Speech-language pathology assistant scope of practice. Retrieved from www.asha.org/policy/SP2013-00337/

American Speech-Language-Hearing Association. (2015a). History of ASHA. Retrieved from http://www.asha.org/about/history/

American Speech-Language-Hearing Association. (2015b). Model bill of rights for people receiving audiology or speech-language pathology services. Retrieved from http://www.asha.org/public/outreach/bill_rights.htm

American Speech-Language-Hearing Association. (2017). About the American Speech-Language-Hearing Association (ASHA). Retrieved from http://www.asha.org/about/

Arnold, L., & Stern, D. T. (2006). What is medical professionalism? In D.T. Stern (Ed.), *Measuring Medical Professionalism* (pp. 15-38). New York, NY: Oxford University Press.

Association of American Medical Colleges. (2002). *A guide to the preparation of the Medical Student Performance Evaluation*. Washington, DC: Association of American Medical Colleges.

Association of American Medical Colleges. (2017). Retrieved from https://www.aamc.org/

Atwal, A., & Caldwell, K. (2006). Nurses' perceptions of multidisciplinary team work in acute health-care. *International Journal of Nursing Practice, 12*(6), 359-360.

Bruder, M. B. (1994). Working with members of other disciplines: Collaboration for success. In M. Wolery & J. S. Wilbers (Eds.), *Including children with special needs in early childhood programs* (pp. 45-70). Washington, DC: National Association for the Education of Young Children.

Bullock, A., & Trombley, S. (Eds.). (1999). *The new Fontana dictionary of modern thought*. London: Harper-Collins.

Center for Advancement of Interprofessional Education. (2008). Retrieved from http://www.caipe.org.uk

Chalmers, R. K. (1997). Contemporary issues: Professionalism in pharmacy. *Tomorrow's Pharmacist*, (March), 10-12.

Choi, B. V., & Pak, A. W. (2006). Multidisciplinarity, interdisciplinarity and transdisciplinarity in health research, services, education and policy: 1. Definitions, objectives, and evidence of effectiveness. *Clinical Investigative Medicine, 29*(6), 351-364.

Commission on Accreditation of Physical Therapy Education. (2015). What we do. Retrieved from http://www.capteonline.org/WhatWeDo/

Duchan, J. F. (2002). What do you know about your profession's history? *The ASHA Leader, 7*, 4-29.

Duchan, J. F. (2011). History of speech-language pathology: Twentieth century. Retrieved from http://www.acsu.buffalo.edu/~duchan/history.html

Falk-Kessler, J. (2014). Professionalism, communication & teamwork. In B. Schell, G. Gillen, & M. Scaffa (Eds.), *Willard and Spackman's Occupational Therapy*, (12th ed., pp. 452-465). Philadelphia, PA: Lippincott, Williams & Wilkins.

Gilbert, J. H., Yan, J., & Hoffman, S. J. (2010). A WHO report: Framework for action on interprofessional education and collaborative practice. *Journal of Allied Health, 39*(1), 196-197.

Hammer, D., Anderson, B. M., Brunson, D. W., Grus, C., Heun, L., Holtman, M., … & Frost, J. (2012). Defining and measuring a construct of interprofessional professionalism, *Journal of Allied Health, 41*(2), e49-e53.

Holtman, M. C., Frost, J. S., Hammer, D. P., McGuinn, K., & Nunez, L. M. (2011). Interprofessional professionalism: Linking professionalism and interprofessional care. *Journal of Interprofessional Care, 25*(5), 383-385. doi:10.3109/13561820.2011.588350.

Horowitz, B. P. (2002). Ethical decision-making challenges in clinical practice. *Occupational Therapy in Health Care, 16*(4), 1-15.

Interprofessional Education Collaborative Expert Panel. (2011). *Core competencies for interprofessional collaborative practice: report of an expert panel*. Washington, DC: Interprofessional Education Collaborative.

Interprofessional Education Collaborative. (2016). *Core competencies for interprofessional collaborative practice: 2016 update*. Washington, DC: Interprofessional Education Collaborative.

Institute of Medicine. (2001). *Crossing the quality chasm*. Washington DC: National Academy Press.

The Joint Commission. (2015). About the Joint Commission. Retrieved from http://www.jointcommission.org/about_us/about_the_joint_commission_main. Aspx

Lingard, L., Vanstone, M., Durrant, M., Fleming-Carroll, B., Lowe, M., Rashotte, J., … Tallett, S. (2012). Conflicting messages: Examining the dynamics of leadership on interprofessional teams. *Academic Medicine: Journal of the Association of American Medical Colleges, 87*(12), 1762-1767. doi:10.1097/ACM.0b013e318271fc82.

Margalit, R., Thompson, S., Visovsky, C., Geske, J., Collier, D., Birk, T., & Paulman, P. (2009). From professional silos to interprofessional education: Campus wide focus on quality of care. *Quality Management in Health Care, 18*(3), 165-173. doi:10.1097/QMH.0b013e3181aea20d.

Melvin, J. L. (1989). Status report on interdisciplinary medical education. *Archives of Physical Medicine and Rehabilitation, 70*, 273-276.

Mitchell, R.J., Parker, V., & Giles, M. (2011). When do interprofessional teams succeed? Investigating the moderating roles of team and professional identity in interprofessional effectiveness. *Human Relations, 64*(10), 1321-1343.

Moyers, P. A. & Metzler, C. A. (2014). Interprofessional collaborative practice in care coordination. *The American Journal of Occupational Therapy, 68*(5), 500-505.

National Resident Match Program. (2015). Retrieved from www.nrmp.org/

NCCPA, ARC-PA, AAPA, PAEA. (2012). Competencies for the physician assistant profession. Retrieved from http://www.nccpa.net/Uploads/docs/PACompetencies.pdf

The Pennsylvania Code. (2012). Functions of the LPN. Retrieved from http://www.pacode.com/secure/data/049/chapter21/s21.145.html

"Pharmacy." (2015). In Merriam-Webster dictionary. Retrieved from http://www.merriam-webster.com/dictionary/pharmacy

Physician Assistant History Society. (n.d.). Timeline. Retrieved from http://www.pahx.org/timeline.html

Popovich, N. G., Hammer, D. P., Hansen, D. J., Spies, A. R., Whalen, K. P., Beardsley, R. S., ... & Athay, J. L. (2011). Report of the AACP professional task force. *American Journal of Pharmaceutical Education, 75*(10), 1-4.

Reeves, S., Perrier, L., Goldman, J., Freeth, D., & Zwarenstein, M. (2013). Interprofessional education: Effects on professional practice and healthcare outcomes (update). *The Cochrane Database of Systematic Reviews*, 3CD002213. doi:10.1002/14651858.CD002213.pub3.

Rothberg, J. (1981). The rehabilitation team: Future direction. *Archives of Physical Medicine and Rehabilitation, 62*, 407-410.

Thistlethwaite, J., & Nisbet, G. (2007). Interprofessional education: What's the point and where we're at. *The Clinical Teacher, 4*, 67-72.

U.S. National Library of Medicine. (2013). Doctor of medicine profession (MD). Retrieved from https://www.nlm.nih.gov/medlineplus/ency/article/001936.htm

Vanderhoff, M. (2010). Maximizing your role in early intervention. Retrieved from http://www.apta.org/AM/Template.cfm?Section=Home&TEMPLATE=/CM/HTMLDisplay.cfm&CONTENTID=8534

Whelan, J. C. (n.d.). American Nursing: An introduction to the past. Retrieved from http://www.nursing.upenn.edu/nhhc/Pages/AmericanNursingIntroduction.aspx.

World Health Organization. (2010). *Framework for action on interprofessional education & collaborative practice*. Geneva: World Health Organization. Retrieved from http://whqlibdoc.who.int/hq/2010/WHO_HRH_HPN_10.3_eng .pdf

Zeiss, A. M. & Steffer, A. M. (1996). Interdisciplinary healthcare teams: The basic unit of geriatric care. In L. L. Carstensen, B. A. Edelstein, & L. Dornbrand (Eds.), *The practical handbook of clinical gerontology* (pp. 423–449). Thousand Oaks, CA: Sage Publications.

4

The Professionalization of the Occupational Therapy Profession

Elizabeth D. DeIuliis, OTD, OTR/L

INTRODUCTION

*"The professional student should at least have
a fair knowledge of this history of his profession"*
—Edward Kremers, 1892
AphA Section of Pharmaceutical
Education and Legislation
(Worthen, 2005)

So far, you have learned about basic terms associated with professionalism, and have seen the role that professionalism plays in other health care and social care professions. We will now examine these and other key concepts specifically relative to the occupational therapy profession. This chapter will briefly review the history of the professionalization of occupational therapy, identify key documents and contexts that greatly influenced professional practice, and discuss various elements within clinical practice that enforce and regulate professional responsibility, behavior, and conduct.

KEY WORDS

Accreditation Council for Occupational Therapy Education: Accrediting body for schools that train occupational therapy practitioners and occupational therapy assistants; sets educational standards that must be met and maintained for accreditation

American Occupational Therapy Association (AOTA): The nonprofit organization in America dedicated to expanding and refining the knowledge base of occupational therapy, providing support to research and education; has existed in its current form since 1923

National Society for the Promotion of Occupational Therapy: Founded March 15, 1917, this organization arose from the push toward moral treatment, social reform, and scientific medicine, as well as a belief in the therapeutic value of arts and crafts; became the AOTA in 1923

The Joint Commission: Accrediting body for hospitals and health care facilities; sets standards to monitor quality of care, as well as many components of professional and ethical conduct such as leadership standards specifically geared toward enforcing institutional leadership structure, hospital culture, and system performance

OBJECTIVES

By the end of reading this chapter and completing the learning activities, the reader should be able to:

1. Identify events in the formative years in the history of the occupational therapy profession that led to its professionalization

2. Name the occupational therapy profession's official documents regarding professionalism and ethics

3. Demonstrate a knowledge and understanding of the American Occupational Therapy Association Code of Ethics

4. Name the values of the occupational therapy profession

5. Distinguish the role that professionalism plays at the international, national, and regional level in occupational therapy practice.

BRIEF HISTORY OF THE PROFESSIONALIZATION OF OCCUPATIONAL THERAPY

Some of the major events in the history of the occupational therapy profession that led to its professionalization are: moral treatment, formation of the National Society for the Promotion of Occupational Therapy (NSPOT) and later the American Occupational Therapy Association (AOTA), post-war eras, rehabilitation movement, and medical model movement. The root of the occupational therapy profession began to materialize in the era of moral treatment (Figure 4-1). Although tragic, the wars in which the United States participated were consistently a driving force in the evolution of rehabilitation (Eldar & Jelić, 2003). Due to the overwhelming number of war-time injuries, "reconstruction aides" were recruited by the Surgeon General. Reconstruction aides or occupational nurses were the first descriptors used to describe members of what would become the occupational therapy profession (Low, 1992). .

On March 15, 1917, the NSPOT was founded in Clifton Springs, New York. Charter members included; Eleanor Clarke Slagle (a partially trained social worker), George Edward Barton (a disabled architect), Adolf Meyer (a psychiatrist), Susan Johnson, Thomas Kidner, Isabel G. Newton (Barton's secretary who later became his wife), and Susan Tracy (Dunton, 1925). This society was created from a push toward incorporation of the moral treatment of people, scientific medicine, and arts and crafts into health care. It also included a push toward social reform (Schwartz, 2009).

Shortly after the founding of the NSPOT, World War I broke out. This war forced the new profession of occupational therapy to clarify its role in the medical domain, and to standardize training and practice. Occupational therapy practitioners established clinics, workshops, and training schools nationwide. The onset of World War I was important for occupational therapy because:

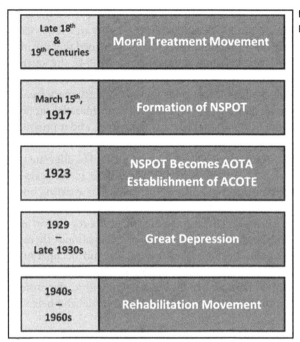

Figure 4-1. A timeline of occupational therapy professionalization.

Box 4-1

The AOTA is a nonprofit organization which still exists today and has unconditionally been dedicated to expanding and refining the knowledge base of occupational therapy by providing support to research and education.

---

it made the founders articulate the therapy they were providing; three of the founders belonged to countries engaged in the war; it validated the success of occupational therapy; it influenced who would provide services; and the idea of the patient-practitioner relationship became the popular model for treatment (Peloquin, 1991, p. 734). The first official definition of occupational therapy was: "an activity, mental or physical, definitely prescribed for the distinct purpose of contributing to and hastening recovery from disease or injury" (Pattison, 1922).

Post-war, however, there was a struggle to keep people in the profession. Emphasis was shifted from the altruistic wartime mentality to the financial, professional, and personal satisfaction that comes with being an occupational therapy practitioner. The NSPOT was renamed the AOTA in 1923 (Box 4-1). Entry and exit criteria were established, and the AOTA advocated for steady employment, decent wages, and fair working conditions for the profession. The era between 1940s and 1960s brought on the "Rehabilitation Movement," which promoted the profession as a medical entity, where occupational therapy practitioners were in greater demand to treat not only the mentally ill, but individuals with physical disabilities as well. During this time, there was a simultaneous shift in occupational therapy services toward focusing on medical outcomes as opposed to the original humanitarian and societal benefits (Friedland, 1998). However, the push for scientific research in the field of occupational therapy was not significantly revisited until the 1950s.

Since the 1960s, conceptualizations of the word "profession" changed as many occupations, particularly those with a service focus, sought out a professional identity. An occupation must have certain characteristics to substantiate its claim to professional status; the most common of these are that practitioners within the field have ownership of a knowledge base, the authority and autonomy to practice according to this knowledge, and altruism that their practice is for the pur-pose of social good (Freidson, 1988). The medical model, developed in the 1950s and 1960s gave occupational therapy practitioners a "loftier status" (Friedland, 1998, p. 378). It turned therapy into a service that could be more readily understood, and it caught the public eye. In 1947, the journal *Occupational Therapy and Rehabilitation* and the first major textbook, *Willard & Spackman's Principles of Occupational Therapy*, were published. Occupational therapy practitioners finally achieved military status. This recognition provided other opportunities to gain financial support from the federal government for the education of occupational therapy personnel, and it provided leadership training skills for members of the AOTA.

In 1956, the Certified Occupational Therapy Assistant (COTA) role was created to alleviate the demand for occupational therapy practitioners, who were required to attend four to six years of schooling. The COTA role required only minimal training, and was utilized as an assisting body and aide. In the 1960s and 1970s, there was a continued demand for more scientific evidence and research in the occupational therapy field, as well as specialization, including more regulation and governance over education and rehabilitation practice. The profession of occupational therapy continued to grow. During the 1960s, as medicine became "specialized," so did occupational therapy. Occupational therapy practitioners were called upon and became qualified to treat in the fields of pediatrics and developmental disabilities. This change lead to tension within the profes-sion, as there were those who believed in generalization of the profession and those who believed in specialization.

It was during this time in the 1960s where initial concern grew about professionalism in occupational therapy. Many felt that the profession had lost sight of the value and meaning of occupation, the concept that had led to the creation of the profession, and that this had led to role confusion and loss of identity for occupational therapy practitioners. Although at this time, the occupational therapy profession had been established for nearly 50 years, it was not until 1969 when the AOTA adopted the first formal definition of occupational therapy. This definition stated that "occupational therapy is the art and science of directing man's response to selected activity to promote and maintain health, to prevent disability, to evaluate behavior and to treat or train patients with physical and psychosocial dysfunction" (AOTA, 1969, p. 185). Furthermore, with de-institutionalization came an even greater need to help individuals with intellectual disabilities and psychiatric disorders to become independent and productive members of society.

During the 1980s and 1990s, the occupational therapy profession began to focus more heavily on a person's quality of life, thus becoming more involved in education, prevention, screenings, and health maintenance. Clearly, the profession of occupational therapy is a product of, and dependent on, a social environment that values the individual and believes that each person has the capacity to act on his or her own behalf, to achieve a better state of health through occupation. The role of the occupational therapy practitioner, as well as the professional expectations of the role, have evolved from that of a craft-oriented medical technician to that of a professional clini-cian, researcher, educator, advocate, and consultant (AOTA, 1993).

HISTORY OF THE OCCUPATIONAL THERAPY CODE OF ETHICS

A professional code supports moral understanding by connecting the profession to a moral purpose, thereby helping professionals to see their practices as "performance for public good"
—Robert K. Fullinwider, 1996

The AOTA has evolved into the driving force that dictates the profession's beliefs, philosophies, and values in America. Since its inception, the AOTA has endorsed many official documents, often called "white papers," as public statements used to communicate the national organization's posi-tion on various topics. In 1970s, several writers suggested that the occupational therapy profession needed to consider whether they valued the idea of occupational therapy becoming a "true profession." As a result, several steps toward professionalization were taken. The AOTA has been committed to both educating practitioners about ethical occupational therapy practice and enforcing the ethical standards of the profession.

The AOTA developed a professional code of ethics that codified professional values and beliefs about practice to its receipts of service, colleagues, and society. A code of ethics is a formal, written, public expression of principles and ethics of the profession, and emulates the tenets of the Hippocratic Oath (discussed in Chapter 2).

There are two main components of a code of ethics:

1. Prescription concerning what professionals or the profession as whole ought to do and what they ought to aim to be (in terms of performance/behavior). This may include:

   a. Goals in which its members should aspire to

   b. Patient care issues (i.e., provide services in a fair/equitable manner, patient rights)

   c. Professional relationships (including a framework for professional behavior and responsibilities)

2. Consequences and sanctions that follow noncompliance

Therefore, although the essence of ethics and humanistic and moral values has been at the core of the occupational therapy profession since its inception in 1917, it was not explicitly written until April 1977—nearly 60 years later! This document written in 1977 provided guidelines to occupational therapy practitioners to help them recognize and resolve ethical dilemmas, practice at the expected standards using guided principles, and educate the public. In general, it was meant to inspire professional conduct for quality and empathetic occupational therapy practice, while also respecting the rights of and diversity of our consumers. The original code has since been revised in the following years: 1979, 1999, 1994, 2005, 2010, and most recently, 2015. Along with the *Occupational Therapy Code of Ethics*, two additional complementary documents were developed: *Core Values and Attitudes* (1993) and *Guidelines to the AOTA Code of Ethics* (1998). The 2010 and subsequent editions combined these three previous documents. The *AOTA Occupational Therapy Code of Ethics and Ethics Standards* (2010) was a public statement to all of the AOTA's members of ideals, values, or rules used to promote and maintain high standards of conduct within the profession, aimed to inform and protect current and potential consumers, and protect the integrity of the profession. This commitment extends beyond service recipients to include professional colleagues, students, educators, businesses, and the community.

The *Core Values of the Profession* (1993) was based on humanism, which derived from the era of moral treatment. This white paper was designed to complement the code of ethic and codified the beliefs and ideals of the occupational therapy profession.

Throughout the various revisions of this document, there has been seven long-standing core values within the occupational therapy profession (Table 4-1).

The purpose of the *Occupational Therapy Code of Ethics* (AOTA, 2015b) is to:

- Identify and describe the principles supported by the occupational therapy profession

- Educate and protect the general public and members regarding established principles to which occupational therapy personnel are accountable

- Socialize occupational therapy personnel new to the practice to expected standards of conduct

- Assist occupational therapy personnel in recognition and resolution of ethical dilemmas in all aspects of their diverse roles

Within this document, there are six Principles and Standards of Conduct, each addressing a different aspect of enforceable professional behavior (Table 4-2).

TABLE 4-1
OVERVIEW OF CORE VALUES OF THE OCCUPATIONAL THERAPY PROFESSION

CORE VALUE	MEANING
Freedom	Allowing the individual to exercise choice, as well as to demonstrate independence, initiative, and self-direction
Altruism	Unselfish concern for others
Justice	Upholding moral and legal principles such as fairness, equity, truthfulness, and objectivity
Prudence	Ability to govern and discipline oneself through the use of reason
Equality	Perceiving all individuals as having the same fundamental human rights and opportunities
Truth	Requires that we be faithful to facts and reality
Dignity	Valuing the inherent worth and uniqueness of each person

TABLE 4-2
SUMMARY OF OCCUPATIONAL THERAPY ETHICAL PRINCIPLES

STANDARD	MEANING
Beneficence	To contribute to the well-being and good health of a client. Treat all clients equally, advocate for client, promote public health, charge reasonable fees for services provided
Nonmaleficence	To do no harm; ensures that occupational therapy practitioners maintain therapeutic relationship and do not exploit the client physically, emotionally, psychologically, socially, sexually, or financially
Autonomy	Freedom to decide and freedom to act; expectation that information shared by patient to the occupational therapy practitioner will be kept private, and only shared with those directly involved. Respect legal right to refuse treatment; informed consent, voluntary agreement, right to benefits, as well as risks and costs
Justice	Fair and equitable, appropriate treatment of individuals.
Veracity	Truth; accurately representing qualifications, education, training, and competence
Fidelity	Trust; relationship and interactions between occupational therapy practitioners, colleagues, and clients; maintaining confidentially, accurately representing qualifications, reporting misconduct to appropriate entities

TABLE 4-3
REVIEW OF POTENTIAL DISCIPLINARY ACTIONS FOR AN ETHICAL OR PROFESSIONAL CONDUCT VIOLATION

DISCIPLINARY ACTION	DEFINITION
Reprimand	Written, formal letter of disapproval of misconduct—this is non-disclosable and non-communicative to other bodies. All actions other than reprimand are publicized
Censure	Formal expression in public—for example, as a statement in a newsletter or posted on a licensure board website
Probation	Subject to terms. Continued membership is conditional; found guilty, then followed to see if complicit with disciplinary actions and/or sanctions
Suspension	Removal of membership for a period of time, or removal of practice privileges
Revocation	Permanent removal of membership or practice privileges

Although occupational therapy practitioners certainly rely on their own values and morals in clinical practice, professional decision making does rely on clear clinical decision-making skills, as well as a professional code of ethics. As stated earlier, an integral element of having a code of ethics is having an infrastructure in place to support and enforce it. The Ethics Commission (EC) is an advisory commission of the Representative Assembly that is responsible for the development and revision of the AOTA Code of Ethics and related ethics standards. Their primary role is ethics education, as well as reviewing and investigating ethical complaints filed by AOTA members, including making recommendations for disciplinary action in the event of ethical violations. The AOTA and the EC only have governance over its members; therefore, acceptance of AOTA membership commits individuals to adherence to the Code of Ethics Standards and its enforcement procedures. If a person has behaved in an unethical manner and he or she are not an AOTA member, the AOTA would not be able to sanction him or her. However, this would most likely carry over to the other credential agencies that oversee occupational therapy practice, including State Licensure Boards or National/Specialty Certification Boards such as for hand therapist certification, and/or NBCOT.

As a professional, it is essential that you are knowledgeable about best practices in dealing with an ethical compliant. The Enforcement Procedures for the Occupational Therapy Codes of Ethics and Standards (2014) states the procedures that are followed by the EC to enforce the code of ethics. This document is accessible to the public and available to all members of the profession, State Regulatory Boards, consumers, and others.

Disciplinary Actions/Sanctions Process

If the EC determines that an unethical conduct has occurred, it may impose sanctions upon the individual.

The potential sanctions are discussed in Table 4-3.

Conduct Violation

There is an appeal process if a sanction has been imposed. Either the EC or the respondent of the sanction may appeal within 30 days after notification of the EC decision. If no appeal is filed within that time frame, those disciplinary sanctions that are censured are published in accordance with these procedures and other notifications are made (such as published on the AOTA website, or State Regulatory Boards newsletter). Full description of the appeals process can be found in Enforcement Procedures for the Occupational Therapy Code of Ethics (AOTA, 2015b).

OTHER PROFESSIONAL ORGANIZATIONS' GOVERNANCE ON ETHICS/CONDUCT

International

At the international level, The World Federation of Occupational Therapy (WFOT) Code of Ethics was designed to offer broad guidelines for the practice of occupational therapy worldwide. Last revised in 2005, this document describes the general categories of personal attributes, responsibility toward the consumer, appropriate conduct for occupational therapy practitioners in any professional circumstance, and expectations for promotion and development (WFOT, 2005). This public statement declared at the international level a demand from occupational therapy practitioners for a combination of ethical standards, moral values, and professional conduct.

National

National Board for Certification in Occupational Therapy, Inc

National Board for Certification in Occupational Therapy (NBCOT) is a non-profit credentialing agency that provides certification for the occupational therapy profession. As the credentialing agency for the profession of occupational therapy, NBCOT serves to assure the public that persons practicing as occupational therapy practitioners have entry-level competence. The NBCOT is centrally concerned with "safe, proficient and/or competent practice in occupational therapy practice" (NBCOT, 2016a). Prior to sitting for an NBCOT certification examination, certification candidates must agree to abide by the NBCOT Code of Conduct. In its Candidate/Certificant Code of Conduct, NBCOT defines and clarifies the professional responsibilities, saying:

> as certified professionals in the field of occupational therapy, NBCOT certificants will at all times act with integrity and adhere to high standards for personal and professional conduct, accept responsibility for their actions, both personally and professionally, continually seek to enhance their professional capabilities, practice with fairness and honesty, abide by all federal, state, and local laws and regulations, and encourage others to act in a professional manner consistent with the certification standards and responsibilities set forth below. (NBCOT, 2016b)

The NBCOT Candidate/Certificant Code of Conduct contains many principles that reflect expectations of ethical practice. The importance of being a professional during the initial and re-credentialing process is discussed in Chapter 10.

State/Regional Level

Occupational therapy practice is regulated in all 50 states, the District of Columbia, Puerto Rico, and Guam. Different states have various types of regulation. State Regulatory Boards are responsible for monitoring and enforcing the continued competence, qualifications, licensure requirements, and credentialing process at the state level, scope of practice, and supervision. State laws and regulations significantly affect the practice of occupational therapy professionals. State practice guidelines are developed by regulators who are appointed public officials in state government. The overall purpose of these regulations is to protect consumers in a state from unqualified or unethical practitioners. Some state regulations stipulate clear guidelines regarding developing continued competence or receiving ethical training. For example, the state of Ohio requires occupational therapy practitioners to receive at least one contact hour of ethics education per licensure renewal. The North Dakota State Board of Occupational Therapy Practice requires new license holders in the state to complete and submit a jurisprudence exam, regarding North Dakota-specific scope of practice and licensure requirements. The North Carolina Board of Occupational Therapy also has requirements for an ethics continued competence activity. Their law states that for each renewal period, each licensee shall document completion of at least one contact hour of an ethics course related to the practice of occupational therapy. It is a professional's responsibility to be knowledgeable and abide by both state and national regulations regarding occupational therapy practice. You can visit www.aota.org for greater details on state policy and regulations.

Institutional Level

Outside of professional organizations and credentialing bodies, individual employers or work sites most likely dictate guidelines for professional behavior, conduct, and performance. Institutional Review Boards, which may take place in an academic or clinical setting, are ethical review committees that are formally designed to approve, monitor, and review research, specifically aimed at protecting the rights and welfare of research participants. More information regarding ethics in scholarship and research will be discussed in Chapter 15.

More specifically, individual employers and work settings have specific expectations for professionalism in occupational therapy clinical practice. Many employers have "zero tolerance" policies, which are aimed at controlling undesirable, unprofessional, and unethical behavior and conduct. For example, The Joint Commission, which accredits hospitals and health care facilities, sets standards to monitor quality of care, which are called national patient safety standards. However, these standards enforced by The Joint Commission are not only focused upon the care of the patient. There are also leadership standards that are specifically geared toward enforcing institutional leadership structure, hospital culture, and system performance, which encompass many components of professional and ethical conduct. For example, The Joint Commission leadership standard (LD.03.01.01) addresses disruptive and inappropriate behaviors in two of its elements of performance (Schyve, 2009):

- The hospital/organization has a code of conduct that defines acceptable, disruptive, and inappropriate behaviors.

- Leaders create and implement a process for managing disruptive and inappropriate behaviors.

Therefore, unprofessional behavior and conduct has ramifications that could occur at the institutional, state, national, and international level.

FORMAL DOCUMENTS RELATED TO OCCUPATIONAL THERAPY

White Papers

White papers are formal documents that are written to inform readers about key issues or present an official body's overall philosophy or mindset. In health care, white papers are traditionally written by formal organizations, committees, or regulatory bodies and may in turn become policy or position papers. The AOTA lists many official documents or white papers on their website, such as the Occupational Therapy Code of Ethics (2015b). Although there has never been a white paper from the AOTA exclusively geared toward professionalism, there have been other key documents that have added to the professionalization of occupational therapy.

Standards of Practice

This document, revised in 2015, defines the minimum standards of occupational therapy practice for occupational therapy and occupational therapy assistants. It includes standards related to:

- Credentials such as education, examination, and licensure requirements to practice
- Professional responsibility including adherence to state, federal, and other regulatory requirements
- Stipulations of the occupational therapy process including screening, evaluation, intervention, and discharge (AOTA, 2015a)

Scope of Practice

The purpose of the Scope of Practice (2014) is to:
- Define the scope of occupational therapy by delineating the domain of services including evaluation and intervention, describe education and certification requirements needed to practice
- Inform consumers, health care providers, educators, and other stakeholders regarding the scope of occupational therapy

Standards for Continued Competency

This document, revised in 2015, discusses the necessity of ongoing professional development and lifelong learning within the occupational therapy profession. The requirement of continued competence is discussed related to five key standards (AOTA, 2015c):

- Knowledge
- Critical reasoning
- Interpersonal skills
- Performance skills
- Ethical practice

Guidelines for Supervision, Roles and Responsibilities During the Delivery of Occupational Therapy Services

This 2014 document provides a set of guidelines describing the supervision, roles, and responsibilities of occupational therapy practitioners, including occupational therapy practitioners, occupational therapy assistants, and occupational therapy aides. Principles related to frequency, type and scope of supervision are discussed, as well as role delineations between the different levels of practitioners. It is the professional responsibility of an occupational therapy professional to comply with these guidelines to provide safe, effective and ethical services (AOTA, 2014).

BOX 4-2

The Pledge and Creed states:

REVERENTLY AND EARNESTLY do I pledge my whole-hearted service in aiding those crippled in mind and body.

TO THIS END that my work for the sick may be successful, I will ever strive for greater knowledge, skill and understanding in the discharge of my duties in whatsoever position I may find myself.

I SOLEMNLY DECLARE that I will hold and keep inviolate whatever I may learn of the lives of the sick.

I ACKNOWLEDGE the dignity of the cure of disease and the safeguarding of health in which no act is menial or inglorious.

I WILL WALK in upright faithfulness and obedience to those under whose guidance I am to work, and I pray for patience, kindliness, and strength in the holy ministry to broken minds and bodies.

Adapted from American Occupational Therapy Association. (1942). Occupational therapy notes. *Occupational Therapy and Rehabilitation, 21*(5), 314-320; Reed, K. L. & Sanderson, S. N. (1999). *Concepts of occupational therapy.* Philadelphia, PA: Lippincott Williams & Wilkins.

BOX 4-3

Here is a more contemporary example of an oath that represents the moral, ethical, and professional principles of the occupational therapy profession.

Occupational Therapy Creed

Respectfully and enthusiastically, I do hereby promise my whole-hearted service to care for those who are entrusted to me. I assure competence in my work and will strive for greater knowledge, skill and understanding in the discharge of my duties in whatever role I embrace: practitioner, educator, researcher or manager. I solemnly declare that I will hold and keep sacred whatever I may learn in lives of those I enter. In embracing the responsibilities and the challenges of working with persons of diverse backgrounds, I will uphold a person's right to self-determination and always endeavor to provide quality care. I pledge from this day forth to forever soar ethically, compassionately and hope for patience, gentleness and understanding in all therapeutic partnerships.

Occupational Therapy Pledge and Creed

It is often a rite of passage during graduation ceremonies for new graduates to recite an oath or pledge for their respective profession. It may encompass a pinning, white-coat, or hooding ceremony, depending on the degree. This ritual symbolizes a student's official transition into professional life. The oath serves as a commitment to model and foster professionalism and ethical practice, as well as to engage in personal and professional growth. The Occupational Therapy Pledge and Creed was submitted by the Boston School of Occupational Therapy and adopted by the AOTA in 1926. Since its inception in 1926, there have been several variations of this pledge (Boxes 4-2 and 4-3). Perhaps this creed should not be limited to new practitioners starting their career, but stand as an expectation for all occupational therapy practitioners to read, reflect, and embody routinely?

Eleanor Slagle Lectureships

"The integrity of the profession is in your hands"
—Eleanor Slagle, 1937

In addition to these important documents, which guide the future and direction of the occupational therapy profession, the Eleanor Slagle Lectureship is another flagship mainstay in this realm. As noted previously, Eleanor Clarke Slagle was one of the most influential founders of the occupational therapy profession. Often referred to as the "mother of occupational therapy," in her time, Slagle set the stage for the growth and development of a new profession. The first Eleanor Slagle lectureship was awarded in 1955 as an academic honor established as a memorial to the late Slagle. This lectureship became the foundation for documenting the advancement of occupational therapy, and to this day is still the highest honor given by the American Occupational Therapy Association. The lectureship acknowledges a vision for the future including the advanced theory, standards and improved methods that enhance occupational therapy practice and service. The honor is awarded annually to a member of the association who has "creatively contributed to the development of knowledge of the profession through research, education and/or clinical practice" (AOTA, n.d.).

The first lectureship was given in 1954 to Florence M. Stattell, who spoke on equipment designed for occupational therapy. Major themes presented in Slagle lectures include occupational therapy practice, education, philosophy, and theory. DeBeer (1987) completed a meta-analysis and examined 27 Slagle lectures between 1955 and 1985, and indicated that professionalism (related to concepts such as role delineation, professional validation, and professional identity) was a common theme in over one-third of them. Furthermore, four lecturers have specifically attempted to validate occupational therapy as a profession (Ackley, 1962; Fiorentino, 1975; Gilfoyle, 1984; Yerxa, 1967). Other, more recent recipients of the Slagle recognition have delivered a message with a strong undertone of professionalism (Table 4-4).

Relationship Between Occupational Therapy Theory and Professionalism

The occupational therapy profession has always been driven by a philosophy of morals, ethics, and duty to mankind. In addition to ethical behavior being a hallmark of the occupational therapy profession, one could also infer a strong connection between occupational therapy theory, its models of practice, and professional behavior expectations. Following suit with many occupational therapy models of practice and frames of reference, performance is a product of interaction between the person, occupation, and the environment. If the desired performance is professionalism, this would infer that a meaningful interaction of the person, occupation, and context is required.

Intentional Relationship

Dr. Renee Taylor, PhD, a distinguished occupational therapy clinician and scholar, is the creator of the Intentional Relationship Model (IRM). While this model provides a framework for developing relational skills between a practitioner and client, the IRM also emphasizes the need for occupational therapy professionals to remain "self-aware" of behavior, to be "self-disciplined" and to exhibit "empathy" (Gorenberg & Taylor, 2014, p. 2). Taylor (2008) further discusses how practitioners need to act deliberately and thoughtfully to successfully establish and maintain a therapeutic

TABLE 4-4
SNAPSHOT OF ELEANOR SLAGLE LECTURES WHICH EMPHASIZED PROFESSIONALISM

YEAR	LECTURER	TOPIC
1967	Wilma L. West	• Professional Responsibility in a Time of Change • Encouraged the profession to look ahead, and seek innovative approaches to meet societal needs.
1972	Jerry A. Johnson	• Occupational Therapy: A Model for the Future • Current practitioners must strive to ensure that new practitioners, who will one day represent occupational therapy, are competent, knowledgeable, and strive for professional excellence.
1984	Elnora M. Gilfoyle	• Transformation of a Profession • Concerned about and questioned the internal values of the profession.
1985	Anne Cronin Mosey	• A Monistic or Pluralistic Approach to Professional Identity? • Occupational therapy practitioners have long been concerned with the process of articulating their identity. Mosey addressed two approaches to the process of articulating the identity of the profession, monism and pluralism, and expressed a preference for adopting the latter.
2009	Kathleen Barker Schwartz	• Reclaiming Our Heritage: Connecting Our Founding Vision to the Centennial Vision • Encouraged the profession to remember and embody the vision, beliefs, and values that the founders of our profession established.

relationship with the client. Developing student professionals can benefit from using the IRM in identifying and developing their individual therapeutic use of self and professional identity, in response to the interpersonal characteristics of clients, colleagues, and individuals in society.

The IRM describes six therapeutic modes, emphasizes the importance of self-reflection, and directs significant attention to the range of interpersonal skills needed to establish and maintain the therapeutic relationship (Taylor, 2008). Taylor believes that practitioners naturally select and employ therapeutic modes that are consistent with their personalities. Critical and ongoing self-awareness and interpersonal discipline are underlying principles key to the IRM, as well as important intrinsic qualities of being a professional. Similar to the sophisticated combination of intrinsic and extrinsic qualities of professionalism, therapeutic use of self is a blending of professional knowledge and interpersonal skills. Table 4-5 provides an example of IRM's therapeutic modes, and how they can contribute to the development of professional skills.

TABLE 4-5
SIX THERAPEUTIC MODES

THERAPEUTIC MODE	DESCRIPTION, APPLICATION, AND ROLE
Advocating	Understands and emphasizes barriers to participation. Ensures client rights Approaches interpersonal difficulties by adjusting and accommodating to the needs of the client
Collaborating	Client-centered practice and client empowerment Expects active and equal participation between client and practitioner Encourages confidence, autonomy and independence
Empathizing	Fully understands the client's inner world and personality Involves being a good listener and to adjust and adapt based upon client's behavior and response Attend to client's expression of emotion
Encouraging	Instills hope and courage Positive reinforcement, encouragement, humor, motivation Goal-oriented Convey an entertaining, cheerful and playful attitude
Instructing	Clear education and feedback about performance Be skilled at sharing information Unafraid to share professional opinions or set limits Assumes a high level of responsibility for learning
Problem-Solving	Reason and logic Exploration of options and consequences Technical skill, creativity Programmatic and strategic

Adapted from Taylor, R. R. (2008). *The Intentional relationship: Occupational therapy and use of self.* Philadelphia, PA: F.A. Davis.

SUMMARY

Ethics and morality have been deeply rooted in the heart of the occupational therapy profession since its origination in the United States, as well as throughout the wider world. Many of the foundational principles of occupational therapy embody a specific focus on humanistic values and ethics. The Occupational Therapy Code of Ethics, other white papers, and occupational therapy theories help to support the continued dialogue of ethical and professional issues in the profession. Regardless of being a professionally-minded profession for nearly 100 years, a more explicit definition and guidelines to promote professionalism for current and future practitioners is needed. The formation and development of a professional identity in occupational therapy is paramount to the journey of becoming an occupational therapy practitioner. As occupational therapy professionals, our primary role has always been toward the patient or client. Our secondary role should be toward our profession.

LEARNING ACTIVITIES

1. Provide an example of an unethical or unprofessional behavior associated with the six Ethical standards in the Occupational Therapy Code of Ethics.

2. Have you come into contact with any ethical dilemmas while on fieldwork or during shadowing experiences? What was the ethical dilemma? What did you do? What was the outcome?

3. Select one of the Eleanor Slagle Lectureships discussed in this chapter. Write a one page paper summarizing the main constructs of the Lecture and its relationship to professionalism. Describe the effect that this lectureship had on occupational therapy practice.

4. Search for your state's practice act and/or licensure board. Identify what is required to become an occupational therapy practitioner in the state where you reside. Discuss which requirements pertain to professionalism.

REFERENCES

Ackley, N. (1962). The challenge of the sixties [Eleanor Clarke Slagle Lecture]. *American Journal of Occupational Therapy, 44*, 273-281.

American Occupational Therapy Association. (n.d.). Eleanor Clarke Slagle Lectures. Retrieved from http://www.aota.org/Education-Careers/Awards/Slagle.aspx

American Occupational Therapy Association. (1942). Occupational therapy notes. *Occupational Therapy and Rehabilitation, 21*(5), 314-320.

American Occupational Therapy Association. (1969). Definition of occupational therapy. *American Journal of Occupational Therapy, 23*, 185.

American Occupational Therapy Association. (1993). Occupational therapy roles. *American Journal of Occupational Therapy, 47*(12), 1087-1099.

American Occupational Therapy Association. (2014). Guidelines for supervision, roles, and responsibilities during the delivery of occupational therapy services. *American Journal of Occupational Therapy, 68*(Suppl. 3), S16-S22.

American Occupational Therapy Association. (2015a). Standards of practice for occupational therapy. *American Journal of Occupational Therapy, 69*(Suppl 3), S1-S6.

American Occupational Therapy Association. (2015b). Occupational therapy code of ethics. Retrieved from http://www.aota.org/-/media/corporate/files/practice/ethics/code-of- ethics.pdf

American Occupational Therapy Association. (2015c). Standards for continuing competence. *American Journal of Occupational Therapy, 69*(Suppl. 3), 6913410055.

DeBeer, F. (1987). Major themes in occupational therapy: A content analysis of the Eleanor Clarke Slagle lectures, 1955-1985. *American Journal of Occupational Therapy, 41*(8), 527-531.

Dunton, W. R. (1925). *Standards of the National Society for the Promotion of Occupational Therapy.* Bethesda, MD: AOTA Press.

Eldar, R., & Jelić, M. (2003). The association of rehabilitation and war. *Disability & Rehabilitation, 25*(18), 1019-1023.

Fiorentino, M. R. (1975). Occupational therapy: Realization to activation [1974 Eleanor Clarke Slagle Lecture]. *American Journal of Occupational Therapy, 29*, 15-21.

Friedland, J. (1998). Occupational therapy and rehabilitation: An awkward alliance. *American Journal of Occupational Therapy, 52*(5), 373-380.

Freidson, E. (1988). *Profession of medicine: A study of the sociology of applied knowledge.* Chicago, IL: University of Chicago Press.

Fullinwider, R. K. (1996). Professional codes and moral understanding. In M. Coady & S. Block (Eds.), *Codes of Ethics and the Professions* (pp. 72-87). Melbourne, Australia: Melbourne University Press.

Gilfoyle, E. M. (1984). Eleanor Clarke Slagle Lectureship, 1984: Transformation of a profession. *American Journal of Occupational Therapy, 38*(9), 575-584.

Gorenberg, M. D., & Taylor, R. R. (2014). The intentional relationship model: A framework for teaching therapeutic use of self. *OT Practice, 19*(17), CE1-CE6.

Johnson, J. A. (1972). 1972 Eleanor Clarke Slagle Lecture: Occupational therapy: A model for the future. Retrieved from http://www.aota.org/-/media/Corporate/Files/Publications/\AJOT/Slagle/1972.pdf

Low, J. F. (1992). The reconstruction aides. *American Journal of Occupational Therapy, 46*, 38-43.

Mosey, A. C. (1985). Eleanor Clarke Slagle Lecture, 1985: A monistic or a pluralistic approach to professional identity? *American Journal of Occupational Therapy, 39*(8), 504-509.

National Board for Certification in Occupational Therapy. (2016a). About the NBCOT. Retrieved from http://www. nbcot.org/about-us

National Board for Certification in Occupational Therapy. (2016b). Code of conduct. Retrieved from http://www. nbcot.org/code-of-conduct

Pattison, H.A. (1922). The trend of occupational therapy for the tuberculous. *Archives of Occupational Therapy, 1,* 19-24.

Peloquin, S. M. (1991). Occupational therapy service: Individual and collective understandings of the founders, part 2. *American Journal of Occupational Therapy, 45*(8), 733-744.

Reed, K. L. & Sanderson, S. N. (1999). *Concepts of occupational therapy.* Philadelphia, PA: Lippincott Williams & Wilkins.

Schwartz, K. B. (2009). Reclaiming our heritage: Connecting the Founding Vision to the Centennial Vision. *American Journal of Occupational Therapy, 63*(6), 681–690.

Schyve, P. M. (2009). Leadership in healthcare organizations: A guide to Joint Commission leadership standards. Retrieved from http://www.jointcommission.org/assets/1/18/ WP_Leadership_Standards.pdf

Slagle, E. C. (1937). Editorial: From the heart. *Occupational Therapy and Rehabilitation, 16*(5), 343-345.

Taylor, R. R. (2008). *The Intentional relationship: Occupational therapy and use of self.* Philadelphia, PA: F.A. Davis.

West, W. L. (1967). 1967 Eleanor Clarke Slagle Lecture: Professional responsibility in times of change. Retrieved from http://www.aota.org/-/media/Corporate/Files/Publications/AJOT/Slagle/1967.pdf

World Federation of Occupational Therapists. (2005). Code of ethics (revised 2005). Retrieved from http://www.wfot. org/ResourceCentre.aspx

Worthen, D. B. (2005). Edward Kremers (1865-1941): Pharmaceutical education reformer. *Journal of the American Pharmacists Association, 45*(4), 517-520.

Yerxa, E. J. (1967). 1966 Eleanor Clark Slagle Lecture: Authentic occupational therapy. *American Journal of Occupational Therapy, 21,* 1-9.

Part II

Professionalism in the Classroom

Although professional development begins in an individual's formative years (as we learned with generational and societal influences), the process of becoming a professional continues with admission into a professional school or program. This section (Chapters 5 and 6) will emphasize the importance of professionalism specifically in the classroom environment. Expectations of the occupational therapy student and best practice teaching approaches to promote professionalism for occupational therapy educators will also be discussed. In addition, vignettes will be used to depict common professional behavior blunders that occur in the classroom; strategies will be provided for how to handle them. Resources, including professional development plans and sample policies will also be provided as appendices.

Emphasis on Professionalism in Occupational Therapy Education

Elizabeth D. DeIuliis, OTD, OTR/L

INTRODUCTION

Although not always explicitly stated, professionalism is a core value and expectation of health care provider educational programs, including those of the occupational therapy profession. The pillars of occupational therapy education are congruent with the pillars of occupational therapy as a profession, and occupational therapy education includes both didactic and experiential learning components (American Occupational Therapy Association [AOTA], 2015a). This education promotes critical reasoning and the integration of technical and professional knowledge, skills, and attitudes, as well as development of a professional identity. Therefore, occupational therapy education must consistently reinforce the development of new knowledge supporting the use of occupation, the application of clinical reasoning based on evidence, the necessity for lifelong learning, and the improvement of professional knowledge and skills (AOTA, 2007). The AOTA (2015a) also holds that the values of occupational therapy education include active and diverse learning, a collaborative process, continuous professional judgement, evaluation and self-reflection, and lifelong learning. Entities such as the Accreditation Council for Occupational Therapy Education (ACOTE) and the Commission on Education (COE) are key stakeholders in the emphasis of professionalism in occupational therapy education.

KEY WORDS

Accreditation Council for Occupational Therapy Education: Accrediting body for schools that train occupational therapy practitioners and occupational therapy assistants; sets educational standards that must be met and maintained for accreditation (AOTA, n.d.)

Asynchronous Learning: Courses and material delivered and accessed at the student's convenience, with no predetermined pace, e.g. completion of independent readings and subsequent online discussion board participation

DeIuliis, E.D.
Professionalism Across Occupational Therapy Practice (pp 107-136).
© 2017 Taylor & Francis Group.

Bloom's Taxonomy: Hierarchical classification of objectives in education across three domains of learning: cognitive, affective, and psychomotor; categorizes intellectual skills and behavior required for holistic teaching, learning, and assessment (Bloom, Engelhart, Furst, Hill, and Krathwohl, 1956)

Mentoring: A communication process and relationship in which a more experienced or more knowledgeable person helps to guide one who is less experienced or less knowledgeable; develops over time and can be an effective resource to strengthen clinical skills as well as professionalism (National Mentoring Partnership, 2016)

Pedagogy: A philosophy or framework to help the educator guide the experience of teaching and learning; associated with the art, science, craft of teaching ("Pedagogy," 2016)

Synchronous Learning: Involves real-time interaction between student(s) and instructor(s), e.g. students watching a live web stream of a class and simultaneously participating in a discussion via web-conferencing

OBJECTIVES

After reading this chapter and completing the learning activities, the reader should be able to:

1. Understand the role of the ACOTE within occupational therapy education

2. Identify educational pedagogies that can help foster professionalism

3. Evaluate best practice teaching approaches to promote professional behavior and attitudes

4. Discuss the role of student and faculty mentoring in developing professionalism

ACCREDITATION COUNCIL OF OCCUPATIONAL THERAPY EDUCATION

The ACOTE is the professions' official accreditation agency for occupational therapy education. Although ACOTE currently operates as a separate entity, in 1923, accreditation of educational programs became a function of the American Occupational Therapy Association (AOTA). The original educational standards were developed in 1927. When the guiding document, *Essentials of an Acceptable School of Occupational Therapy*, was adopted in 1935, four schools were initially accredited (Council on Medical Education and Hospitals, 1936). In 1958, the AOTA assumed responsibility for approval of educational programs for the occupational therapy assistant. The standards on which accreditation was based were modeled after the *Essentials of an Acceptable School of Occupational Therapy* established for baccalaureate programs. The curricular standards go through a review, update, and adoption process every five years, in response to changes in health care, national educational trends, and other higher education accrediting bodies. When the *Essentials of an Acceptable School of Occupational Therapy* were updated in 1983, they included, for the first time, a definition of occupational therapy, and added research and professional development (ethics, standards of care, continued learning of professionals, and promotion of the profession) to the areas that were required within an occupational therapy curriculum (AOTA, 1983). Clinical training expectations were divided between Level I and Level II fieldwork. This shows that curricular mandates related to professionalism and ethics were not stipulated in occupational therapy education until 1983, nearly 66 years after the inception of our profession.

Box 5-1

SNAPSHOT OF ACOTE STANDARDS RELATED TO PROFESSIONALISM

- B.9.2 Discuss and justify how the role of a professional is enhanced by knowledge of and involvement in international, national, state, and local occupational therapy associations and related professional associations

- B.9.4 Identify and develop strategies for ongoing professional development to ensure that practice is consistent with current and accepted standards

- B.9.6 Discuss and evaluate personal and professional abilities and competencies as they relate to job responsibilities

- B.9.8 Explain and justify the importance of supervisory roles, responsibilities, and collaborative professional relationships between the occupational therapy practitioner and the occupational therapy assistant

- B.9.11 Demonstrate a variety of informal and formal strategies for resolving ethical disputes in varying practice areas

Adapted from Accreditation Council for Occupational Therapy Education. (2012). 2011 Accreditation Council for Occupational Therapy Education (ACOTE) standards. *American Journal of Occupational Therapy, 66*(Suppl. 1), S6-S74.

The accreditation standards for educational programs for occupational therapy practitioners delineate expected learning outcomes to ensure that graduates achieve entry-level competence as a generalist. This requires an individual that can respond to the changing and dynamic nature of contemporary health and human services delivery, which requires occupational therapy practitioners to possess basic skills as a direct care provider, consultant, educator, manager, researcher, and advocate for the profession and the consumer. According to ACOTE (2012), minimum competence must be demonstrated in the following areas:

- Foundation requirements
- Basic tenets of occupational therapy
- Occupational therapy theoretical perspectives
- Screening, evaluation, and referral
- Intervention plan, formulation, and implementation
- Context of service delivery
- Research
- Professional ethics, values, and responsibilities

Within each of these areas, standards or learning objectives are established by ACOTE to serve as the minimum level of expectations for occupational therapy assistant programs, master's level occupational therapy programs, and entry-level occupational therapy doctorate programs. Currently, there are no ACOTE standards set for post-professional occupational therapy doctorate programs.

You may notice that there is a section of curricular mandates devoted to professional ethics, values, and responsibilities. Let's review a few of the educational standards of this section. Standards B.9.0 to B.9.13 are all devoted to the development of performance criteria in professional ethics, values, and responsibilities (Box 5-1).

Although all accredited occupational therapy educational programs are required to meet these standards, the manner in which they demonstrate compliance as well as the depth and breadth within the curriculum can vary. Occupational therapy educational programs can assess

| | TABLE 5-1 | |
| | **EDUCATION-RELATED WHITE PAPERS** | |
YEAR	PAPER TITLE	PURPOSE
2007	A Descriptive Review of Occupational Therapy Education	Written for practitioners, academicians, and potential occupational therapy program applicants to augment their understanding of occupational therapy education, including different levels of occupational therapy education
2014	The Philosophy of Occupational Therapy Education	This white paper formally discusses the fundamental beliefs and values of occupational therapy education.
2015	The Importance of Interprofessional Education in Occupational Therapy Curricula	This white paper describes the history of interprofessional education, and provides evidence for the benefits of including interprofessional education in professional curricula. Additionally, serves to define key concepts and core competencies associated with interprofessional education, to address implications of including interprofessional education in entry-level occupational therapy curricula, and to provide resources for faculty.
2015	The Value of Occupational Therapy Assistant Education to the Profession	Discusses the value of the professional roles that occupational therapy assistant hold within contemporary practice.

*There are also white papers published that are specific to fieldwork education; these will be discussed in Chapter 6.

Adapted from American Occupational Therapy Association. (2007). A descriptive review of occupational therapy education. *American Journal of Occupational Therapy, 61*(6), 672-677; American Occupational Therapy Association. (2015a). Philosophy of occupational therapy education. *American Journal of Occupational Therapy, 69*(Suppl. 3), 6913410053; American Occupational Therapy Association. (2015b). Importance of interprofessional education in occupational therapy curricula. *American Journal of Occupational Therapy, 69*(Suppl. 3), 6913410020; American Occupational Therapy Association. (2015c). Value of occupational therapy assistant education to the profession. *American Journal of Occupational Therapy, 69*(Suppl. 3),6913410070.

the student's ability to meet curriculum standards using various measures. Objective test questions, essays, assignments, projects, presentations, and laboratory practicals are all examples of pedagogical approaches that occupational therapy educators can use to measure student learning outcomes.

COMMISSION ON EDUCATION

The COE is the AOTA's official committee regarding education. The COE, an advisory commission of the representative assembly, is a visionary group that identifies, analyzes, and anticipates issues in education. The COE generates education-related policy recommendations to the Representative Assembly for deliberation. The COE works in conjunction with the Education Special Interest Section and has interactions with ACOTE. The COE is responsible for authoring many white papers guiding the educational philosophy of the profession (Table 5-1).

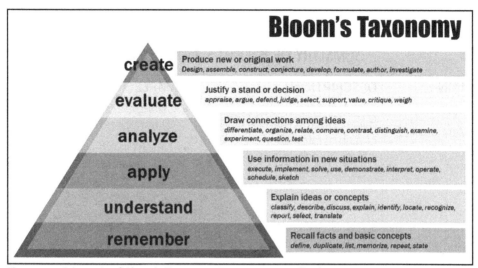

Figure 5-1. Schematic of Bloom's Taxonomy. (Armstrong, P. (n.d.). Bloom's taxonomy. Retrieved from https://cft.vanderbilt.edu/guides-sub-pages/blooms-taxonomy/ This image can be shared, reproduced, or otherwise used, as long as it is attributed to the Vanderbilt University Center for Teaching.)

EDUCATIONAL PEDAGOGIES TO TEACH PROFESSIONALISM AND ETHICS

Although ACOTE standards set the blueprint for occupational therapy education, the manner in which that curriculum is delivered varies based upon the educator, institution, and the context of the teaching/learning interaction. One of these essential variables used by the educator or set forth by the institution is the educational pedagogy. The word pedagogy is associated with the art, science, and craft of teaching ("Pedagogy," 2016). It is more than just an explicit set of instructional methods or teaching techniques—it is a philosophy or framework to help the educator guide the experience of teaching and learning. Although accreditation standards exist regarding exposing students to the teaching and learning process, occupational therapy teaching-scholars indicate that experience in the clinical role does not necessarily prepare the practitioner for the role of an educator (Stutz-Tannenbaum & Hooper, 2009). Here is a brief summary of the work of a few of the more well-known pioneers in teaching and learning who have influenced many of the commonly used pedagogies in education today.

Benjamin Bloom

As an educational psychologist, Benjamin Bloom is most well known for his development of *Bloom's Taxonomy* (Bloom et al., 1956). Bloom created a classification of different objectives that educators set for students to categorize intellectual skills and behavior important for creating a more holistic form of teaching, learning, and assessment. He proposed three domains of learning in a hierarchical design: these were the cognitive, affective, and psychomotor domains. Therefore, learning at the higher levels is dependent on having attained prerequisite knowledge and skills at lower levels.

In 2001, The Revised Taxonomy was published. This version focused more on the active and dynamic process of teaching and learning (Anderson & Krathwohl, 2001). An overview of Bloom's hierarchical domains can be found in Figure 5-1 and Table 5-2.

TABLE 5-2 SUMMARY OF BLOOM'S TAXONOMY		
DOMAIN	**DESCRIPTION**	**EXAMPLE**
Cognitive • Mental skills	This domain includes every-thing from the memorization of factual information to using information from several sources to form new hypoth-eses, or to judge the value of information.	• Listing the signs and symptoms of a myocardial infarction • Determining a diagnosis from evaluation results
Affective • Attitude • Values • Appreciation • Motivations • Self	Some of these values are learned during a student's formative years, during child-hood and shaped by society. Others are the result of con-scious examination. In occu-pational therapy, affective behaviors include nonverbal communication, honesty, active listening, ethical prac-tice, independent reading, learning, and attention to a client's oral and/or non-verbal responses.	• Engaging in a semi-struc-tured interview such as the Occupational Performance History Interview • Eliciting the client's occupation-al profile by using open-ended questions
Psychomotor • Manual skills • Motor skills • Physical skills	Encompasses everything from recognition of motor skills to the ability to design a new technique or piece of adap-tive equipment. Sometimes, no knowledge is assumed and person can simply per-form a motor skill.	• Discriminating by palpation, between a normal and a subluxed shoulder joint

Correlation to Occupational Therapy Education

Similar to the occupational therapy profession, Bloom's Taxonomy proposes a holistic approach to education. The hierarchical domains show a deep connection between the mind (cognitive and affective) and the body (psychomotor), and emphasize how parts of a whole relate to each other to form the whole. Furthermore, the overall classification system presented by Bloom and his colleagues has greatly influenced the curriculum development of occupational therapy educa-tion, providing means for determining the congruence of educational learning objectives and assessment. An educator should attempt to 'move students up' the taxonomy as they progress in their knowledge. Test questions that are written solely to assess knowledge and memory recall are unfortunately very common; to create critical thinkers as opposed to students who simply recall information, we must incorporate the higher levels into assessment. This will also better prepare students to be successful on Level II Fieldwork and to take the national certification examina-tion, which both require students to synthesize, evaluate and apply critical information to various

TABLE 5-3
CORRELATION OF BLOOM'S TAXONOMY TO ACOTE STANDARDS

COGNITIVE DOMAIN

B.2.1. Explain the history and philosophical base of the profession of occupational therapy and its importance in meeting society's current and future occupational needs.

B.5.10. Articulate principles of and be able to design, fabricate, apply, fit, and train in assistive technologies and devices (e.g., electronic aids to daily living, seating and positioning systems) used to enhance occupational performance and foster participation and well-being

PSYCHOMOTOR DOMAIN

B./.3. Demonstrate knowledge of applicable national requirements for credentialing and requirements for licensure, certification, or registration under state laws.

B.1.7. Apply quantitative statistics and qualitative analysis to interpret tests, measurements, and other data for the purpose of establishing and/or delivering evidence-based practice.

AFFECTIVE DOMAIN

B.5.20. Effectively interact through written, oral, and nonverbal communication with the client, family, significant others, communities, colleagues, other health providers, and the public in a professionally acceptable manner

B.5.22. Refer to specialists, both internal and external to the profession, for consultation and intervention.

Adapted from Accreditation Council for Occupational Therapy Education. (2012). 2011 Accreditation Council for Occupational Therapy Education (ACOTE) standards. *American Journal of Occupational Therapy, 66*(Suppl. 1), S6-S74.

clinical scenarios. ACOTE (2012) standards are intentionally written using the three domains. A critical review of the standards will showcase many verbs synonymous with Bloom's hierarchy (Table 5-3).

John Dewey

John Dewey was an American philosopher and psychologist, and is often described as a pedagogical inspiration and an education reformer. His ideas about education sprang from a philosophy of pragmatism, instrumentalism, and progressive education. Dewey was an important catalyst for active and experiential learning, arguing that education and learning are social and interactive processes (Shook, n.d.). He believed that students thrive in an environment where they are allowed to experience learning, have hands-on interactions within the curriculum, and that all students should have the opportunity to take part in their own learning—not just as a way to gain knowledge, but also as a way to learn how to live. Dewey's philosophy focused on the interaction between the learner and what is being learned, shifting the emphasis on the learner's interest. He viewed schools as a community where students should be active members, and that curriculum should be relevant and meaningful to the learner's life.

Correlation to Occupational Therapy Education

Deweyan philosophy has a great affinity with occupational therapy, particularly because both aspire to a holistic worldview that is centered on activity and the importance of active engagement to facilitate learning. Dewey's educational philosophy went on to inspire pedagogies such as problem-based learning (PBL), which is widely used in occupational therapy education, and experiential learning, seen in occupational therapy curriculum as fieldwork education and the doctoral experiential component (Cutchin, 2004).

Maslow and Rogers

Carl Rogers and Abraham Maslow were influential American psychologists, and were among the founders of the humanistic approach to psychology, also known as humanism. Rogers is widely considered to be one of the founding fathers of psychotherapy research, and was honored for his pioneering research with the Award for Distinguished Scientific Contributions by the American Psychological Association in 1956. Humanism originated in response to limitations of Freud's psychoanalytic theory and B.F. Skinner's behaviorism. Humanistic education is a holistic approach that views the learner, or person, as a sum of their parts. This person-centered framework is a unique approach to understanding personality and human relationships, and is widely used in many social disciplines such as psychotherapy and counseling (Cain, 2002).

Correlation to Occupational Therapy Education

Maslow and Rogers' educational philosophy influenced many components of both the occupational therapy profession and its education. They emphasize the importance of being a student-centered educator, and to view the learner as a holistic being; these tenets mirror the foundation of client-centered therapy. Humanism also incorporates psychosocial aspects, such as spiritual aspiration and self-actualization, as important components of a human and learner's psyche (Rogers, 1966). Self-actualization, which was derived from humanistic psychological therapy created by Maslow, represents the ongoing growth of an individual toward fulfillment of one's highest need or greatest potential. Self-actualization can be seen as similar to concepts such as self-discovery, self-reflection, self-realization, and self-exploration—language used in many occupational therapy theories and models of practice.

David Kolb

David Kolb, an educational theorist, had a significant effect on education with the creation of the experiential learning theory. Kolb was an early advocate for active and engaged learning. He proposed that learning occurs not just by doing (the primary event), by also reflecting (the secondary event) on the engaged experience. Learning is the process whereby knowledge is created through the transformation of experience. Knowledge results from the combination of grasping experience and transforming it (Kolb, D. A., 1984). Kolb's model is related to, but not synchronic with, other pedagogies and theories of active learning such as cooperative learning or service learning. Kolb's model includes four elements as follows.

1. Concrete experience (Do)
2. Observation of and reflection on that experience (Observe)
3. Formation of abstract concept based upon reflection (Think)
4. Testing of new concepts (Plan)

Kolb describes this process of experiential learning as continual, which symbolizes the importance of lifelong learning. He also discusses certain skills and qualities that are important for the learner to possess in order to be engaged and to reflect. Students in higher education must have and use analytical skills to conceptualize experiences, and must have decision-making and problem-solving skills to execute a learned action.

Connection to Occupational Therapy Education

Kolb's effect on the world of education influenced many signature pedagogies of occupational therapy education, such as service-learning or community-engaged learning. His experiential learning theory model emphasized concepts that echo those familiar to occupational therapy, in that it is based upon the dynamic process between the person and the environment through the use of selected learning styles. Service learning is a pedagogy that integrates meaningful community service with instruction and structured reflection, aimed to enrich the learning experience, teach civic responsibility, and strengthen communities ("Service-Learning," 2017). These pedagogies differ from fieldwork because they innately require reflection on the experience. In 1984, Kolb proposed a Learning Style Inventory, which can be a useful tool for academics, fieldwork educators, and managers to explore the way students, learners, and employees learn—and how they deal with day-to-day situations, as well as to predict performance (Landa-Gonzalez, Velis, & Greg, 2015). The experiential learning theory went on to influence the development of occupational therapy theories, such as the cognitive orientation to daily occupational performance approach in cognitive rehabilitation (Polatajko & Mandich, 2004).

Lev Vygotsky

The work of Lev Vygotsky has become the foundation of much research and theory in cognitive development over the past several decades, particularly with what has become known as Social Development Theory. Vygotsky's theories stress the fundamental role of social interaction in the development of cognition, as he believed strongly that community plays a central role in the process of "making meaning" (Vygotsky, 1978). Vygotsky's work is frequently referred to as the collaborative learning theory. Collaborative learning has been practiced and studied since the early 1900s. The principles are based on the theories of Dewey, Vygotsky, and Bloom. Their collective work focusing on how students learn has led educators to develop more student-focused learning environments that put students at the center of instruction. Collaborative learning occurs when two or more people learn or attempt to learn something together. Unlike individual learning, people engaged in collaborative learning capitalize on one another's resources and skills—asking one another for information, evaluating one another's ideas, monitoring one another's work, and so on.

Correlation to Occupational Therapy Education

Collaboration is a familiar term within occupational therapy literature. The importance of working together with our clients and colleagues is a part of our training. Educators may aim to foster collaborative learning through group projects or assignments, which encourage students to work together and learn from one another. This reinforces learning and helps to develop professional skills such as communication, teamwork, and conflict resolution. Furthermore, this notion of collaborative learning is emphasized in occupational therapy literature, specifically within non-traditional supervision models in fieldwork, where two or more fieldwork students are paired with one fieldwork educator. More will be discussed regarding fieldwork education and supervision models in Chapter 7.

Summary

It is evident that there are shared philosophical tenants of higher education pedagogy and occupational therapy education. Recognizing learning styles and adjusting the approach to the learning conditions have relevance for maximizing outcomes. Educators in health care professional programs should consider designing instructional activities that advance students' awareness of their preferences and support the use of diverse approaches for success in various learning contexts, as well as to develop professionalism (Landa-Gonzalez et al., 2015).

COMMON PEDAGOGIES IN OCCUPATIONAL THERAPY EDUCATION

Occupation is defined as "doing."

—David L. Nelson, 1988

A fundamental pillar of the occupational therapy profession is that human beings learn best by doing, which is why we believe in active engagement in occupations that are meaningful and satisfying, to influence health, quality of life, and well-being. Our clients learn skills and develop abilities by physically performing and actively engaging in tasks and activities—not just by listening to oral instruction or reading a patient education handout. This same philosophy is true for teaching and learning for occupational therapy students. Nolinske and Mills (1999) stated that "lecture-based pedagogical approaches cannot adequately prepare students in professional and technical occupational therapy programs" (p. 31). Pedagogical experts are also in agreement with this sentiment, and invite more active learning approaches to be used in education. Here is a brief summary of some of the commonly used pedagogies in occupational therapy education.

Relational Learning

Key Words

- Human connection
- Apprenticeship
- Mentorship model

This learning approach centers on the relationship of the teacher and the student. It allows teachers and learners to learn together. Relational learning deconstructs the hierarchy of the traditional teacher/student relationship, and creates opportunity for collaboration and sharing of ideas. "This relational learning models a professional identity that exemplifies a human connection, empathy, and respect while seeing the patient as a whole person" (Schaber, 2014, p. S42).

Using Relational Learning to Teach Professionalism

A great deal of "teaching" about professionalism occurs informally during the educational process. The manner in which you interpersonally interact, both verbally and nonverbally, with students and colleagues provides clear messages and teachable moments about professionalism. Professionalism should be demonstrated during all communication and correspondence with your peers and students. For example, even a simple email could be a way to model professionalism. Instead of writing "Hey, Julie, you didn't come to class. Get it together. From, Dr. Smith". You could write "Dear Julie, I noted that you were not present in class today. According to our attendance policy, you are responsible for any missed information. Please let me know if you have any questions. Respectfully, Dr. Smith". Occupational therapy educators are role models to their students, and should exhibit strong intrinsic and extrinsic qualities of professionalism to guide students into becoming professionals.

Affective Learning

Key Word

- Transformative

This pedagogy involves a transformation between the teacher and the student. At its core, such transformative learning is defined by an individual making meaning of the world through his or her experiences. Affective learning involves a change in attitudes, beliefs, and values in both the teacher and the student. "For students, educators open the door and usher them into an exploration of events that have an impact on the occupational life of the individual, difficult topics such as death, pain, loss, grief, stigma, and oppression that profoundly transform personal identity and build professionalism" (Schaber, 2014, p. S42). Educators who successfully use the affective learning pedagogy challenge students to move beyond their knowledge comfort level. For the teacher, it entails accepting emotional vulnerability as well as engaging in the conveying of knowledge. It also requires the highest ethical integrity (Patience, 2008).

Using Affective Learning to Teach Professionalism

Teaching professionalism must involve the whole student; their values, beliefs, and assumptions. Academic and fieldwork educators play crucial roles in the development of an occupational therapy student's professional identity. Educators who practice affective pedagogy must be self-aware, self-confident, and selfless in ways that enable them to engage in close and healthy relationships with their students. Learning experiences that stimulate transformative learning provides a context for best practice "because it promotes professional development among students as competent, entry-level practitioners" (Crist, 2011). Fieldwork students can "develop or construct personal meaning from their experiences and validate it through interaction and communication with their fieldwork educators" (Santalucia & Johnson, 2010, p. CE-2). Being professional means being your best self.

Active Engagement

Key Words

- Experiential learning
- Shadowing
- Fieldwork
- Simulation

Active engagement is a model of instruction that involves learning by doing. Some examples of active engagement will be discussed later on in this chapter, which include cognitive orientation to daily occupational performance learning, project based learning (PBL), and the flipped classroom. Each of these are examples in which the instructor designs the learning environment and activities to allow the student to actively participate, which shifts the responsibility of learning to the student. Active learning has been known to improve knowledge acquisition and retention, which is of important value to occupational therapy educators as application of knowledge and skill is required to be successful in fieldwork and to pass the national certification exam (DeBourgh, 2008; Patterson, Kilpatrick, & Woebkenberg, 2010).

Using Active Engagement to Teach Professionalism

Active learning can be a successful teaching approach for more than just clinical skill development. PBL, case-based learning, role-playing, and simulation can also be used to develop a student practitioner's professionalism. PBL is an educational method that is used to facilitate students' effective learning of critical occupational therapy content and professional processes, including self-directed learning habits and integration of foundation clinical knowledge to scenarios. Teaching methods that operate under a "think aloud, talk aloud nature" like PBL require students to interact and explain professionally with their peers and faculty, which prepares students for clinical practice. PBL affords students the opportunity to develop or remediate non-cognitive professional behaviors that have been recognized as important predictors of their future success in fieldwork (McNulty, Crowe, & VaneLeit, 2004, p. 71). Formalized clinical education such as fieldwork allows students a direct opportunity to observe and engage in real-world scenarios to develop their clinical and professional skill set (Crist & Scaffa, 2012).

Academic and fieldwork educators should consider the learner as an occupational being and design and structure active learning based upon the learner's needs and characteristics. Purposeful observation, active engagement, and critical reflection allow the learner to make meaning of the experience. While active learning is a preferred pedagogical approach for both clinical and professional skill development, there are opportunities where a student may be asked to actively observe, particularly early in their educational experience. During these occasions, observation logs can be useful for the learner. An observation log encourages clinical observations via structured questions. Questions may be designed to generate a clinical discussion, facilitate communication among the cohort, or assist students in clinical observation acuity and ability to connect theory and practice (Hanson & DeIuliis, 2015). Observation logs can be incident or skill-specific (Queensland Occupational Therapy Fieldwork Collaborative, 2007). For example, they might be used during a role-play of a team meeting, patient interview scenario, or ethical dilemma to encourage the development of critical reasoning and professionalism. See Appendix A for an example.

Service Learning

Key Words

- Community-engaged learning
- Civic-oriented
- Reflection

Service learning, also known as community engaged learning, is another active learning pedagogy that combines learning outcomes with service to the community and society to enhance both student growth and the common good. Through service learning, students are able to meet course objectives, engage in personal and professional growth, and develop a sense of responsibility as active citizens in society. This pedagogy challenges learners to develop many qualities of professionalism such as (civic) responsibility, problem solving, critical thinking, and ethical reasoning. The primary outcome of civic-oriented learning is to create individuals capable of making significant ethical and value-laden contributions to the community, practice, and professional knowledge (Jones, Valdez, Nowakowski, & Rasmussen, 1994).

Using Service Learning to Teach Professionalism

Instructors design learning opportunities in the real-world community contexts, such as homeless shelters, correctional facilities, not-for profit organizations, and students develop important skills of community engagement with diverse cultures and communities. An important component of service learning is the reflection, where students develop a deeper understanding of the skills they are developing and the effect they have on society. Hoppes, Bender, and DeGrace (2005) discuss how service learning not only contributes to society and communities, but also to the professional preparation of the student involved. Service learning requires students to think differently, promote an attitude of caring, and expand their professional role in a variety of settings. The emphasis that service learning has on diversity, and cultural and generational competence, can be a critical factor in the development of a health care student's professional identity (Greene, 1997).

Situational Learning

Key Words

- Apprenticeship
- Authenticity
- Context

Situational learning takes place in the same context in which it is applied. This instructional approach involves learning in a specific context, and combines real-world activities with cognitive learning such as beliefs, values, and attitudes. Situational learning explicitly teaches the intrinsic foundation of professionalism by allowing the student to experience and reflect how knowledge is obtained and applied in real-world situations. "The situated learning theory underscores the social dimension of learning and advocates for an authentic context to promote learning" (Sladyk, Jacobs, & MacRae, 2010, p. 223). It is through this pedagogy that the teaching-learning environment is often referred to as a community (Greene, 1997).

Using Situational Learning to Teach Professionalism

Situated learning is an experiential pedagogy that has influenced the development of occupational therapy curriculum. Situated learning emphasizes higher order thinking (or deep learning) rather than the acquisition of knowledge. It focuses on application rather than retention. Fieldwork education and the doctoral experiential component are specific examples which require occupational therapy student to apply knowledge and skills and reflect on their experience in real-world contexts. The use of situated learning in health care education enhances the employability of its students (Inelmen & Inlemen, n.d.).

Summary

> *"What I hear, I forget. What I see, I remember. What I do, I understand."*
> —Chinese Proverb 451 BC

Occupational therapy students are taught to and learn to be a professional by various methods. Occupational therapy literature has emphasized student learning preferences to be active and engaged for decades (Stafford, 1986). Beyond teaching about what is and what is not professional, much of what is learned about being a professional is something that is modeled, experienced, and reflected upon. It is essential for occupational therapy educators to design and implement learning activities that foster professionalism, both in formal and informal ways. Formal ways can occur through active learning such as service learning or fieldwork education as part of a required curriculum. Informal ways include designing learning activities that offer time for reflection and modeling qualities of a professional. There are various pedagogies or teaching approaches that can be used to promote dynamic, collaborative, and reflective learning environments to develop professionalism. Both occupational therapy educators and students are responsible for constructing a culture of professionalism.

ROLE OF OCCUPATIONAL THERAPY EDUCATOR AND PROFESSIONALISM

Student learning is the primary goal of occupational therapy educators. Occupational therapy education should aim to initiate student practitioners to think, to perform, and to conduct themselves not just as clinicians, but also as professionals. This specific aim is not just about how to remain ethical and professional in clinical practice, but in the student practitioners' overall behavior and attitudes. This acculturation to the expectations of the profession should begin on day one of occupational therapy school. In Chapter 1, you became familiar with the knowledge, skills, intrinsic and extrinsic attitudes, behaviors, and clinical reasoning necessary for professionalism. Knowledge and one's mindset have been discussed as significant components of professionalism, and the classroom and formal education process is where this process of professional development begins.

An occupational therapy educator or faculty role is multifaceted. Besides being a teacher, these individuals may also be clinicians, researchers, scholars, service leaders, administrators, and so on. Professionalism, and compliance with standards set forth by the profession such as in the *Occupational Therapy Code of Ethics* (AOTA, 2015d) and *Scope of Practice* (AOTA, 2014), are expectations to be met within all of these roles. For example, as an educator, one needs to maintain confidentiality with student academic records, be fair and equitable in student assessment (such as assigning grades), and model professional behavior and attitudes. As a researcher, one needs to be ethical and fair in their process of obtaining informed consent from their participants. (More information regarding professionalism and ethics in scholarship will be discussed in Chapter 15.) Furthermore, occupational therapy educators are responsible for passing on this "sense of ethos, professionalism and core values" to the future practitioners of the profession (Kanny & Kyler, 1999, p. 72). Simpson and Dyer (1997) stated that the role of the educator "is changing from a performer on a stage or in a laboratory to one who creates the circumstances from which learning occurs" (p.2). Academic and fieldwork educator roles are more than just instruction and teaching. Coaching, facilitating, guiding, and advising are other important components of the educator role that greatly influence professional development. A common way that this ethos is passed on is by the use of mentoring.

Professionalism and Mentoring

Mentoring is both a process and a relationship. It is a personal and/or professional relationship, in which the more experienced or more knowledgeable person (mentor) helps to guide a less experienced or less knowledgeable person (mentee) (National Mentoring Partnership, 2016). The mentor can be older or younger than the mentee, but must possess a certain area of expertise. This process involves communication and is relationship-based. Roles of a mentor can include teaching, advising, or guiding the mentee. However, effective mentors are more than just teachers; they are role models, consultants, problem solvers, and supporters. They provide constructive feedback, guidance, networking, information, and opportunities. The mentor-mentee relationship is something that develops over time. For this relationship to be meaningful, it requires effective communication, and accessibility.

Whereas a mentorship role can be an effective resource to develop clinical skills, it can also be used to develop professionalism. Many occupational therapy educational programs have a faculty/student mentorship program throughout their curriculum. For example, within the Department of Occupational Therapy at Duquesne University, each student is assigned a faculty mentor at their inception into the program. The student retains the same mentor throughout the duration of the program. A student is required to meet with their mentor at least once a semester, more often if needed. During this meeting, the mentor and mentee collaborate on setting self-directed professional development goals to transform the occupational therapy student into a professional. Goals can be geared toward increasing initiative and participation in classroom activities, such as "raising hand at least once a class;" communication skills such as a student-led presentation; or organization, such as "using a planner or calendar system to keep track of academic and personal appointments." As the student progresses through the academic program, goals become more directed toward preparation for fieldwork, doctoral experiential component, the National Board for Certification in Occupational Therapy (NBCOT) exam preparation, or job searching.

Box 5-2

CHARACTERISTICS OF EFFECTIVE MENTORS

- Altruistic, honest, trustworthy, active listeners
- Have professional experience that can facilitate mentee development
- Display patience and tolerance; give encouragement
- Value ongoing learning; act as a role model
- Exhibit enthusiasm

Adapted from Cooper, D. L., & Miller, T. K. (1998). Influence and impact: Professional development in student affairs. *New Directions for Student Services, 84,* 55-69; Place, N. T., & Bailey, A. (2006). Mentoring: Providing greatest benefit to new and seasoned faculty In an extension organization. *Proceedings of the Association for International Agricultural and Extension Education, 22,* 498-507; Straus, S. E., Johnson, M. O., Marquez, C., & Feldman, M. D. (2013). Characteristics of successful and failed mentoring relationships: A qualitative study across two academic health centers. *Academic Medicine: Journal of the Association of American Medical Colleges, 88*(1), 82-89.

Box 5-3

Professional mentoring can be used to accrue NBCOT Professional Development Units. PDU ID # 9

Description: Mentor, an occupational therapy colleague or other professional, improves skills of the protégé, and also acts as a disciplinary monitor (mentor must be currently certified with NBCOT)

Accrual: 2 hours = 1 unit (maximum of 18 units)

Documentation Required: Goals, objectives, and analysis of mentee performance. Both the mentor and the mentee can seek to obtain professional development units from a documented mentee/mentor relationship.

*Mentoring Guidelines and Log are available on the NBCOT website. Adapted from National Board for Certification in Occupational Therapy. (n.d.). Guidelines for mentoring. Retrieved from http://www.nbcot.org/assets/candidate-pdfs/practitioner-pdfs/mentoring-guidelines-log.

See Appendix B for a Sample Student Professional Development Plan. In addition to the professional development plan, the mentor and mentee relationship can also be used to discuss, plan, and organize a professional portfolio. More information on the importance and creation of the portfolio can be found in Chapter 11. Being an effective mentor is more than just listening to and advising your mentee. A mentor should be a role model and promote a strong example of professionalism to the mentee (Box 5-2).

In 2009, educational leaders in the occupational therapy profession articulated desirable attributes of occupational therapy educators in the document *Specialized Knowledge and Skills of Occupational Therapy Educators of the Future* (AOTA, 2009), which included Innovator/visionary, Scholar/explorer, Leader, Integrator, and Mentor. The AOTA indicates that occupational therapy educators (including faculty members, academic fieldwork coordinators and fieldwork educators) should aim to be a "trusted role model, who inspires, encourages, influences, challenges and facilitates the growth and development" (p. 805) (Box 5-3).

Role Modeling

A role model is a person whose behavior, example, or success is or can be emulated by others, especially by younger people ("Role Model," 2016). Along with mentoring, the use of role-modeling is a powerful contributor to one's professional development (Paice, Heard, & Moss, 2002). Role

---

Box 5-4

ROLE MODELING THROUGH STUDENT OCCUPATIONAL THERAPY ASSOCIATION

The use of a Student Occupational Therapy Association chapter can be an excellent method to role-model professionalism. A Student Occupational Therapy Association is typically a student-led organization that allows occupational therapy students to assume leadership roles in both undergraduate and graduate phases of education. The mission and vision behind a Student Occupational Therapy Association is geared toward facilitating opportunities for camaraderie among students, as well as provide meaningful, productive, and professional interaction among students, faculty, and individuals in the community. Students have the opportunity to take on leadership roles that allow them to develop deeper professional behaviors.

*See more at http://www.aota.org

Adapted from Mernar, T. J. (2000). Handbook for developing or modifying a student occupational therapy association: An organizational approach. [Master's thesis.] South Orange, NJ: Seton Hall University; Simons, S., Georgen, M., Fay, S., Landgraf, E., & Matlock, C. (2013). Participation in student Occupational therapy associations. [Master's thesis.] Saint Louis, MO: Saint Louis University.

Box 5-5

CHARACTERISTICS OF GOOD ROLE MODELS

- Passion
- Integrity
- Relationship-focused
- Excellence
- Positive choice making
- Demonstrate confidence
- Optimism
- Resilience/ability to overcome obstacles
- Generous
- Community-focused

Adapted from Johnson, J. A. (2015). Nursing professional development specialists as role models. *Nurses in Professional Development, 31*(5), 297-299.

---

models differ from teachers in that role models are people who are admired for the way they act and whose behavior is considered as a standard of excellence toward which to aspire. Role models for occupational therapy students can be individuals in positions they would like to reach, who possess qualities they would like to have, and/or people whom they can identify with. Therefore, students can learn to act, behave, and perform professionally when they interact with their role models. Occupational therapy students should be exposed to role models across various levels, including their peers, staff, faculty, and practicing professionals. In order to continue to enhance the professionalization of occupational therapy, all levels of occupational therapy practitioners should strive to be a positive role model (Côté & Leclère, 2000). Characteristics of good role models and qualities of professionalism can be found in Boxes 5-4 and 5-5.

TABLE 5-4 **LEARNING STYLE INVENTORIES**	
INVENTORY	**DESCRIPTION**
VARK Questionnaire	Fleming and Mills (1992) suggested four modalities that seemed to encompass the experiences of the students and teachers. The acronym VARK stands for the Visual, Aural, Read/Write, and Kinesthetic sensory modalities that are used for learning information.
TLSI 3.1	Developed by Kolb and Kolb (2005), this computerized assessment allows students to discover their learning style, expand their strengths, and provides information on how educators can use this information to best serve students as well as possible strategies for accommodating different learning styles.
National Association of Secondary School Principals Learning Style Profile	The National Association of Secondary School Principals (NASSP) Learning Style Profile is an instrument for the diagnosis of student cognitive styles, perceptual responses, as well as study and instructional preferences such as study time preference, posture, mobility, and climate preferences such as sound, lighting, and temperature (Keefe & Monks, 1986).
Jackson's Learning Style Profile	Jackson's model suggests that learning styles are influenced by a variety of factors including experience, personal choice, and biology. The Learning Style Profile is based on a neuropsychological model of learning, modeled on principles of approach and avoidance, and argues for the division of personality into temperament and character (O'Connor & Jackson, 2008).
Grasha-Reichmann Learning Style Scale (GRLSS)	The Grasha-Reichmann Learning Style Scale (GRLSS) defines learners according to the type and level of interaction. The learning styles are avoidant, participative, competitive, collaborative, dependent, and independent. The Grasha-Reichmann model focuses on student attitudes toward learning, classroom activities, teachers, and peers (Grasha & Reichmann, 2003). The Grasha-Reichmann Learning Style Scale also has a teaching style survey that instructors can complete to see how their instruction matches or conflicts with their learners, so they can adapt and diversify to meet more learners' needs.

Learning Style Inventories

As an educator, increasing a learner's awareness of his or her learning style is crucial. Learning style inventories can be fairly quick and easy strategies to inform students of how they learn, as well as predict what kind of instructional strategies or method will be most effective for an individual learner, group of learners, or for a particular learning activity. These inventories typically take the form of a questionnaire that focuses on how people prefer to learn. Respondents choose the answers that most closely resemble their own preferences. To promote optimal and meaningful learning experiences, educators need to match their teaching styles to the needs of their learners (Tables 5-4 and 5-5).

TABLE 5-5 TYPES OF LEARNERS AND STRATEGIES		
LEARNER TYPE	**STRATEGIES FOR LEARNING**	**EXAMPLE FOR PROFESSIONALISM**
Visual/Non-Verbal Learner	• Illustrations • Videos • Charts • Pictures • Designs	Looking at pictures of professional dress attire
Visual/Verbal Learner	• Written words • Handouts • Note-taking	Learning the Occupational Therapy Code of Ethics by re-writing the ethical principles
Tactile/Kinesthetic Learner	• Hands-on • Movement • Role-play • Simulation	Engaging in mock interview role-play scenarios with classmates
Auditory/Verbal Learner	• Oral strategies • Tape recorder • Discussion	Engaging in small group discussions regarding effective strategies to provide constructive feedback to peers

CURRENT EDUCATIONAL TRENDS

Not unlike occupational therapy clinical practice and health care in general, the context and demands of higher education have constantly been transforming. The student profile is evolving and becoming more diverse, as well as the methods for teaching.

Contemporary Educational Delivery Models

The days of 100% classroom-based, lecture-only learning are over. According to the National Center for Education Statistics (2014), approximately one in four students have taken at least one distance education course. The technology-savvy millennial generation have and will continue to influence education (Allen & Seaman, 2013). As students, they have forced learning institutions and employers to communicate and educate in new ways. Online, hybrid, or blended learning environments are becoming more of the norm in higher education. Online education, sometimes referred to as distance learning, is when curriculum is delivered over the Internet and can be accessed from a web platform for an academic institution, such as Blackboard or Moodle. Online education can be asynchronous or synchronous. Asynchronous courses are delivered and accessed at the student's convenience and pace. An example of asynchronous learning would involve students doing independent reading about a topic and then posting a reflection on an online discussion board. Synchronous learning involves real-time interaction between the student(s) and the

TABLE 5-6
COMMON INSTRUCTIONAL TECHNOLOGIES

INSTRUCTIONAL TECHNOLOGY	DESCRIPTION
Smart Board	Line of interactive whiteboards produced by the Calgary-based company Smart Technologies
Click-Share	Collaborative software and technology that allows individuals to share content wirelessly on individual laptops
Student Response Systems	Wireless response system that allows faculty to request information, and for students to respond by using a "clicker" or hand-held response pad to send his or her information to a receiver

instructor(s). An example of a synchronous learning event would involve students watching a live web stream of a class, while simultaneously taking part in a discussion or participating in a class discussion via web-conferencing. Most forms of distance education involve a blending of these two types of learning.

Occupational therapy educational programs can be face-to-face, hybrid (involving face-to-face and online education), or strictly online. Although online education can provide flexibility in terms of time and place of study, to be successful, students need to take charge and be responsible for their learning. Being successful in an online or blended curriculum requires strong organization and time management skills, self-motivation, initiative, and independent learning. During an asynchronous course, students have to be able to start and work on tasks on their own, without someone keeping them focused, and they have to be self-disciplined to follow the class schedule and meet deadlines. In addition, strong interpersonal communication, especially written communication, is a key professional skill needed to network and meaningfully connect with others in the online learning environment. Professional online students must be active learners and self-starters who are not afraid to ask questions when they do not understand or need clarification. Since the course instructor cannot "see" the student, students need to be proactive and as explicit as possible when communicating concerns or questions. Furthermore, the online instructor isn't the only source of information. Online learners are encouraged to be team-oriented and collaborative and reach out to their classmates to problem solve as needed.

Instructional Technology

In response to the growing technology skill set of the Millennials and Generation Z, the use of technology in the classroom is booming. Products such as SMART boards, bamboo pads, click-share, and student response systems are just a few examples of educational technology that are on the rise. Student response systems, also known as "clickers," are an interactive educational tool that allow instructors to create a dynamic learning environment and capture real-time assessment data (Bojinova & Oigara, 2011; Cain, Black, & Rohr, 2009; Mula & Kavanagh, 2009). According to research, a student response systems can be used to engage students, elicit and address prior understanding (including misconceptions), identify areas of difficulty, obtain feedback, facilitate peer instruction and discussion, collect multiple trials of data from experiments conducted during class, and improve attendance in class (Cain, Black, & Rohr, 2009; Sevian & Robinson, 2011) (Table 5-6).

BOX 5-6

EXAMPLE OF SHARED TEAM-BASED LEARNING ACTIVITY FOR PROFESSIONALISM

Create a dynamic case study of an unprofessional and/or ethical dilemma. Break up the class into small groups. Provide each group the same set of questions. Instruct each group to explore and problem-solve the case. After each small group has completed their questions, have each group report their conclusions to the large group.

Novel Educational Methodologies

Group learning, also known as cooperative or shared learning, is a teaching strategy in which small teams, each with students of different levels of ability, use a variety of learning activities to improve their understanding of a common task. The ownership of teaching and learning is shared by groups of students, and is no longer the sole responsibility of the teacher. The authority of setting goals, assessing learning, and facilitating learning is shared by all parties involved. Students have more opportunities to actively participate in their learning, question and challenge each other, share and discuss their ideas, and internalize their learning. Along with improving academic learning, cooperative learning helps students to engage in thoughtful discourse and examine different perspectives, and increases students' esteem, motivation, and empathy. According to Johnson and Johnson (1990), there are five basic elements that allow successful small-group learning:

- Positive interdependence: Students feel responsible for their own and the group's effort
- Face-to-face interaction: Students encourage and support one another; the environment encourages discussion and eye contact
- Individual and group accountability: Each student is responsible for doing their part; the group is accountable for meeting its goal
- Group behaviors: Group members gain direct instruction in the interpersonal, social, and collaborative skills needed to work with others
- Group processing: Group members analyze their own and the group's ability to work together

Research indicates that collaborative learning has several benefits which may positively influence professional development and better prepare students for collaborative practice in health care environments, such as increasing critical reasoning skills, team-building skills, and communication (Box 5-6) (Laal & Ghodsi, 2012).

Process-Oriented Guided Inquiry Learning

Process-oriented guided inquiry learning (POGIL) is a student-centered, group-learning instructional pedagogy that involves a learning cycle of exploration, concept invention, and application. Students work in small groups with individual roles to ensure that all students are fully engaged in the learning process. Since students are using the content to solve a structured problem or set of questions, rather than being given the content via a lecture, they are more likely to grasp the relevance of the content (Hanson, 2006). Research indicates that POGIL improves long-term retention of information, which is useful to occupational therapy educators who are ultimately preparing students to demonstrate competency during fieldwork experiences and the national certification exam. The suggested group size for POGIL is three to five students, with specific roles assigned to each member per session. See Table 5-7 for a sample group setup.

TABLE 5-7	
SAMPLE GROUP ROLES AND RESPONSIBILITIES FOR PROCESS-ORIENTED GUIDED INQUIRY LEARNING	

ROLE	RESPONSIBILITY
Manager	Manages and directs the group
Time-Keeper	Ensures participation in roles, ensures continued flow, interfaces with facilitator
Recorder	Records the names and roles of the group, takes notes according to topics and flow of discussion
Presenter	Presents concise oral report of discussion or findings to the class
Reflector	Observes and comments on the group's performance; a key aspect of Process Oriented Guided Inquiry Learning is that the learning session ends with shared critical thinking questions
Additional roles might include: Technician, Encourager, Fact-Checker	

POGIL develops process skills such as critical thinking, problem solving, group process skills, and communication through cooperation and reflection, helping students become lifelong learners and preparing them to be more competitive in a global market (Hanson, 2006; Jaffe, Gibson, & D'Amico, 2015).

Simulation

Historically, simulation has been used in the training of pilots, armed forces, and astronauts, as a medium to imitate a real-world act or scenario. The use of simulation in health care student's education and training is on the rise. Simulation provides a safe, interactive, virtual environment to transition knowledge into practice (Baird et al., 2015). The use of simulation as an education modality taps into a combination of various learning styles: visual, auditory, and tactile. While most commonly used for clinical skill development and competency, recent evidence indicates that simulation can be used to teach skills related to professionalism and ethics such as communication, decision-making, teamwork, and leadership skills (Baird et al., 2015). There are both hi-tech and low-tech methods to incorporate simulation. High-tech simulation can be used via clinical simulation laboratories, which mirror actual clinical environments. Clinical simulation labs may include the use of mannequins to replicate patient encounters, and/or clinical equipment to mimic a health care setting. Low-tech simulation options can include the use of role-play learning activities and standardized patients. Besides appealing to various learning styles, the use of simulation also allows educators to work toward the acquisition of higher-order thinking. According to Bloom's taxonomy, this can be promoted by allowing learners to apply, demonstrate, evaluate, and synthesize knowledge learned in the classroom to a safe, simulated, clinical environment. Lastly, the use of simulation allows for more interactive learning, which is a desired characteristic of learning among Generations Y and Z (Box 5-7) (Faust, Ginno, Laherty, & Manuel, 2001).

Box 5-7

TOPICS FOR ROLE-PLAY SIMULATION TO DEVELOP PROFESSIONALISM

Scenarios to practice include:

- Patient/therapist boundaries
- Handling a challenging patient encounter
- Handling a patient complaint
- Handling an incorrect patient encounter

Box 5-8

TIPS FOR TEACHING GENERATIONS Y AND Z

1. Become a learning facilitator to foster self-directedness
2. Embrace the use of educational technology and edutainment
3. Use guided discovery to promote student metacognition and self-awareness
4. Allow learning to incorporate self-expression and individuality
5. Model the way for professionalism

Adapted from Edutainment. (n.d.) In Oxford Dictionaries. Retrieved from http://www.oxforddictionaries.com/us/definition/american_english/edutainment; Kouzes, J. M., & Posner, B. Z. (2008). *The leadership challenge* (4th ed.). Hoboken, NJ: Wiley.

Summary

Occupational therapy educators are responsible for promoting a student's ability to think "critically and make ethical decisions that are based on sound core values and professional attitudes" (Kanny & Kyler, 1999, p. 72). Therefore, it is vital that these educators have the necessary skills and abilities to educate students' in this realm of professionalism. In response to the current trends in higher education discussed previously in this chapter, the following is a summary of best practice teaching approaches and how they relate to teaching professionalism (Box 5-8).

SUMMARY

"Educating the mind, without educating the heart is no education at all"

—Aristotle

In Chapter 1, we discussed the general characteristics and stereotypes associated with generations. The future of the occupational therapy profession lies within Generations Y and Z, because these are current undergraduate occupational therapy students, as well as the students in middle and high school who are deciding on their career path. Educators who merely follow the textbook, and use a lecture only format in their teaching are likely to be perceived as "old school," which contributes to a decreased perception of teaching effectiveness among Generation Y and Z learners. Occupational therapy educators need to understand the nature of these generations, and adopt teaching strategies that work with them—in other words, be student-centered educators. A greater emphasis on active learning pedagogies, blended learning environments, team and collaborative learning, and the use of educational technology including simulation, are all strategies to enhance the learning outcomes of this generation and foster their professional development.

LEARNING ACTIVITIES

1. Take at least one of the learning style inventories identified in this chapter. What type of learner are you? What are the advantages and disadvantages of your learning style? What strategies do you use to help you learn and remember information?

2. Think about your learning style as it relates to clinical practice and future employment. How can knowing how you learn help you to make important decisions to be successful in both fieldwork and the workforce?

3. Think about courses you have taken thus far in your training. What types of pedagogies have you seen your instructors use? What types of pedagogies kept you most engaged?

4. Identify an individual from your personal or professional life who could serve as a role model for you. What qualities do they have that you look up to, and why?

REFERENCES

Accreditation Council for Occupational Therapy Education. (2012). 2011 Accreditation Council for Occupational Therapy Education (ACOTE) standards. *American Journal of Occupational Therapy, 66*(Suppl. 1), S6-S74.

Allen, I. E., & Seaman, J. (2013). *Changing course: Ten years of tracking online education in the United States.* Newburyport, MA: Sloan Consortium.

American Occupational Therapy Association. (n.d.). Overview of ACOTE. Retrieved from http://www.aota.org/education-careers/accreditation/overview.aspx

American Occupational Therapy Association. (1983). Essentials of an accredited education program for the occupational therapist. *American Journal of Occupational Therapy, 37*(12), 817-823.

American Occupational Therapy Association. (2007). A descriptive review of occupational therapy education. *American Journal of Occupational Therapy, 61*(6), 672-677.

American Occupational Therapy Association. (2009). Specialized knowledge and skills of occupational therapy educators of the future. *American Journal of Occupational Therapy, 63*(6), 804-818.

American Occupational Therapy Association. (2014). Scope of practice. *American Journal of Occupational Therapy, 68*(Suppl. 3), S34-S40.

American Occupational Therapy Association. (2015a). Philosophy of occupational therapy education. *American Journal of Occupational Therapy, 69*(Suppl. 3), 6913410053.

American Occupational Therapy Association. (2015b). Importance of interprofessional education in occupational therapy curricula. *American Journal of Occupational Therapy, 69*(Suppl. 3), 6913410020.

American Occupational Therapy Association. (2015c). Value of occupational therapy assistant education to the profession. *American Journal of Occupational Therapy, 69*(Suppl. 3),6913410070.

American Occupational Therapy Association. (2015d). Occupational therapy code of ethics.Retrieved from http://www.aota.org/-/media/corporate/files/practice/ethics/code-of-ethics.pdf

Anderson, L. W., & Krathwohl, D. (Eds.). (2001). *A taxonomy for learning, teaching, and assessing: a revision of Bloom's taxonomy of educational objectives.* New York, NY: Longmans.

Baird, J. M., Raina, K. D., Rogers, J. C., O'Donnell, J., Terhorst, L., & Holm, M. B. (2015). Simulation strategies to teach patient transfers: Self-efficacy by strategy. *American Journal of Occupational Therapy, 69*(Suppl. 2), 6912185030.

Bloom, B., Englehart, M., Furst, E., Hill, W., & Krathwohl, D. (1956). *Taxonomy of educational objectives: The classification of educational goals. Handbook I: Cognitive domain.* New York, NY: Longmans.

Bojinova, E., & Oigara, J. (2011). Teaching and learning with clickers: Are clickers good for Students? *Interdisciplinary Journal of E-Learning and Learning Objects, 7*(1), 169-184.

Cain, D. J. (2002). *Humanistic psychotherapies: Handbook of research and practice.* Washington, DC: American Psychological Association.

Cain, J., Black, E. P., & Rohr, J. (2009). An audience response system strategy to improve student motivation, attention, and feedback. *American Journal of Pharmaceutical Education, 73*(2), 1-21

Cooper, D. L., & Miller, T. K. (1998). Influence and impact: Professional development in student affairs. *New Directions for Student Services, 84*, 55-69.

Côté, L., & Leclère, H. (2000). How clinical teachers perceive the doctor-patient relationship and themselves as role models. *Academic Medicine: Journal of the Association of American Medical Colleges, 75*(11), 1117-1124.

Council on Medical Education and Hospitals. (1936). Medical education in the United States and Canada: Data for the academic year 1935-1936. *Journal of the American Medical Association, 107*(9), 661-692.

Crist, P. (2011). Transformative learning in fieldwork. Retrieved from http://occupational-therapy.advanceweb.com/Columns/Issues-in-Fieldwork/Transformative-Learning-in-Fieldwork.aspx

Crist, P., & Scaffa, M. (2012). *Best practices in occupational therapy education.* Abingdon, UK: Routledge.

Cutchin, M. P. (2004). Using Deweyan philosophy to rename and reframe adaptation-to-environment. *American Journal of Occupational Therapy, 58*(3), 303-312.

DeBourgh, G. A. (2008). Use of classroom "clickers" to promote acquisition of advancedreasoning skills. *Nurse Education in Practice, 8*(2), 76-87.

Edutainment. (n.d.). In Oxford Dictionaries. Retrieved from http://www.oxforddictionaries.com/us/definition/american_english/edutainment

Faust, J. E., Ginno, J., Laherty, J., & Manuel, K. (2001). Teaching information literacy to Generation Y: Tested strategies for reaching the headphone-wearing, itchy mouse-fingered, and frequently paged. Retrieved from: http://library.csueastbay.edu/acrl2001/

Fleming, N. D., & Mills, C. (1992). Not another inventory, rather a catalyst for reflection. *To Improve the Academy, 11*, 137-155.

Grasha, A. F., & Riechmann, S. W. (2003). Grasha-Riechmann student learning style scales. Retrieved from http://www.angelfire.com/ny3/toddsvballpage/Cognitive/GR.pdf

Greene, D. (1997). The use of service learning in client environments to enhance ethical reasoning in students. *American Journal of Occupational Therapy, 51*(10), 844-852.

Hanson, D. M. (2006). *Instructor's guide to process-oriented guided-inquiry learning.* Lisle, IL: Stony Brook.

Hanson, D. M., & DeIuliis, E. D. (2015). The collaborative model of fieldwork education: A blueprint for group supervision of students. *Occupational Therapy in Healthcare, 29*(2), 223-239.

Hoppes, S., Bender, D., & DeGrace, B. W. (2005). Service learning is a perfect fit for occupational and physical therapy education. *Journal of Allied Health, 34*(1), 47-50.

Inelmen, E., & Inelmen, E. M. (n.d.). "Situated learning" as an enhancer for the employability of the undergraduate student. Retrieved from http://www.sefi.be/wp-content/abstracts/1206.pdf

Jaffe, L. E., Gibson, R., & D'Amico, M. (2015). Process-oriented guided-inquiry learning: A natural fit for occupational therapy education. *Occupational Therapy in Health Care, 29*(2), 115-125.

Johnson, J. A. (2015). Nursing professional development specialists as role models. *Nurses in Professional Development, 31*(5), 297-299.

Johnson, D. W., & Johnson, R. T. (1990). *Learning together and alone: Cooperative, competitive and individualistic learning.* Englewood Cliffs, NJ: Prentice-Hall.

Jones, B., Valdez, G., Nowakowski, J., & Rasmussen, C. (1994). *Designing learning and technology for educational reform.* Oak Brook, IL: North Central Regional Educational Laboratory.

Kanny, E. M., & Kyler, P. L. (1999). Are faculty prepared to address ethical issues in education? *American Journal of Occupational Therapy, 53*(1), 72-74.

Keefe, J. W., & Monks, J. S. (1986). *Learner Style Profile: Examiner's manual.* Reston, VA: National Association of Secondary School Principals.

Kolb, D. A. (1984). *Experiential learning: Experience as the source of learning and development.* Englewood Cliffs, NJ: Prentice-Hall.

Kolb, A. Y., & Kolb, D. A. (2005). *The Kolb learning style inventory—Version 3.1 2005 technical specifications.* Boston, MA: Hay Resource Direct.

Kouzes, J. M., & Posner, B. Z. (2008). *The leadership challenge* (4th ed.). Hoboken, NJ: Wiley.

Laal, M., & Ghodsi, S. M. (2012). Benefits of collaborative learning. *Procedia - Social and Behavioral Sciences, 31*, 486-490.

Landa-Gonzalez, B., Velis, E., & Greg, K. (2015). Learning styles as predictors of fieldwork performance and learning adaptability of graduate non-traditional occupational therapy students. *Journal of Allied Health, 44*(3), 145-151.

McNulty, T. M., Crowe, T. K., & VanLeit, B. (2004). Promoting professional reflection through problem-based learning evaluation activities. *Occupational Therapy in Healthcare, 18*(1-2), 71-82.

Mernar, T. J. (2000). Handbook for developing or modifying a student occupational therapy association: An organizational approach. [Master's thesis.] South Orange, NJ: Seton Hall University.

Mula, J. M., & Kavanagh, M. (2009). Click go the students, click-click-click: The efficacy of astudent response system for engaging students to improve feedback and performance. *e-Journal of Business Education and Scholarship of Teaching, 3*(1), 1-17.

National Board for Certification in Occupational Therapy. (n.d). Guidelines for mentoring. Retrieved from http://www.nbcot.org/assets/candidate-pdfs/practitioner-pdfs/mentoring-guidelines-log

National Center for Education Statistics. (2014). Enrollment in distance education courses, by state: Fall 2012. Retrieved from http://nces.ed.gov/pubs2014/2014023.pdf

National Mentoring Partnership. (2016). Home page. Retrieved from http://www.mentoring.org/

Nelson, D. L. (1988). Occupation: Form and performance. *American Journal of Occupational Therapy, 42*(10), 633-641.

Nolinske, T., & Millis, B. (1999). Cooperative learning as an approach to pedagogy. *American Journal of Occupational Therapy, 53*(1), 31-40.

O'Connor, P. J., & Jackson, C. J. (2008). The factor structure and validity of the learning styles profiler (LSP). *European Journal of Psychological Assessment, 24*(2), 117-123.

Paice, E., Heard, S., & Moss, F. (2002). How important are role models in making good doctors? *British Medical Journal, 325*, 707-710.

Patience, A. (2008). The art of loving in the classroom: A defence of affective pedagogy. *Australian Journal of Teacher Education, 33*(2), 54-67.

Patterson, B., Kilpatrick, J., & Woebkenberg, E. (2010). Evidence of teaching practice: The impact of clickers in a large classroom environment. *Nurse Education Today, 30*(7), 603-607.

Pedagogy. (2016, January 1). In Merriam-Webster dictionary. Retrieved from http://www.merriam-webster.com/dictionary/pedagogy

Place, N. T., & Bailey, A. (2006). Mentoring: Providing greatest benefit to new and seasoned faculty in an extension organization. *Proceedings of the Association for International Agricultural and Extension Education, 22*, 498-507.

Polatajko, H. J., & Mandich, A. (2004). *Enabling occupation in children: The cognitive orientation to daily occupational performance (CO–OP) approach.* Ottawa, ON: CAOT Publications.

Queensland Occupational Therapy Fieldwork Collaborative. (2007). The clinical educator's resource kit. Retrieved from http://www.qotfc.edu.au/resource/index.html?page=65335&pid=65377

Rogers, C. R. (1966). *Client-centered therapy.* Washington, DC: American Psychological Association.

Role Model. (2016, January 1). In Dictionary.com. Retrieved from http://dictionary.reference.com/browse/role-model

Santalucia, S., & Johnson, C. (2010, October 25). Transformative learning: Facilitating growth and change through fieldwork. *OT Practice, 15*(19), CE-1-CE-8.

Schaber, P. (2014). Keynote address: Searching for and identifying signature pedagogies in occupational therapy education. *American Journal of Occupational Therapy, 68*(Suppl. 2), S40-S44.

Service-Learning. (2017). In Dictionary.com. Retrieved from http://www.dictionary.com/browse/service-learning?s=t

Sevian, H., & Robinson, W. E. (2011). Clickers promote learning in all kinds of classes—Small and large, graduate and undergraduate, lecture and lab. *Journal of College Science Teaching, 40*(3), 14-18.

Shook, J. (n.d.). John Dewey, American pragmatist. Retrieved from http://dewey.pragmatism.org/

Simpson, R. D., & Dyer, T. G. (1997). The American professoriate in transition. Retrieved from http://podnetwork.org/content/uploads/96_97_v8.pdf

Simons, S., Georgen, M., Fay, S., Landgraf, E., & Matlock, C. (2013). Participation in student Occupational therapy associations. [Master's thesis.] Saint Louis, MO: Saint Louis University.

Sladyk, K., Jacobs, K., & MacRae, N. (Eds.). (2010). *Occupational therapy essentials for clinical competence.* Thorofare, NJ: SLACK Incorporated.

Stafford, E. M. (1986). Relationship between occupational therapy student learning styles and clinic performance. *American Journal of Occupational Therapy, 40*(1), 34-39.

Straus, S. E., Johnson, M. O., Marquez, C., & Feldman, M. D. (2013). Characteristics of successful and failed mentoring relationships: A qualitative study across two academic health centers. *Academic Medicine: Journal of the Association of American Medical Colleges, 88*(1), 82-89.

Stutz-Tannenbaum, P., & Hooper, B. (2009). Creating congruence between identities as a fieldwork educator and a practitioner. *AOTA Special Interest Section Quarterly: Education, 19*(2), 1-4.

Vygotsky, L. (1978). *Mind in society.* Cambridge, MA: Harvard University Press.

APPENDIX A: SAMPLE OBSERVATION LOG

	SESSION OBSERVED	STUDENT OBSERVATIONS	STUDENT REFLECTIONS
What were the primary goal(s) or problem(s) addressed in the treatment session?			
What underlying client factors (physical, cognitive, psychosocial) contributed to the problem? How?			
Give an example of preparatory method(s), purposeful activities, and/or occupation-based interventions used in the session.			
What elements of the session were client-centered?			
How did the lead practitioner attend to safety?			
What therapeutic strategies were used by the lead practitioner professional? In what ways were they effective or not?			
What frame of reference(s) was the practitioner using as a conceptual framework? Justify this choice with observations made during the session			
Additional Comments			

Adapted from: Hanson, D., & Deluliis, E. (2015). The Collaborative Model to Fieldwork Education: a blueprint for group supervision of students. OT in Healthcare: Special Issue in Education, 29(2), 223-239.

APPENDIX B: SAMPLE PROFESSIONAL DEVELOPMENT PLAN OUTLINE FOR A 6-YEAR ENTRY LEVEL OCCUPATIONAL THERAPY DEPARTMENT PROGRAM

1st YEAR PROFESSIONAL DEVELOPMENT PLAN

At the beginning of each semester:

1. Students write at least two or three goals for themselves that can be completed this semester and post on BlackBoard

2. Identify specific strategies you will use to measure whether you have accomplished each goal

3. Schedule a brief meeting with your faculty mentor to discuss your goals

4. Post your revised goals on your BlackBoard personal page and self-monitor your goal attainment

At the end of the semester:

1. Document evidence that have met each goal

2. Generate a brief reflection on this semester's professional development goals and begin thinking about creating a new plan for next semester

Check your goals: Are they SMART Goals?

S = Specific, M = Measurable, A = Attainable, R = Realistic, T = Time-specific

Professional Service Goal(s)
Measurable Strategies to Accomplish this Goal:
Evidence that I accomplished this Goal:

Practitioner Goal(s)
Measurable Strategies to Accomplish this Goal:
Evidence that I accomplished this Goal:

Leadership Goal(s)
Measurable Strategies to Accomplish this Goal:
Evidence that I accomplished this Goal:

Practice Scholar Goal(s)
Measurable Strategies to Accomplish this Goal:
Evidence that I accomplished this Goal:

End of Semester Reflection

2nd YEAR PROFESSIONAL DEVELOPMENT PLAN

Professional Service Goal(s)
Measurable Strategies to Accomplish this Goal:
Evidence that I accomplished this Goal:

Practitioner Goal(s)
Measurable Strategies to Accomplish this Goal:
Evidence that I accomplished this Goal:

Leadership Goal(s)
Measurable Strategies to Accomplish this Goal:
Evidence that I accomplished this Goal:

Practice Scholar Goal(s)
Measurable Strategies to Accomplish this Goal:
Evidence that I accomplished this Goal:
End of Semester Reflection

3rd YEAR PROFESSIONAL DEVELOPMENT PLAN

Professional Service Goal(s)
Measurable Strategies to Accomplish this Goal:
Evidence that I accomplished this Goal:

Practitioner Goal(s)
Measurable Strategies to Accomplish this Goal:
Evidence that I accomplished this Goal:

Leadership Goal(s)
Measurable Strategies to Accomplish this Goal:
Evidence that I accomplished this Goal:

Practice Scholar Goal(s)
Measurable Strategies to Accomplish this Goal:
Evidence that I accomplished this Goal:

Fieldwork Preparation Goal(s)
Measurable Strategies to Accomplish this Goal:
Evidence that I accomplished this Goal:
End of Semester Reflection

4th YEAR PROFESSIONAL DEVELOPMENT PLAN

Professional Service Goal(s)
Measurable Strategies to Accomplish this Goal:
Evidence that I accomplished this Goal:

Practitioner Goal(s)
Measurable Strategies to Accomplish this Goal:
Evidence that I accomplished this Goal:

Leadership Goal(s)
Measurable Strategies to Accomplish this Goal:
Evidence that I accomplished this Goal:

Practice Scholar Goal(s)
Measurable Strategies to Accomplish this Goal:
Evidence that I accomplished this Goal:

Fieldwork Preparation Goal(s)
Measurable Strategies to Accomplish this Goal:
Evidence that I accomplished this Goal:

NBCOT Certification Exam Preparation Goal(s)
Measurable Strategies to Accomplish this Goal:
Evidence that I accomplished this Goal:
End of Semester Reflection

5th YEAR PROFESSIONAL DEVELOPMENT PLAN

Professional Service Goal(s)
Measurable Strategies to Accomplish this Goal:
Evidence that I accomplished this Goal:

Practitioner Goal(s)
Measurable Strategies to Accomplish this Goal:
Evidence that I accomplished this Goal:

Leadership Goal(s)
Measurable Strategies to Accomplish this Goal:
Evidence that I accomplished this Goal:

Practice Scholar Goal(s)
Measurable Strategies to Accomplish this Goal:
Evidence that I accomplished this Goal:

Fieldwork Preparation Goal(s)
Measurable Strategies to Accomplish this Goal:
Evidence that I accomplished this Goal:

NBCOT Certification Exam Preparation Goal(s)
Measurable Strategies to Accomplish this Goal:
Evidence that I accomplished this Goal:

    End of Semester Reflection

6th YEAR PROFESSIONAL DEVELOPMENT PLAN

Professional Service Goal(s)
Measurable Strategies to Accomplish this Goal:
Evidence that I accomplished this Goal:

Advanced Practitioner Goal(s)
Measurable Strategies to Accomplish this Goal:
Evidence that I accomplished this Goal:

Professional Leadership Goal(s)
Measurable Strategies to Accomplish this Goal:
Evidence that I accomplished this Goal:

Practice Scholar Goal(s)
Measurable Strategies to Accomplish this Goal:
Evidence that I accomplished this Goal:

Doctoral Experiential Component Goal
Measurable Strategies to Accomplish this Goal:
Evidence that I accomplished this Goal:

    End of Semester Reflection

    End of Occupational Therapy Department Program Reflections

From http://www.duq.edu/assets/Documents/occupational-therapy/Fieldwork-Education/ OT%20student%20handbook%206.28.16.pdf

Socializing Students to Professional Expectations in the Classroom

Elizabeth D. DeIuliis, OTD, OTR/L

INTRODUCTION

Teaching students and health care providers about professionalism and ethics is more than just providing them with a document on the code of ethics, or having them read an academic integrity policy. Occupational therapy educators have a multi-faceted role in developing professionalism in occupational therapy students. In addition to the various educational pedagogies discussed in Chapter 5, several key steps are suggested by Kirk (2007) in teaching professionalism in the classroom:

- Setting expectations (i.e., have clear policies)
- Performing assessments (gather baseline and ongoing results)
- Remediating inappropriate behaviors
- Preventing inappropriate behaviors
- Implementing a cultural change

Through this process, educators are responsible to teach, motivate, and empower students to think about their values, attitudes, and beliefs to shape their own professional identity. This chapter will discuss strategies to promote professionalism in the classroom.

KEY WORDS

Academic Integrity: Honesty, trust, fairness, respect, and responsibility within the academic community, applying to both the educators and the learners; academic integrity extends into clinical and community learning, as well as any interaction or relationship connected to the teaching-learning process

Plagiarism: Claiming another person's work as your own; can be intentional or unintentional, resulting from not citing sources in paraphrasing, or direct copying

DeIuliis, E.D.
Professionalism Across Occupational Therapy Practice (pp 137-159).
© 2017 Taylor & Francis Group.

OBJECTIVES

By the end of reading this chapter and completing the learning activities, the reader should be able to:

1. Identify the relationship between academic integrity and professionalism
2. Discuss specific approaches to promote professionalism in the classroom
3. Evaluate strategies to address unprofessional behaviors

ACADEMIC INTEGRITY

It is impossible to talk about professional behavior, attitude, and responsibility for the occupational therapy student without discussing academic integrity. Academic integrity is truly the moral code or ethical testament in an academic setting. It is directly linked to intellectual honesty and responsibility in scholarship. The foundation of academic integrity encompasses many of the signature attributes of professionalism, including honesty, trust, fairness, respect, and responsibility within the academic community, applying to both the educators and the learners. In allied health professional education, academic integrity extends beyond the classroom learning environment to include clinical and community learning, and ultimately any interaction or relationship connected to the teaching-learning process. It is the professional responsibility of occupational therapy students and faculty members to be knowledgeable about the academic integrity policy of their institution, including procedures for reporting and the process of dealing with academic misconduct (Box 6-1).

Reporting Procedures for Academic Misconduct

As much as it a student's duty to display academic integrity, it also necessary that they properly report any observed or potentially observed academic misconduct (Table 6-1; Boxes 6-2 to 6-5).

BOX 6-1
EXAMPLES OF ACADEMIC MISCONDUCT

- Cheating
- Unauthorized collaboration: intentionally or unintentionally working with another student(s) on assignments or examinations
- Plagiarism: not citing sources in direct copying or paraphrasing
- Academic misconduct in online learning environment—logging in another student, having another student take your exam, using notes when asked not to
- Fabrication, forgery, alteration of documents
- Destruction of property

TABLE 6-1
DO'S AND DON'TS FOR ACADEMIC INTEGRITY

DON'T	• Copy answers from another student
	• Allow another student to copy your answers
	• Take an exam or complete an assignment as another student
	• Use electronic devices during exams
	• Collaborate with another student beyond the extent specifically approved by the course instructor
DO	• Trust your instinct
	• Be ethical
	• Be professional in reporting

BOX 6-2

GENERAL CONSEQUENCES FOR ACADEMIC MISCONDUCT

- Earn a zero on the project, assignment, exam
- Failure of the course
- Dismissal from the program and/or institution
- Legal ramifications

BOX 6-3

TIPS FOR OCCUPATIONAL THERAPY EDUCATORS

- Keep all student exams: Hand them back in class for review, but be sure they are returned and properly secured
- Mix up exam room seating: Or use two testing areas, each with a proctor
- Consider multiple exam forms
- Group assignments: Ask students to state and describe their input and contribution (See Box 6-4)
- For writing-intensive projects: Require drafts and references prior to due date
- Use of rubrics: Set clear expectations of performance

Box 6-4

GROUP ASSIGNMENT REFLECTIONS

1. What personal insight or contribution did I make to the group during this project?
2. What did I learn from the group experience that I probably wouldn't have without it?

Box 6-5

SAMPLE GROUP GRADING POLICY

Group Project Grading Policy: Unless otherwise specified in the assignment guidelines, group assignments receive one total group grade with each member of the team receiving an identical grade. Team members may propose an alternative distribution of the group assignment grade. Proposals for an alternative grade distribution must be made in writing. The proposal should specifically define an alternative distribution of the group assignment grade and provide a rationale for the proposed change. After the group presents their proposal to the instructor, the instructor will determine the final distribution of the group assignment grades. The group will be notified by the instructor as to his/her decision.

STRATEGIES TO PROMOTE ACADEMIC INTEGRITY IN THE OCCUPATIONAL THERAPY CLASSROOM

In promoting integrity as a quality held by a professional, it is critical to make it a part of your learning environment, not just during disciplinary action (Box 6-6).

Online Courses

Learning activities and assessment methods for online courses should not just be simply "face-to-face" classroom activities transferred to the Internet. Learning assessments and test items should be designed specifically for an online environment. This means that the medium and delivery has been considered and designed into the actual assessment. Strategies such as passwords, browser security and other options can help support student authenticity and academic integrity in the online environment (Box 6-7).

STRATEGIES TO BUILD A STUDENT'S PROFESSIONAL IDENTITY IN THE CLASSROOM

Direct/Formal Strategies

Have you ever noticed how handbooks and policy manuals seem to be getting thicker and thicker every year? In my time as an occupational therapy educator and an academic fieldwork coordinator, I can attest to the increase in number and type of policies within the department

Box 6-6

FACE-TO FACE/HYBRID COURSE

- Create clear academic integrity statements, policies, and procedures that are consistently implemented across the curriculum.

- Educators should formally address academic integrity policies during student orientation events and require students to read and sign an agreement to the policy (keep this signed form in their student file). Educators should provide examples to help students understand the difference between collaboration on assignments and cheating, and identify plagiarism.

- Inform and educate the entire community regarding the academic integrity policies and procedures (post on your website, list on course syllabi, display it on a cover page of each exam, show it on a lecture slide before each test). Make academic integrity a part of your culture, not just when an issue arises.

- Providing a writing style sheet or handbook regarding plagiarism

- State whether the instructor/institution uses a plagiarism detection service; i.e., many of the existing educational web-platforms such as Blackboard, Moodle, etc. have the means to check student work authenticity against their own work, their peers, and other resources on the Internet.

Box 6-7

ONLINE COURSES

- Password-protect exams: This option requires students to have and apply a personal identification code or password to take exams, as a method to ensure that the student enrolled in the course is the student taking the exam.

- Use browser security features: This is an additional application that is used to literally "lock down" the student's browser so that when the student opens an assessment item, that item is the only thing that can be accessed on the computer. A student cannot navigate to any other pages on the Internet or browse the computer for local files.

- Show exam/quiz questions one at a time instead of all at once, or use a randomization option.

and fieldwork manual. As an occupational therapy educator, there are both direct/formal and indirect/informal strategies that can be used to help build an occupational therapy student's professional identity and begin to socialize them to the expectations of the profession. Having clear and consistent policies is an important direct strategy to promote professionalism in occupational therapy students. Common policies that promote aspects of professionalism include the following.

Student Dress Code

One way to teach students the importance of professional image is to enforce a dress code policy. The guidelines or policy should clearly state the expectations regarding attire for didactic and laboratory class sessions. Policies should be included in the student handbook, as well as listed on course syllabus (Box 6-8).

Box 6-8

SAMPLE POLICY FOR STUDENT DRESS CODE

Students contribute to the professional image of the occupational therapy department and the profession. This requires special attention to your appearance and clothing choices. Dress and be groomed professionally. Revealing clothing will not be allowed. This includes very low cut tops, tight or provocative clothes, very short skirts, or very short shorts. Revealing sleeveless shirts, blouses, or dresses will not be allowed. Shorts must be at least mid-thigh length when standing. Sweatshirts, sweatpants, T-shirts, and jeans are allowed when neat and clean, without holes and/or tears. Fingernails should be trimmed close to fingertips for lab activities. Shirts or clothing with profanity or obscene statements are not allowed. Do not wear long necklaces, excessive finger rings, earrings, or bracelets and remove eyebrow, nose, and tongue piercings. Non-compliance with this stated dress code will result in deduction of your overall professional behavior points.

Figure 6-1. Unprofessional lab attire 1.

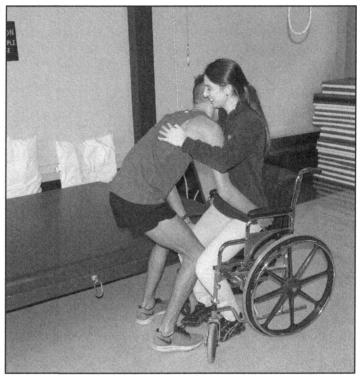

Figure 6-1 illustrates an in-class lab session focused on transfer training. The student performing the transfer is not in compliance with appropriate and professional lab attire, wearing clothing that is too revealing.

Figure 6-2 demonstrates an in-class lab session focused on establishing competency with taking vital signs. The student practicing taking blood pressure is not in compliance with appropriate and professional lab attire and is wearing clothing that is too revealing.

Figure 6-3 depicts an in-class lab session focused on pediatric developmental milestones. The student on the left in the prone position is not in compliance with a professional student dress code. The student on the right, acting as the practitioner, is wearing appropriate lab attire.

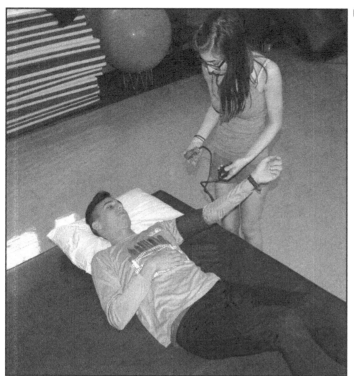

Figure 6-2. Unprofessional lab attire 2.

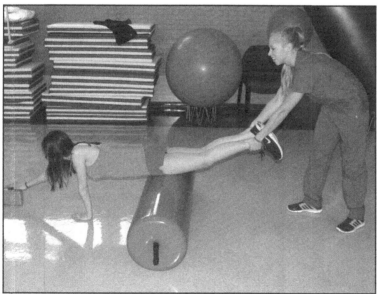

Figure 6-3. Unprofessional lab attire 3.

Figure 6-4. Professional student uniform.

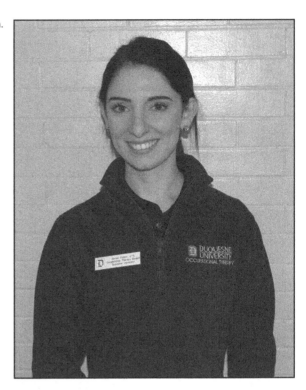

Figure 6-5. Professional student uniform.

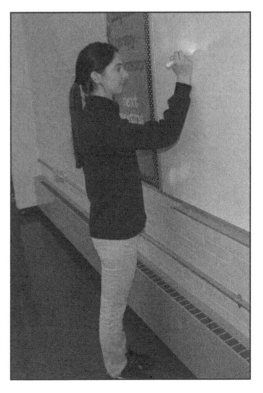

Some educational programs have a uniform such as an official shirt, or scrubs, and a nametag or photo ID badge (Figures 6-4 and 6-5).

Box 6-9

SAMPLE POLICY FOR GENERAL CLASSROOM EXPECTATIONS

Professional behavior includes objective and respectful student/instructor/peer inter-actions, refraining from personal discussions during lectures and presentations, and maintaining appropriate dress attire to class and lab sessions. Professional behaviors are expected both inside and outside the classroom. Participation includes coming to class on time and prepared (i.e., having read the assigned materials, completed homework/assignments, etc.) and to actively contribute to the discussions/lab activities, asking questions or providing comments or examples that facilitate total class discussion, assuming equal responsibility in group projects, as well as returning supplies/equipment and class furniture to their proper location/storage places. Appropriate and assertive verbal and nonverbal communication is a requisite. Determination of professional behavior and participation is based upon the judgment of the course instructor. Please note that lab participation accounts for 10% of total grade.

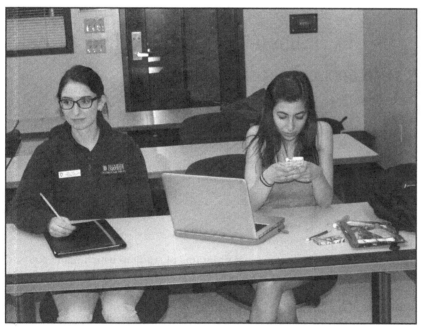

Figure 6-6. Professional behaviors in the classroom.

General Classroom Expectations

Professionalism and the demonstration of professional behaviors can be a component of a student's overall grade in a course. Setting clear expectations surrounding student's attitude, behaviors, and performance is key in modeling real-world demands such as preparedness, and interpersonal communication (Box 6-9).

In Figure 6-6, the student on the left is demonstrating professionalism via her image, attire, and body language. The student on the right is demonstrating a lack of professionalism exhibited by her inappropriate use of technology, poor eye contact, and closed body posturing.

Box 6-10

SAMPLE POLICY FOR ATTENDANCE

Attendance is an essential and required part of being an occupational therapy student professional. Work and outside obligations are to be managed by the student in a way that does not hinder or limit educational expectations. Work, medical, dental, or other appointments should not be scheduled during class time and will not be considered an excused absence. Students who are unable to attend class because of serious illness, hospitalization, a serious accident or other extenuating circumstance are responsible for notifying their instructor or department mentor. Students are expected to supply any required written verifications as soon as possible. Repeated unexcused absences (three or more during Fall and Spring semesters and two or more during summer semester) and/or frequent tardiness to class or community-based sessions (three or more during Fall and Spring semesters and two or more during summer semester) will result in a deduction of up to 10% of a student's total course grade and each subsequent unexcused absence will result in an additional 2% deduction.

Box 6-11

SAMPLE POLICY FOR USE OF TECHNOLOGY

Courses may require the use of laptops for class sessions, including exams, quizzes, or other classroom activities. When laptops are used in class, it is expected to be for school and classroom activities only. Laptops may not be used during class for personal use. If you are found emailing, tweeting, accessing the internet, Facebooking, or using your technology in ways not expressly related to the topic assigned by the instructor during class time, you will be excused from the classroom and lose the privilege of using a laptop during class for the rest of the semester.

Time and Attendance

Occupational therapy curriculums are professional programs of study in which many courses taken later in the curriculum build on and deepen knowledge, skills, and behaviors addressed earlier in the curriculum. In a similar manner, content and learning activities within a course build on and deepen knowledge, skills, and behaviors acquired earlier in that same course. Students are unable to learn and deepen their learning if they are not present in class. Students have an obligation to attend every class listed on the course schedule. Timeliness and accountability are important traits to ensure in a professional-in-training. Tardiness is unprofessional and disruptive. Occupational therapy educators should take attendance, and enforce department policies regarding lateness and absenteeism (Box 6-10).

Use of Technology and Smart Devices

In society today, the use of technology is the daily norm. In educational settings, students have access to computers, laptops, and various other smart devices to use in the learning process, including taking notes, downloading lectures, and retrieving necessary online resources. However, it can be challenging for the occupational therapy educator to regulate who is using technology appropriately and who is not during class and/or lab sessions (Box 6-11).

Box 6-12

SAMPLE POLICY FOR CELL PHONES

Turn off all electronic devices (cell phones, pagers, etc.) BEFORE the start of class and during all meetings with faculty. Vibrate setting is not considered silenced. In the rare case of an emergency, the student is to ask for permission from the faculty member in charge of a given class or meeting to keep a cell phone turned on the vibrate setting to receive the emergency call. Texting during class or group meetings is never acceptable.

Box 6-13

SAMPLE POLICY FOR RECORDING

Refrain from using any recording device in any didactic or clinical course or experience, without prior written permission by the course instructor/supervisor AND the subjects being recorded. When permitted to record, the student must understand that a single recording is to be made, that it is NOT to be duplicated, excerpted, transferred, placed on the internet, or shared with others, all HIPAA standards must be followed, and that the recording is to be erased at the end of the semester or before, as requested by any of the interested parties mentioned above.

Cellphones in Class/Lab

The use of cellphones during classroom and laboratory activities is unprofessional, disruptive, and can be viewed as being academically dishonest. Therefore, students must not answer phones, text messages, or emails during class or lab sessions. During class all phones should be turned off (Box 6-12).

Audio/Video Recording

The lecture and laboratory curriculum that is delivered by occupational therapy educators is considered to be their intellectual property. Occupational therapy students must receive the educator's permission prior to engaging in audio and/or video recording of classroom/lab content (Box 6-13).

Social Media/Networking

Social networking can be defined as "the use of a website to connect with people who share personal or professional interests, place of origin, education at a particular school, etc" (Bemis-Dougherty, 2010, p. 42). Occupational therapy students should be held accountable for information shared on social networking and media websites. Students, faculty, and staff must be aware that posting certain information is illegal. Violation may expose the offender to criminal and civil liability. Offenses may be considered non-academic misconduct and be subject to the appropriate policies and procedures (Box 6-14).

When in doubt about whether material will put you at risk of violating the above criteria, do not send it until you've consulted with a trusted colleague, faculty advisor, or someone more knowledgeable about legal and ethical professional matters.

Box 6-14

SAMPLE POLICY FOR SOCIAL MEDIA

Students are responsible and accountable for what they post or discuss via social media. The content of postings, messaging, chats, etc. should always be respectful. Disclosure of any information about your clinical experience is strictly forbidden. Students must comply with all HIPAA standards and violation of such may result in legal action against the student, automatic failure of a class or clinical rotation, and possibly dismissal from the program. Postings must not include any references to: patients, their conditions, treatment, characteristics, etc.; clinical sites or clinical instructors (no criticism about a site or instructor); associated personnel at a clinical rotation (including other students); or, any information about what is happening during a clinical experience. Do not ask your teacher, supervisor or fieldwork educator to "friend" you. This puts them and you in a potentially awkward and inappropriate situation. Compliance with the social media policy is expected at all times. There is a zero tolerance for any violation of this policy. Any violation is considered unprofessional and will result in disciplinary action, up to and including dismissal from the program. These guidelines are not stagnant and may change as new social networking tools emerge.

Box 6-15

SAMPLE POLICY FOR HIPAA COMPLIANCE

The student is required to respect the dignity, individuality, privacy, and personality of each and every individual. Information about a client should be shared on a "need to know" basis only, and not for reasons of personal interest. In other words, to provide services, it is necessary for various professional personnel to know personal information about a client. If a client's information is discussed related to official class business (e.g., during seminars, classes), the client's identity must remain anonymous; and information about the client that is not necessary to the learning situation must not be shared (e.g., identity of known relatives, legal or moral issues not related to occupational therapy services being rendered). This is also true about personal discussions that students participate in during class time. Students are expected to respect the confidentiality and privacy of their classmates.

Adherence to Health Insurance Portability and Accountability Act

As discussed in Chapters 3 and 5, confidentiality is an ethical principle that covers both verbal and written communication. Knowledge and demonstration of compliance with Health Insurance Portability and Accountability Act (HIPAA) is required of both health care students and practitioners (Box 6-15).

Occupational therapy educators should verify completion of student HIPPA training and keep records in their student files. See Appendix A for sample HIPPA training acknowledgment forms.

Policies Regarding Membership to Professional Organization

Professionals are expected to be lifelong learners. They are also expected to participate in their respective professional organizations. Occupational therapy educators can increase students' professional development and engagement in professional service by requiring occupational therapy students to become student members to the American Occupational Therapy Association or their state association.

Professional Behavior Policy and Remediation Plan

Many occupational therapy educational programs have a "professional behavior" policy and enlist student help in crafting professional behavior expectations. A professional behavior policy should outline specific plans for remediation when unprofessional behavior, attitudes, or actions occur. See Appendix B for sample professional behavior policy and remediation plan.

Summary

In developing policies to promote professionalism, it is necessary to have clear and specific language that defines the expected behavior, processes of how it is evaluated, and remediation processes. As they enter the occupational therapy education program, students and the faculty that teach them should receive a list of expected behaviors and policies for which they will be evaluated and held accountable. The consequences of acting inappropriately should also be explained.

INDIRECT/INFORMAL STRATEGIES FOR PROFESSIONALISM

"We learn by practice and the best practice is to follow a model of the virtuous person."
—Aristotle

Having clear policies and procedures to govern occupational therapy student's behavior and actions is important, yet there are also more indirect strategies to enculturate students to professionalism. As an occupational therapy educator, you are a direct role-model to your students, not just for education on clinical and technical skills, but the development of professionalism as well. Reflect on your attitudes, values and actions as an educator. Are you on time and prepared for class? Do you dress appropriately, according to your institution's dress code? Do you use your cell phone and text during breaks in class? Do you model professional communication in your nonverbal, verbal, and written communication—including emails or postings on a web platform for instruction? Do you maintain composure during challenging situations? Students also observe your communication and interactions with peers, colleagues, and other professionals. As an educator, is it very important to be aware of how you set the foundation for building a student's professional identity. Modeling professionalism and discussing it with students are key strategies to promote the professional development.

Professional Behavior Inventories

To successfully implement clear and specific professional behavior policies, it is recommended to have means to assess student behaviors, attitudes, and performance. Occupational therapy programs can develop their own criteria and measurement tools to measure behaviors and attitudes surrounding professionalism, or use those that are published (Box 6-16).

Box 6-16

PROFESSIONAL BEHAVIOR TOOLS*

- Professional Behavior Assessment (Koenig, Johnson, Morano, & Ducette, 2003)
- Professional Development Evaluation (Smith-Randolph, 2003)

*Other disciplines such as nursing, physical therapy, medicine, and pharmacy all have professional behavior scales geared for students and endorsed by their professional organizations.

Clinical Vignettes

This section includes common professional behavior blunders that can occur in the classroom, as well as strategies to handle them.

Unprofessional Use of Social Media

A professor gives a student a bad grade on an assignment. In turn, the student posts a disrespectful and inappropriate post about the professor on social media where it is public to his or her "friends" and "followers".

How to Prevent the Situation From Occurring

Prevent the situation by only posting about positive events or happenings to social media. If you are concerned over whether something is appropriate to post on social media, consider if you would be okay with your grandma seeing the post. If not, it is probably not appropriate to post on social media for future employers, professors, and friends to see. Remember that social media is a public forum. Occupational therapy educators can prevent this situation by having clear policies regarding the use of social media and professional behavior which are enforced throughout the curriculum.

How to Handle the Situation

Remove (delete) the post immediately from social media. Although it might feel good to vent negative emotions on social media, the posts will not be viewed as appropriate by professionals. Instead of posting for the public, vent negative emotions from stressful situations to a trusted friend in private and have them help you determine steps to mediate the stress. Occupational therapy students should also be encouraged to voice specific concerns with their respective faculty in a professional manner. Occupational therapy educators should comply with their policies regarding inappropriate use of social media, which may include a remediation plan.

Unprofessional Use of Technology in Class

A student is observed by their professor to be using his or her laptop to do online shopping during an in-class lecture.

How to Prevent the Situation

Students, if you are easily distracted in class, it may be advised to avoid using your laptop during lectures. Although laptops can be a powerful tool for some to use during note-taking, it is not the best option for everyone. Instead, come prepared to class by printing out posted PowerPoint presentations or lecture notes and take notes by hand. Often, students find that handwriting notes not only encourages their sustained attention, but it also kinesthetically helps to retain the information they are writing. Occupational therapy educators should have clear policies regarding the use of technology in the classroom.

How to Handle the Situation

The professor can suggest that all students hand-write notes, as opposed to using technology in the classroom. However, the use of technology in the classroom should not be banned completely, as many students are able to use it appropriately in class and benefit greatly from it. From the perspective of the student, he or she must realize that using technology for activities other than note-taking and learning in class can be distracting for others sitting around him or her. The student must find a more beneficial way to participate and encourage the participation of their peers in the classroom. Occupational therapy educators can be more cognizant of using classroom space for teaching and walk around the room during lecture, which will keep students more engaged, and allow for more direct observation of student performance and attention. Educators should comply with the stated policy on noncompliance with use of technology in the class, which may include remediation.

Tardiness/Absenteeism

A student is repeatedly tardy to her 8 o'clock course due to sleeping through her alarm in the morning.

How to Prevent the Situation

Although it is sometimes difficult to find motivation early in the morning to attend an 8 o'clock course, the student should not use the early start time as an excuse for repeated tardiness. Tardiness can be prevented by waking up early enough to allow for plenty of time in the morning to prepare for the day. Try placing your alarm on your desk, away from your bed. This will force you to wake up and get out of bed to walk over to your desk and turn it off. You can also try preparing for the next day the night before. For example, pack your backpack with all the necessary supplies, pick out an outfit to wear, or pack your lunch during the evening so you will not have to spend time doing it the next morning. Occupational therapy departments should have clear policies regarding how excessive tardiness and/or absenteeism is handled.

How to Handle the Situation

To handle the situation of repeated tardiness, the student should understand how tardiness is a poor reflection of her motivation, work ethic, and professionalism. She should first apologize to the professor for her unprofessional behavior. The student should also assure her professor that she will employ strategies to prevent tardiness from occurring in the future. From the perspective of the professor, the expectations for class attendance should be made clear in the beginning of the course. If absences or tardiness become an issue for individual students, the professor should address the problem with the student after class to ensure steps are being taken to prevent the behavior from continuing. Occupational therapy educators should maintain records of student attendance and/or instances of tardiness, such as follow-up emails to students to support policies.

Academic Integrity

A student is best friends with another student in the previous cohort. The younger student is struggling with an assignment, and the older student kindly offers to allow her friend to look at the same assignment from last year. The younger student accepts the offer and heavily bases her work from her friend's previous assignment.

How to Prevent the Situation

To prevent a situation that challenges academic integrity, the younger student can simply deny the older student's offer to use her work. It helps to realize that although it may be more difficult, the benefits of learning are greater when you take the time to complete the assignment alone. If the student is struggling with the assignment, it is best to seek assistance from the professor instead of peers to finish the assignment. Occupational therapy educators should have clear policies regarding unsanctioned sharing and/or collaborating among students in the occupational therapy program.

How to Handle the Situation

If the situation was brought to the professor's attention, the professor should follow the school's standard policy regarding academic integrity to discipline the student. Many educational web platforms such as Blackboard or Moodle allow educators to run originality reports, which shows overlap between current and previous student cohorts as well as plagiarism. Occupational therapy educators should consider using educational technologies such as these to obtain objective data to support concerns regarding the authenticity of student work. From the perspective of the student, it is best to be honest when explaining the situation and intent of the actions to the professor.

SUMMARY

Education is a key factor in any profession. Some may argue that traits of professionalism cannot be taught—that they are inherently present in varying degrees when students enter educational programs. While this may be true to a certain extent, the process of professional socialization posits that students learn the values, behaviors, and traits of their professions during their training. Metaphorically, it takes a village to develop a student's professional identity; educators, peers, mentors, and positive role-models all have a direct and indirect influence on an occupational therapy student's professional development. In closing, developing professionalism in occupational therapy students involves more than just teaching. Role-modeling, mentoring, and facilitating are all essential actions for educators to implement in order to develop the professionalism of occupational therapy students.

LEARNING ACTIVITIES

1. Identify one of your most memorable teachers. What characteristics do you feel make them a good educator? How did this person demonstrate and teach you about professionalism?

2. Review the teaching approaches discussed in this chapter. Think about a learning experience you have had in your occupational therapy education. Provide an example of how these learning approaches were used in your own education.

3. Think about an experience in the classroom where you had difficulty learning or had a challenge grasping new material. Can you provide an example of how maybe you would adapt this learning activity using the best practice approaches presented in this chapter that may have helped you increase your understanding of the material or concept?

4. Locate the academic integrity policy at your institution. Review examples of academic misconduct, potential consequences, and the reporting process. Identify an example of misconduct for each of the principles discussed in your institution's policy.

REFERENCES

Bemis-Dougherty, A. (2010). Professionalism and social networking. *PT in Motion, 2*(5), 40-47.

Kirk, L. M. (2007). Professionalism in medicine: Definitions and considerations for teaching. *Baylor University Medical Center Proceedings, 20*(1), 13-16.

Koenig, K., Johnson, C., Morano, C. K., & Ducette, J. P. (2003). Development and validation of a professional behavior assessment. Retrieved from http://jdc.jefferson.edu/cgi/viewcontent.cgi?article=1012&context=otfp

Smith-Randolph, D. (2003). Evaluating the professional behaviors of entry-level occupational therapy students. *Journal of Allied Health, 32*(2), 116-121

APPENDIX A: STATEMENT OF ADHERENCE TO HIPAA POLICIES AND PROCEDURES

I, the undersigned, who has a "need to know" in regards to patient health information, certify that I have received HIPAA training and will honor all of the entity's policies and procedures as related to HIPAA. I also know that at any time that I do not understand something related to HIPAA that I can request and receive further training.

_____   _____
Signature   Name

_____   _____
Facility/Department   Date

HEALTH INSURANCE PORTABILITY AND ACCOUNTABILITY ACT TRAINING

This certifies that

_____

has completed HIPAA Privacy and Security Training
as required by

45CFR164.530(b)(1) and 45CFR164.308(a)(5)(i)

_____

HIPAA Trainer   Date

APPENDIX B: DEPARTMENT OF OCCUPATIONAL THERAPY PROFESSIONAL BEHAVIOR POLICIES

Identification of Professional Behavior Issue

Standards for professional behavior are described in the Description of Professional Behaviors section of this document. Students are expected to behave according to these standards during academic and clinical learning experiences. If an academic or clinical faculty member identifies and documents a serious problem with a student's professional behavior or inability to maintain a standard within the realm of acceptable professional behavior, the following protocol will be followed:

1. The faculty member will meet with the student to identify the behavior and counsel the student to demonstrate behavior consistent with the professional standard.

2. If the faculty determines that the student has a recurrence of an unprofessional behavior prior to the completion of their professional program, both the student and faculty member will meet with the Professional Behavior Committee (consisting of the department chair, occupational therapy faculty mentor, and one faculty member who does not teach in the occupational therapy program) to determine a remediation plan and contract for the student.

3. The remediation plan and contract will include the following items:

- A description of the specific behaviors that the student is expected to demonstrate

- The specific tasks that the student is expected to accomplish

- Time frames related to accomplishing the tasks and behaviors

- Repercussions for unsuccessful remediation or inability to meet the terms of the contract

- Who will monitor the terms of the contract

- How the terms of the contract will be monitored

4. The committee will meet again, at a time stated in the contract, to determine if the student has successfully completed the remediation plan and has met the terms of the contract.

5. The following are the repercussions resulting from unprofessional behavior.

   a. Immediate dismissal: In addition to felony conviction or pleading no contest for behaviors that would prohibit the granting of an occupational therapy license other behaviors may be determined to be non-remediable.

   b. Probation: Behaviors that the committee has determined are remediable. The terms of the probation and remediation will be outlined in the contract.

   c. Dismissal: Behaviors that the committee has determined are remediable; however, the student has been unable or unwilling to remediate, as defined in the remediation plan and contract.

Description of Professional Behaviors

The American Occupational Therapy Association has developed the *Occupational Therapy Code of Ethics, Standards of Practice for Occupational Therapy, Core Values and Attitudes of Occupational Therapy Practice and the Standards for Continuing Competence,* documents that define specific abilities and behaviors that a graduate of a Masters of Science in Occupational Therapy program should demonstrate. The core values include: altruism, equality, freedom, justice, dignity, truth and prudence. The standards for continuing competence include: knowledge, critical reasoning interpersonal abilities, performance standards, and ethical reasoning. The following represents six essential behaviors that integrate items from these documents with a focus on the academic environment.

1. Integrity: Represents one's own and others' abilities honestly; is truthful and sincere; accepts responsibilities for one's actions; able to reflect on one's personal reactions to encounters with others.

2. Respect: Adheres to confidentiality and professional boundaries; works toward conflict resolution in a collegial way; demonstrates consideration for the opinions and values of others; shows regard for diversity.

3. Responsibility: Present and punctual for all learning experiences; able to cope with challenges, conflicts, and uncertainty; recognize one's limits and seeks help; recognizes the needs of others and responds appropriately; demonstrates willingness to discuss and confront problematic behavior of self and others.

4. Competence: Takes responsibility for one's own learning; participates equally and collegially in groups; demonstrates self-reflection and accurate self-assessment; able to identify personal barriers to learning; works with faculty to manage learning difficulties.

5. Maturity: Demonstrates emotional stability; appropriately confident yet humble; demonstrates appropriate professional dress, demeanor, and language; accepts constructive criticism and applies it in a useful way; inspires confidence in others; displays appropriate emotions; is not hostile, disruptive, confrontational, aggressive, or isolated; does not engage in behavior that endangers or threatens self or others.

6. Communication: Able to communicate effectively with others; demonstrates courteous and respectful communication, even in difficult situations; uses active listening; communicates with empathy and compassion.

Professional Behavior Continuum

The Professional Behavior Continuum is a self-reflective tool for students to use to evaluate their professional behavior during their progression through the professional phase of the occupational therapy program. Students are encouraged to meet with their mentors to review their progress and to seek guidance as needed.

1. Integrity

Lacks honesty	Always honest
Lacks personal responsibility	Accepts responsibility for actions
Lacks self-reflection	Exceptional self-reflection

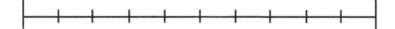

2. Respect

Lacks respect for confidentiality/professional boundaries

Respects confidentiality/professional boundaries

Does not resolve conflict in a respectful/collegial way

Resolves conflict in a respectful/collegial way

Does not respect others' opinions/values

Respects others' opinions/values

Does not respect diversity

Respects diversity

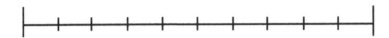

3. Responsibility

Is not present/punctual for learning

Present/punctual for learning

Does not cope with challenge/conflict/uncertainty

Copes with challenge/conflict/uncertainty

Does not recognize limits/seek help

Recognizes limits and seeks help

Does not recognize others' needs

Recognizes/responds to others needs

Does not confront problematic behavior

Confronts problematic behavior

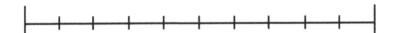

4. Competence

Does not take responsibility for learning

Takes responsibility for learning

Lacks self-reflection

Self-reflective

Unequal/noncollegial participation

Equal/collegial participation

Does not identify learning barriers

Identifies learning barriers

Does not manage learning difficulties

Manages learning difficulties

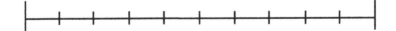

5. Maturity

Lacks emotional stability	Demonstrates emotional stability
Lacks confidence/humility	Confident and humble
Lacks professional dress/language	Professional dress/language
Does not use constructive criticism	Excellent use of constructive criticism
Inappropriate behavior (hostile, aggressive, etc.)	Appropriate behavior

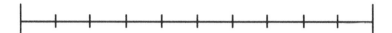

6. Communication

Ineffective communication with others	Communicates effectively with others
Lacks respect/courteousness	Respectful/courteous
Lacks empathy/compassion	Communicates with empathy/compassion
Lacks active listening skills	Uses active listening skills

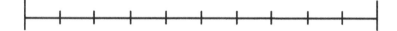

Part III

Professionalism for the Occupational Therapy Fieldwork Student

Providing education about professionalism is not solely the responsibility of the didactic academic community. Every occupational therapy practitioner plays a large part in shaping the future of the profession, specifically those practitioners who are fieldwork educators. A key component in occupational therapy education, and in reaching the goals of the Centennial Vision, is fieldwork education (Crist, Scaffa, & Hooper, 2010; Hanson, 2011; Musselman, 2007; Stutz-Tannenbaum & Hooper, 2009). Fieldwork in occupational therapy has been referred to as integral in providing the student the opportunity to transfer his or her academic knowledge to practice (Crist, Brown, Fairman, Whelan, & McClure, 2007; Meyers, 1989). This section will focus on professional expectations during fieldwork education and doctoral experiential learning experiences. Vignettes will be provided to illustrate common professional behavior problems in fieldwork education, and strategies to prevent and/or handle them.

REFERENCES

Crist, P. A., Brown, L. I., Fairman, A., Whelan, L., & McClure, L. (2007). Entry-level OTR and COTA intervention utilization derived from NBCOT practice analysis: Implications for fieldwork experiences. *Occupational Therapy in Health Care, 21*(1-2), 71-89.

Crist, P. A., Scaffa, M., & Hooper, B. (2010). Occupational therapy education and the centennial vision. *Occupational Therapy in Health Care, 24*(1), 1-6.

Hanson, D. (2011). The perspectives of fieldwork educators regarding level II fieldwork students. *Occupational Therapy in Healthcare, 25*(2-3) 164-167.

Meyers, S. K. (1989). Program evaluation of occupational therapy level II fieldwork environments: A naturalistic inquiry. *Occupational Therapy Journal of Research, 9*(6), 347-361.

Musselman, L. (2007). Achieving AOTA's centennial vision: The role of educators. *Occupational Therapy in Health Care, 21*, 295-300.

Stutz-Tannenbaum, P., & Hooper, B. (2009). Creating congruence between identities as a fieldwork educator and a practitioner. *AOTA Special Interest Section Quarterly: Education, 19*(2), 1-4.

7

What Is Fieldwork Education?

Elizabeth D. DeIuliis, OTD, OTR/L

INTRODUCTION

Like other health care professions, occupational therapy education requires the component of practical application in the curriculum. Other professions use various terminologies to describe this experiential learning, such as clinical education, residencies, or internships. The occupational therapy profession identifies it as fieldwork education. Fieldwork education is often described as a bridge that connects the theoretical didactic classroom instruction to real-world clinical practice, and is an integral piece of the occupational therapy education process (Aiken, Menaker, & Barsky, 2001; Brandenburger-Shasby et al., 1998). Fieldwork is integrated with occupational therapy coursework to apply core values (including professionalism) and curricular threads in practice with mentorship from occupational therapy faculty and fieldwork educators.

KEY WORDS

Academic Fieldwork Coordinator: Full-time faculty member or professional staff member in an occupational therapy program who is principally responsible for developing, coordinating, organizing, and monitoring the entire fieldwork process, including the oversight of the fieldwork educator and the fieldwork student

American Occupational Therapy Association Fieldwork Performance Evaluation of the Level II Fieldwork Student: A 42 item tool designed to measure a student's performance of the occupational therapy process across multiple settings in the context of a Level II Fieldwork placement

Clinical Coordinator of Fieldwork Education: The fieldwork site's formal representative and liaison to the academic institution; this individual is responsible for the development, management, and logistic details of fieldwork education

DeIuliis, E.D.
Professionalism Across Occupational Therapy Practice (pp 163-199).
© 2017 Taylor & Francis Group.

Direct Supervision: Supervision that occurs when a fieldwork educator directly observes a student's performance, either face-to-face or in-line-of-sight contact

Doctoral Experiential Component: A 16 week experiential learning component undertaken as part of an occupational therapy development program in addition to the existing Level I and Level II fieldwork education requirement; the goal of the doctoral experiential component is to develop occupational therapy practitioners with advanced skills (ACOTE, 2012)

Fieldwork Educator: An occupational therapy practitioner with a set minimum amount of clinical experience who serves as a supervisor, mentor, and role model for a student during the course of a fieldwork placement

Indirect Supervision: Supervision that occurs when the fieldwork educator gathers information from the supervisee after performance through a variety of methods such as electronic, written, telephone communications, or interaction with other colleagues who have interacted with the student

Level I Fieldwork: A preparatory placement aimed at introducing students to the fieldwork experience, allowing them to apply knowledge to practice, and to develop understanding of the needs of clients (ACOTE, 2012)

Level II Fieldwork: A 16 or 24 week experience with aim to develop competent, professional, entry-level, generalist occupational therapy practitioners who are capable of clinical reasoning and reflective practice, as well as to transmit the values and beliefs that enable ethical practice (ACOTE, 2012)

Student Evaluation of Fieldwork Experience: A tool through which a fieldwork student can provide feedback to their fieldwork educator or site

Supervision: Intentional intervention by a fieldwork educator aimed at helping fieldwork students develop clinical and professional skills; a mutual process involving participation from both the fieldwork student(s) and the fieldwork educator(s) to establish, maintain, promote, or enhance clinical and professional performance

OBJECTIVES

By the end of reading this chapter and completing the learning activities, the reader should be able to:

1. Describe how fieldwork experiences promote clinical reasoning and reflective practice.
2. Discuss the role of fieldwork educators as facilitators in the educational and professionalization process.
3. Recognize qualities in a fieldwork educator and student communicating and modeling professionalism through role-play scenarios.
4. Identify strategies to address professionalism deficits in fieldwork.

Fieldwork education is undeniably a crucial pedagogy of occupational therapy education, as the Accreditation Council for Occupational Therapy Education (ACOTE) continues to set explicit standards governing the fieldwork component of occupational therapy educational programs. In 1924, the American Occupational Therapy Association (AOTA) published its first standards

TABLE 7-1	
OVERVIEW OF OFFICIAL DOCUMENTS RELATED TO FIELDWORK	
DOCUMENT	**DESCRIPTION**
Occupational Therapy Fieldwork Education: Value and Purpose (AOTA, 2009a)	Describes the overarching purpose of fieldwork education in the occupational therapy profession
Fieldwork Level II and Occupational Therapy Students: A Position Paper (AOTA, 2012)	Describes the desired characteristics of a fieldwork placement for occupational therapy students in Level II fieldwork education and articulates the desired attributes of a fieldwork setting to maximize students' learning in context
COE Guidelines for an Occupational Therapy Fieldwork Experience—Level II (AOTA, 2013a)	Defines the Level II fieldwork experience and clarifies the appropriate conditions and principles that must exist during Level II fieldwork

related to fieldwork education. Initially, these standards were highly managerial and assessment-oriented. Over the next 90 years, the standards became more explicit and descriptive. For example, ACOTE has more recently mandated that at least one fieldwork experience "has as its focus psychological and social factors that influence engagement in occupation" (ACOTE, 2012, p. S34). Furthermore, the AOTA has embraced the need for the occupational therapy profession to be more powerful in the 2017 Centennial Vision which states that "we envision that occupational therapy is a powerful, widely recognized, science-driven, and evidence-based profession with a globally connected and diverse workforce meeting society's occupational needs" (AOTA, 2007, p. 14). The AOTA considers education, including fieldwork, to be a key factor in achieving the "power" aspect of the Centennial vision, and a primary driver in transforming the future of the occupational therapy profession. When occupational therapy fieldwork educators are skilled not only in clinical practice, but also education and supervision, they advance the efficacy of the occupational therapy profession. Here is quick overview of some of the most influential white papers supporting the importance of fieldwork education within the occupational therapy profession today (Table 7-1).

LEVELS OF FIELDWORK EDUCATION

The intention of fieldwork education is to propel each generation of occupational therapy practitioners from the role of a student to that of a practitioner. According to the Accreditation Council for Occupational Therapy Education (ACOTE) (2012), fieldwork is a crucial part of the professional preparation of occupational therapy students, and provides "the opportunity to carry out professional responsibilities" (ACOTE, 2012, p. 33). In occupational therapy education, there are currently two levels of fieldwork education intended to provide students with this opportunity: Level I Fieldwork and Level II Fieldwork. Furthermore, for the entry-level doctoral degree, there is an advanced practical experience called the Doctoral Experiential Component (DEC) (ACOTE, 2012).

Level I Fieldwork

According to the 2011 ACOTE Standards, the goal of Level I fieldwork (FW) is "to introduce students to the fieldwork experience, to apply knowledge to practice, and to develop understanding of the needs of clients" (p. S34). Standard (C.1.8) states that "Level I fieldwork is integral to the program's curriculum design and includes experiences designed to enrich didactic coursework through directed observation and participation in selected aspects of the occupational therapy process" (ACOTE, 2012, p. 34). Compared to Level II FW, Level I FW can be viewed as an introductory clinical learning experience. However, it is still fieldwork, the first official experiential learning for occupational therapy students, and a major stepping stone in the building of their professional identities.

Often, Level I FW is embedded within particular courses and students are placed in specific health care arenas to allow direct connection between the classroom and clinical practice. For example, during the semester where students take a pediatric course, they may simultaneously participate in a pediatric Level I FW experience. It is very important to denote that Level I FW may vary between academic institutions as a result of distinctions in their curriculum philosophy and design. For example, Level I FW could be a concentrated one or two week timespan in a clinic, or a half-day each week over the course of a semester. ACOTE requires that all fieldwork experiences are formally evaluated, however, for Level I FW, there is no standardized evaluation endorsed by the profession. Most academic programs request fieldwork educators to provide input on introductory reasoning skills, basic clinical skills, and professional behaviors during Level I FW, such as time management, communication, organization, and initiative. See Appendix A, Sample Level I FW Evaluation, for further information.

Level II Fieldwork

The goal of Level II fieldwork is "to develop competent, entry-level, generalist occupational therapists," to promote clinical reasoning and reflective practice, to transmit the values and beliefs that enable ethical practice, and to develop professionalism and competence in career responsibilities (ACOTE, 2012, p. S34). Level II FW is more highly regulated by ACOTE than Level I is. ACOTE states that 16 weeks of level II FW are required for occupational therapy assistant educational programs, and 24 weeks for registered occupational therapist programs. The outcome of Level II FW student learning is traditionally evaluated by the AOTA Fieldwork Performance Evaluation of the Level II Student (FWPE) (AOTA, 2002). There are specific items on the AOTA FWPE which require Level II fieldwork students to demonstrate various competencies related to professional behaviors. More information on this will be discussed later in this chapter. In addition to the AOTA FWPE, students provide feedback to the fieldwork site and fieldwork educators using a Student Evaluation of the Fieldwork Experience or an equivalent process approved by ACOTE. See Appendix B, Student Evaluation of Level II FW, for more information.

Doctoral Experiential Component

The potential of moving to an entry-level doctoral degree for occupational therapy practitioners has been a recent subject of debate within the profession. Currently, there are a handful of accredited entry-level occupational therapy development programs, and many more are in the pipeline to develop and become accredited. The entry-level occupational therapy development curriculum varies from the master's degree level in many ways. One of the most significant differences is the addition of a 16-week doctoral experiential component (DEC). This new experiential learning component occurs in addition to the existing Level I and Level II fieldwork education requirements. The goal of the DEC is to develop occupational therapy practitioners with advanced skills, those that are beyond a generalist level (ACOTE, 2012, p. S37). The DEC shall be an integral part of the program's curriculum design, and shall include an in-depth experience in one or more of the following: clinical practice skills, research skills, administration, leadership, program and policy development, advocacy, education, or theory development (ACOTE, 2012). The occupational therapy doctoral student must successfully complete all coursework, Level II FW, and pass a competency requirement prior to the commencement of the DEC.

Since we have reviewed the different levels of fieldwork and experiential learning in occupational therapy education, now let's identify and discuss the key roles involved in fieldwork education and their unique responsibilities: the fieldwork student, fieldwork educator (FWEd), clinical coordinator of fieldwork (CCFW), and the academic fieldwork coordinator (AFWC). Each of these individuals play a significant role in the shaping of an occupational therapy student's professional identity.

Fieldwork Student

Obviously, the fieldwork student is the occupational therapist or occupational therapy assistant participating in the fieldwork experience. During fieldwork, students engage in various tasks, depending on the student, site, and setting. Some examples are assuming patient caseloads, using appropriate assessments and treatment interventions, communicating and documenting information correctly, and practicing interpersonal skills with patients and health care staff to develop characteristics of a professional (Cara, 1998; Vogel, Grice, Hill, and Moody, 2004). Participation in fieldwork education requires students to demonstrate not just clinical skills, but also professionalism. Fieldwork students are responsible for reflecting on their own learning style, clinical interests, and personalities as they counsel with the AFWC and/or faculty mentor in their respective occupational therapy program. Fieldwork students have a professional responsibility to obtain and maintain pre-clinical health or security requirements needed to participate in fieldwork experiences. These requirements are typically determined by the fieldwork site, and are usually the same requirements health care organizations have for their employees in compliance with state and federal standards, such as those dictated by The Joint Commission. Some examples of these clinical requirements may include

- Proof of cardiopulmonary resuscitation training for the health care provider
- Proof of recent physical examination
- Immunization report and/or proof of immunity to vaccines (via blood titer)
- Federal/state background checks and/or fingerprinting
- Drug screening (five or ten panel drug screen)
- Influenza vaccine (especially during flu season)
- Two-step tuberculosis test or blood test

This list is not all encompassing, and fieldwork sites may be more stringent.

Fieldwork students can be suspended, dismissed, and/or terminated from their fieldwork experience if required documentation is not complete. It is beneficial to instruct students to manage these professional clearances and requirements by establishing a professional portfolio as a centralized location to store and organize credentials. See Box 11-12 on page 248 for suggested content for professional portfolios.

Fieldwork Educator or Mentor

Fieldwork education is a supervised learning experience. Fieldwork educators (or mentors for occupational therapy development experiential components) are key facilitators in realizing the purpose of fieldwork education. The term fieldwork educator is an intentional title. It differs from

---

Box 7-1

FIELDWORK EDUCATOR RESPONSIBILITIES

- Supervising: The core process of overseeing and managing the learning process, i.e., regulating that the fieldwork student is complying with site policies and procedures.

- Educating: Fieldwork educators are responsible for providing knowledge to and teaching fieldwork students skills and techniques.

- Mentoring: Fieldwork educators are responsible for fostering personal and professional growth within fieldwork students through role-modeling and taking a personal interest in the student as an occupational being.

- Guiding: Fieldwork educators are responsible for facilitating and nurturing the fieldwork process by challenging the student's thinking and encouraging reflective dialogue.

- Evaluating: Fieldwork educators create expectations and responsibilities; establish goals and learning objectives for the student, and provide feedback to the AFWC on the student's performance both informally and formally. Resources used to assist in the evaluation process include setting up an orientation schedule, week-by-week site-specific objectives, and implementing weekly formal and informal meetings to provide constructive feedback.

---

clinical instructor or preceptor in a variety of ways. Key responsibilities within the fieldwork educator role include supervising, educating, mentoring, guiding, and evaluating the fieldwork student (Box 7-1).

Qualifications for Fieldwork Educators and Mentors

ACOTE sets explicit standards for the fieldwork component of the academic program, including qualifications for fieldwork educators (Costa, 2007).

Level I Fieldwork

ACOTE (2012) dictates that occupational therapy educational programs must "ensure that qualified personnel supervise Level I fieldwork. Examples may include, but are not limited to, currently licensed or otherwise regulated occupational therapists and occupational therapy assistants, psychologists, physician assistants, teachers, social workers, nurses, and physical therapists" (pp. S35-S36).

Level II Fieldwork

ACOTE (2012) states that occupational therapy educational programs must "ensure that the student is supervised by a currently licensed or otherwise regulated occupational therapist who has a minimum of one year full time (or its equivalent) of practice experience subsequent to initial certification and who is adequately prepared to serve as a fieldwork educator. The supervising therapist may be engaged by the fieldwork site or by the educational program" (p. S36).

Doctoral Experiential Component

ACOTE (2012) states that occupational therapy doctoral degree educational programs must "ensure that the student is mentored by an individual with expertise consistent with the student's area of focus. The mentor does not have to be an occupational therapist" (p. S38). As stated in the 2011 ACOTE Standards (C.2.4), the DEC student should be mentored by an individual with expertise consistent with the student's area of focus. Mentoring is defined as a relationship between two people in which one person (the mentor) is dedicated to the personal and professional growth of the other (the mentee). A mentor has more experience and knowledge than the mentee. The fieldwork site will provide supervision to occupational therapy development students on site by a qualified and competent (but not necessarily an occupational therapy practitioner) personnel. This individual assists the occupational therapy development student in applying knowledge to practical situations, developing problem-solving skills, and learning practical competencies. The mentor will instruct and orient the occupational therapy development student as needed to perform specific negotiated learning activities consistent with the student's learning objectives. The student must be mentored by an individual with expertise consistent with the student's area of focus (e.g., if the student's focus is occupational therapy treatment for neonates—they must be mentored by a professional in the Neonatal Intensive Care Unit). The mentor does not have to be an occupational therapy practitioner, thereby allowing for various supervision/mentorship models to be used. A more in-depth review of supervision models will be presented later in this chapter.

Summary

Throughout the continuum of fieldwork education and experiential learning, occupational therapy students spend a lot of time with their fieldwork educators. In fact, it may surprise you that students spend more time with fieldwork educators than their occupational therapy faculty. For example, students enrolled in the entry-level master's program at Duquesne University, spend an average of 150 hours on level I FW and, a minimum of 962 hours of level II FW totaling over 1100 hours during traditional fieldwork education. Compare this with the didactic classroom hours over five semesters in the professional phase of the curriculum, equals approximately 1000 hours. This would indicate that fieldwork educators, as with core occupational therapy faculty, play a tremendous role in preparing future occupational therapy practitioners. Christie, Joyce, and Moeller (1985) confirm that occupational therapy students "encounter recurring interpersonal and attitudinal influences" (p. 674) throughout their professional education.

ROLE COMPETENCIES OF THE FIELDWORK EDUCATOR

In 2006, the AOTA published an official document outlining five standards that are attributed to being a competent fieldwork educator: knowledge, critical reasoning, performance skills, interpersonal skills, and ethical reasoning. Specific components that relate to characteristics of professionalism are seen throughout this document, including the following (AOTA, 2006):

- Demonstrate competency to develop and maintain proficiency through formal education, continuing education, and self-study
- Maintain current knowledge of standards, rules, and regulations
- Evaluate interpersonal dynamics
- Project a positive self-image
- Demonstrate a competent and positive attitude toward practice and supervision
- Demonstrate positive, culturally sensitive interactions
- Plan fieldwork experiences that prepare ethical practitioners
- Act as a role model

CLINICAL COORDINATOR OF FIELDWORK EDUCATION

Many fieldwork sites assign the administrative responsibilities relative to fieldwork to one individual within the discipline or rehabilitation service; however, within larger health care facilities, the role might be assumed by a representative of the education department (Costa, 2011). The individual fulfilling the CCFW role serves as the fieldwork site's formal representative and liaison to the academic institution. This individual is responsible for the development, management, and logistic details of fieldwork education. It is beneficial that this individual is experienced as a fieldwork educator and knowledgeable about the fieldwork site and its resources.

Logistically, the CCFW is responsible for scheduling, providing information, documentation, and orientation of incoming students, as well as maintaining their personnel records. This may include a record of the orientation to the facility and equipment, training and/or competencies, evaluations, and personal student data, including contact information and health and security prerequisites. The CCFW should be knowledgeable of and support the curriculum of individual occupational therapy programs, and be familiar with state practice act and payer regulations regarding student services. In absence of a formal clinical coordinator of fieldwork education position, the above tasks and responsibilities can be completed by the fieldwork educator. Professionally speaking, the clinical coordinator of fieldwork education is often the individual at the fieldwork site to set the first impression to the fieldwork student, in regards to how things are run and handled at the site, via their correspondence and general interpersonal interaction with fieldwork students (Hanson & DeIuliis, 2015).

ACADEMIC FIELDWORK COORDINATOR

As discussed previously in this chapter, fieldwork education is a regulated part of the occupational therapy curriculum. There are explicit ACOTE Standards (Standard A.27) that describe the requirements of the AWFC (ACOTE, 2012). The AFWC is a full-time faculty member or professional staff member principally responsible for developing, coordinating, organizing, and monitoring the entire occupational therapy fieldwork process, including the oversight of the fieldwork educator and the fieldwork student. These responsibilities include addressing the many logistical requirements of fieldwork education, such as ACOTE Standards C.1.2, C.1.4, C.1.6., and C.1.7, as well as regulate the process of compliance by which the academic institution program is held accountable for fieldwork education. To ensure that the fieldwork activities support and enhance the goals of the program, continual collaboration is essential between the FWEd, CCFW, and AFWC. The AFWC is also responsible for preplacement planning, and the assigning of students to fieldwork sites. Beyond the preparation phase, the AFWC is responsible for monitoring the student progress on fieldwork and maintaining contact with the FWEd and CCFW throughout the fieldwork experience.

The AFWC also contributes to the academic institutions program evaluation by facilitating outcome measurement during fieldwork education via the AOTA FWPE, and the Student Evaluation of Fieldwork Experience. The AFWC is responsible for collecting and interpreting data from these required tools and reporting the information to faculty as an important process in curriculum review and evaluation. Depending on the academic institution, the AFWC may have other responsibilities such as teaching fieldwork and nonfieldwork related coursework, participating in service, and engaging in scholarship. Similar to the CCFW, the AFWC is often the primary liaison between the academic program and the occupational therapy community, and often is one of the more visible faculty members of the academic institution to the fieldwork community.

Role Competencies of the Academic Fieldwork Coordinator

The AOTA (2004) addressed the expected roles of the AFWC in the document "Role Competencies for an Academic Fieldwork Coordinator." The purpose of this document is to "assist academic settings in determining and/or evaluating the typical responsibilities for an academic fieldwork coordinator in an occupational therapy or occupational therapy assistant educational program" (p. 653). This document consists of five standards, each with subparts that describe the values, knowledge, skills, and responsibilities expected in fulfilling the role as the AFWC. The standards described in this article are knowledge, critical reasoning, interpersonal skills, performance skills, and ethical reasoning.

Specific excerpts from "Role Competencies for an Academic Fieldwork Coordinator" (AOTA, 2004) are the following, and indicate the strong role played by an AFWC in developing a fieldwork student's professionalism:

- Demonstrate an expertise to be able to facilitate the development of future leaders in occupational therapy
- Facilitate professional development
- Project a positive image
- Demonstrate a competent and positive attitude
- Demonstrate positive interactions
- Act as a role model

The process of fieldwork education is intentionally developmental. To some degree, all stakeholders involved in the fieldwork education process play significant roles in the shaping of professional identity of individual occupational therapy students, as well as the future of the profession. Additional role attributes of the fieldwork educator can be found in "Specialized Knowledge and Skills of the Occupational Therapy Educators of the Future" (AOTA, 2009b). In this article, Padilla and colleagues from the Commission on Education describe the desirable traits of fieldwork educators using the following classifications and the competency spectrum of novice-to-advanced.

- Innovator/visionary
- Scholar/explorer
- Leader
- Integrator
- Mentor

FIELDWORK SUPERVISION

Fieldwork educators must exhibit effective characteristics of supervision to provide quality and meaningful learning experiences for students. Supervision is defined as "the act of supervising, especially a critical watching and directing" ("Supervision," 2016). Learning to become a fieldwork educator is "both an art and science" (Costa, 2007, p. 166). Within fieldwork education, supervision is an intentional intervention used by the FWEd to help fieldwork students develop clinical skills as well as professional skills. It is a mutual process that involves participation from both the fieldwork student(s) and the fieldwork educator(s) to establish, maintain, promote or enhance clinical and professional performance. In fact, the Occupational Therapy Code of Ethics states that all occupational therapy practitioners must "provide appropriate supervision in accordance with AOTA Official Documents and relevant laws, regulations, policies, procedures, standards, and guidelines" (AOTA, 2015, p. 6).

Box 7-2

DOCUMENTATION OF FEEDBACK

Documentation of feedback during fieldwork education is very important. Just like during clinical encounters with patients, if you don't document it, it didn't happen. Fieldwork educators should keep track of feedback sessions as evidence to put forward to midterm and final evaluations, or remediation plans if behavior is unsatisfactory.

Methods of Supervision

Depending on the fieldwork student, fieldwork educator, type of fieldwork site, and population, there are various methods of supervision that can be provided during fieldwork education. Similar to the traditional occupational therapy process, in which occupational therapy practitioners elicit an occupational profile to determine how their client learns best and what they are motivated by, fieldwork educators must consider what supervisory methods will be best for developing the student's skills. Supervision can be described as direct and indirect, as well as informal and formal. Direct supervision is when the fieldwork educator directly observes the student's performance through face-to-face, or in-line-of-sight contact. Indirect supervision is when the information is gathered from the supervisee or fieldwork educator after performance, through a variety of methods such as electronic, written, telephone communications, or interaction with other colleagues who have interacted with the student. Formal supervision takes place in a pre-arranged time and space. It is a mutually agreed upon time by the fieldwork student and FWEd for reflection, feedback, and dialogue, as well as an exploration of what further learning needs to occur. For example, during a Level II FW experience, the FWEd may plan that Thursdays during lunch are routine and regular formal supervision meetings with the fieldwork student. This can be a time to review progress in meeting site-specific objectives, as well as have the student reflect on what their current strengths and areas of growth are. Koski and colleagues (2013) reported on the value of using summative assessments during fieldwork to direct students to reflect upon their strengths and areas of need (see Appendix C for weekly feedback form) (Box 7-2).

Informal supervision can take place at any time and typically allows for feedback and reflection immediately after a learning experience. For example, immediately after a bedside treatment session in an acute care hospital, the FWEd and fieldwork student may convene at the nurses' station to quickly dialogue about the events that occurred during the session. Regardless of the type of supervision provided, it is crucial that the supervision is supportive, developmental, and nonjudgmental to foster growth in the fieldwork student. The one-minute preceptor provides a useful framework to provide constructive feedback in the moment (Neher, Gordon, Meyers, & Stevens, 1992). The one-minute preceptor model was designed to promote clinical reasoning and decision making, as well as offer immediate feedback to the learner. The model consists of five skills that can be used in a time-pressured environment (Table 7-2).

Supervision Continuum

As discussed in Chapter 1, the degree, amount, and pattern of supervision required can vary depending on the practitioner's competence, service demands, state laws and licensure requirements, facility procedures, complexities of clients' needs, and caseload characteristics. Many times, fieldwork educators tend to adopt a style of supervision and teaching which reflects their own learning style and/or the teaching-learning style promoted within their workplace. However, the FWEd must ensure that the type, amount, and competence of occupational therapy supervision match the student's learning style, areas of need, and level of role competence. ACOTE (2012) standard C.1.16 indicates that during Level II FW, "initially, supervision should be direct and then

TABLE 7-2 **STEPS TO IMPLEMENT THE ONE-MINUTE PRECEPTOR**	
STEP	**ACTIONS**
Step 1	Get a commitment from the student related to what he or she thinks about the case Ask the student to devise their own course of action or plan
Step 2	Question the student for evidence that supports the student's commitment Evaluate the student's reasoning or background knowledge, and their ability to defend their clinical opinion
Step 3	Teach a general principle or "take-home points" that are applicable to other scenarios
Step 4	Reinforce what the student did well Give the student immediate positive feedback on specific skills or behaviors, not just general praise
Step 5	Correct errors Ask student to evaluate their performance; then, give student immediate constructive feedback and provide recommendations on how to improve

decrease to less direct supervision as appropriate for the setting, the severity of the client's condition, and the ability of the student" (p. 36). Examples of ways to vary supervision during fieldwork are presented in Table 7-3.

REGULATORY OVERSIGHT AND SUPERVISION

Above and beyond the AOTA guidelines and ACOTE mandates regarding fieldwork and supervision, fieldwork educators and fieldwork students must be knowledgeable about state laws and reimbursement bodies that may have stipulation clauses regarding supervision of students in their setting. State practice acts and licensure boards may specify if there are any requirements for supervision that need to be upheld in that state. For example, state practice acts may dictate that all documentation related to client services provided by the fieldwork student must be reviewed and signed by the supervising occupational therapy practitioner, or the state licensure board may require that the student (supervisee) and fieldwork educator (supervisor) create and submit a formal supervision plan. You can find state regulatory board contact information in the licensure section of the AOTA website.

Another source of supervision guidelines are federal regulations, such as those pertaining to Medicare, that specify what type of supervision must be provided when fieldwork students are working with Medicare-covered patients. The AOTA (2013b) provided an informative resource to its members describing the student supervision requirements when a student is participating in service delivery of a client who has Medicare insurance (Box 7-3).

	TABLE 7-3	
	VARIATIONS OF FIELDWORK SUPERVISION	
TYPE OF SUPERVISION	**DESCRIPTION**	**TIME FRAME**
Continuous supervision	Daily, direct, line of sight, at fieldwork site	May be common during weeks 1-4 on Level II FW
Close supervision	Daily, direct, at fieldwork site, yet not always in line of sight*	May be typical at midterm during Level II FW
General supervision	Daily, direct and indirect supervision*	May be typical around week 8 of a 12-week experience
Remote supervision	Only on an as-needed basis, supervisee/student initiates supervision when needed*	Common during final week(s) of Level II FW

*The supervisor must ensure that there are mechanisms in place for monitoring whether the supervisee is practicing safely.

Adapted from Schell, B. A., Gillen, G., Scaffa, M., & Cohn, E. S. (2009). *Willard and Spackman's occupational therapy* (12th ed.). Philadelphia, PA: Lippincott Williams & Wilkins

BOX 7-3

MEDICARE REQUIREMENTS FOR STUDENT SUPERVISION

According to the Centers for Medicare & Medicaid Services, under Part A regulations in skilled nursing facilities, occupational therapy and occupational therapy assistant students may only provide billable services under "line of sight level of supervision of the professional therapist." As defined by the Centers for Medicare & Medicaid Services, the "professional therapist" is an occupational therapy practitioner, not an occupational therapy assistant. The occupational therapy assistant may not provide supervision to occupational therapy assistant students for billable services provided by the student in skilled nursing facilities settings, although such supervision is allowable in acute care settings. Part B guidelines for student supervision are even more stringent. These regulations have severely limited the availability of skilled nursing facilities Level II fieldwork options for occupational therapy assistant students in many geographic areas.

Adapted from American Occupational Therapy Association. (2013b). OT/OTA student supervision & Medicare requirements. Retrieved from http://www.aota.org/-/media/Corporate/Files/Secure/Advocacy/Reimb/Coverage/ot-ota-student-medicare-requirements.pdf

Occupational therapy students, fieldwork educators, and other practitioners are professionally responsible for being knowledgeable about and complying with all state and federal regulations regarding supervision.

Fieldwork Supervision Models

Fieldwork supervision models are the systematic ways in which fieldwork education is designed and delivered. Due to the effect of managed care on health care delivery systems, as well as a dramatic increase in the number of students needing fieldwork placements, many occupational therapy education programs, specifically their affiliated AFWCs, are pressed to explore and implement non-traditional supervision models and emerging fieldwork placements to ensure quality fieldwork experiences (Gat & Ratzon, 2014).

Traditional/Apprenticeship Supervision Model

Historically, the student learning process during fieldwork education has been supported primarily through the use of an apprenticeship model, which is largely dependent on the skills, expertise, and modeling provided by the fieldwork educator. In this model, one fieldwork student is paired with one fieldwork educator for the duration of the fieldwork experience. The fieldwork educator models clinical reasoning strategies and provides a focus for skills to be learned, while the student observes, practices skills, and performs tasks within an established occupational therapy role (Mulholland & Derdall, 2005). Under this model, the fieldwork educator is directly responsible for role-modeling professional behaviors and attitudes, as well as designing learning activities that provide opportunities for professionalism to be addressed.

Collaborative Supervision Model

The pedagogy and benefits of collaborative/team learning were discussed in Chapter 5; this concept can be applied to fieldwork education as well as classroom learning. The collaborative supervision fieldwork model is employed when two or more occupational therapy students are placed with one fieldwork educator. This model must be carefully designed so that the students work closely together, collaborating to solve problems. The fieldwork educator must develop clear and concise behavioral objectives, teach problem solving skills, and provide learning activities for the students that will foster collaboration and self-directed learning.

Although this model of supervision may appear to be more labor-intensive to the fieldwork educator, in actuality, the fieldwork educator spends less time in supervision than in the one-to-one model. The students are encouraged to use each other as a resource, before taking issues to the fieldwork educator. In addition, students often feel more comfortable engaging in risk-taking behaviors with each other. Feedback tends to be nonthreatening and easier to accept from a peer, than a superior. Students also learn more effective teamwork skills and gain expanded perspective as they use each other's body of knowledge (Hanson & DeIuliis, 2015). It is not surprising that the collaborative approach to learning is also more reflective of students' learning preferences (Grenier, 2015; Martin et al., 2004; Mason, 1998; Vogel et al., 2004). This model closely parallels real-world expectations and allows students to develop healthful professional habits by increasing responsibility in their own learning and professional development.

Intraprofessional Supervision Model

Intraprofessonal roles within health care professions was discussed in Chapter 3. The intraprofessional fieldwork supervision model is when students of the same profession, registered occupational therapists and occupational therapy assistants, are purposefully engaged in learning together and collaborating during the fieldwork experience (Costa, Molinsky, & Sauerwald, 2012). Dillon (2001) interviewed occupational therapy practitioner/occupational therapy assistant teams and found that the essence of the relationship between occupational therapy practitioners and occupational therapy assistants cannot be gained from a textbook, or reading articles on professional role delineation and supervisory guidelines. Themes that emerged from the study included: importance of communication, need for mutual respect, and the importance of professionalism.

TABLE 7-4
EXAMPLES OF INTERPROFESSIONAL LEVEL I FIELDWORK EXPERIENCES

DISCIPLINES INVOLVED	CLINICAL FOCUS OR PROJECT
Occupational Therapy and Speech-Language Pathology	Design and implement a program for occupational therapy and speech-language pathology practitioners focused on the use of apps within a cyber-school setting to enhance communication and social participation of children who have autism
Occupational Therapy and Physical Therapy	Create and implement an evidenced-based fall prevention program at a skilled nursing facility, combining elements of gait training, low vision, and environmental modifications
Occupational Therapy and Pharmacy	In an independent living facility, occupational therapy students and pharmacy students can collaborate on increasing client independence with medication management

Scheerer (2001) also describes benefits of the intraprofessional model involving "practicing interaction, teamwork and collaboration as students should provide a lifetime of habit of partnering as practitioners" (p. 204).

Interprofessional Supervision Model

As discussed in Chapter 3, interprofessional learning occurs when two or more disciplines learn about, from, and with each other to enable effective collaboration and improve health care outcomes (World Health Organization, 2010). This model is similar to collaborative or group learning, which emphasizes peer-to-peer teaching and learning; however, the interprofessional model includes learning about and from peers from different disciplines. Specific to fieldwork education, interprofessional supervision models occur with two or more students from different disciplines— such as an occupational therapy and speech-language pathology student in an early intervention setting working together with feeding and oral motor skills. Grenier (2015) indicates that students identified great value to interprofessional learning models, specially collaborating in a team setting and having the opportunity to learn about various roles and professions that occupational therapy practitioners work with. However, pre-planning is needed among the interprofessional teams in regards to identification of clients who require multidisciplinary services, treatment planning, and collaborative goal setting (Table 7-4).

Shared Supervision Model

Some fieldwork educators and/or clinical sites are conducive to a split fieldwork educator model, which involves two fieldwork educators splitting formal supervision and teaching of a single fieldwork student. This model can be useful for fieldwork educators who work less than full-time. The shared supervision model can benefit fieldwork students by having two practitioners to view as role models and mentors; however, for this model to be successful, the supervising therapists must demonstrate good communication, and have consistent expectations of the fieldwork student (Table 7-5).

TABLE 7-5

SUMMARY OF SUPERVISION MODELS AND INFLUENCE ON PROFESSIONALISM

MODEL NAME	NO. OF STUDENTS	NO. OF FWEds	PROFESSIONAL SKILLS ACQUIRED
Apprenticeship Model	1	1	Direct role-modeling from FWEd
Collaborative Model	2 or more	1	Teamwork skills Communication Conflict resolution Self-awareness Initiative
Intraprofessional Model	1 occupational therapy practitioner 1 occupational therapy assistant	1	Teamwork skills Communication Collaboration Conflict resolution
Interprofessional Model	1 occupational therapy practitioner and/or occupational therapy assistant At least 1 other discipline	1	Teamwork skills Interprofessional collaboration Interprofessional communication Interprofessional professionalism
Shared Model	1	2	Direct role modeling from more than one FWEd

Types of Fieldwork Settings

Fieldwork education can take place in a variety of settings that are meant to expose fieldwork students to different theories, models of practice, patient populations, and professional expectations in authentic contexts. Fieldwork sites are typically categorized as traditional or emerging/nontraditional. Traditional fieldwork sites include medical centers (such as hospitals, long-term acute care facilities, and acute psychiatry), rehabilitation settings (including inpatient, outpatient, and skilled nursing facilities), and community settings (such as school based, home health, and mental health settings). More recently, in conjunction with the Centennial Vision, fieldwork education is occurring in emerging areas of practice such as forensic institutions, homeless centers, telehealth, vocational settings, health and wellness centers, adult day centers, and more (AOTA, 2007). During these types of fieldwork experiences, students may be placed in a site without an occupational therapist. A member of the site's staff typically provides day to day supervision, and a faculty staff member or a working therapist with expertise in the area undertakes formal weekly supervision to meet ACOTE standards.

The ACOTE Standards require that the fieldwork educator provide a minimum of eight hours per week at the site. In addition, the fieldwork educator must be easily accessible by a variety of means during the hours a student is present. Furthermore, the person serving as the fieldwork educator must have a minimum of three years' experience after initial certification, as this is considered advanced supervision. The Commission on Education and Commission on Practice Fieldwork Level II position paper (AOTA, 2012) additionally recommends that supervision of occupational therapy and occupational therapy assistant students in Level II FW settings will be of the quality and scope to ensure protection of consumers, and to provide opportunities for appropriate role modeling of occupational therapy practice. It is also recommended that the supervising occupational therapy practitioner and/or occupational therapy assistant must recognize when direct vs indirect supervision is needed, and ensure that supervision supports the student's current and developing levels of competence (AOTA, 2012).

Typically, role-emerging placements are identified as a result of faculty involvement in community development initiatives; otherwise, students may identify a clinical or project interest; or, an individual, organization, or government entity may contact the university to request a learning partnership. Fieldwork education that takes place in nontraditional settings allows fieldwork students to gain a perspective of professionalism beyond occupational therapy, which is of value, regardless of where the student ultimately practices after graduation. Fieldwork can also occur through an interagency model, meaning that the fieldwork experience is divided between more than one fieldwork site. This may be beneficial when different specialty areas are of interest to the student. For example, the student may be placed in a hand therapy clinic two days a week, and then in an acute care setting three days per week.

Summary

This chapter reviewed the basic make-up of fieldwork education, as well as the value and importance it has in the developmental learning process of an occupational therapy student. Fieldwork education is a critical learning experience where occupational therapy students learn and refine both clinical competency and professional skills. ACOTE provides clear guidelines which are intended to guide the fieldwork student, fieldwork educator, and academic fieldwork coordinator in developing an effective environment for clinical and professional learning. The following chapter will closely examine the role that professionalism has during this important clinical learning experience.

Learning Activities

1. Investigate the fieldwork sites that you will be going to. What clearances and requirements are needed? Review your professional portfolio; do you have evidence of meeting these clearances?

2. Create a list of questions that you will ask your fieldwork educator before your fieldwork experiences to prepare yourself clinically and professionally.

3. Check out the Fieldwork Education section on the AOTA's website. Go to www.aota.org; click on Educator-Careers tab, then click on Fieldwork Education.

   a. Describe two resources that would be useful as a fieldwork student.

   b. Describe two resources that would be useful as a fieldwork educator.

   c. What is the most useful thing that you learned from this website?

References

Accreditation Council for Occupational Therapy Education. (2012). 2011 Accreditation Council for Occupational Therapy Education (ACOTE) standards. *American Journal of Occupational Therapy, 66*(Suppl. 1), S6-S74.

Aiken, F., Menaker, L., & Barsky, L. (2001). Fieldwork education: The future of occupational therapy depends on it. *Occupational Therapy International, 8*(2), 86-95.

American Occupational Therapy Association. (2002). Fieldwork performance evaluation for the occupational therapy student. Retrieved from http://ot.lr.edu/sites/ot.lr.edu/files/AOTA%20FW%20Performance%20Evaluation.pdf

American Occupational Therapy Association. (2004). Role competencies for an academic fieldwork coordinator. *American Journal of Occupational Therapy, 58*(6), 653-654.

American Occupational Therapy Association. (2006). Role competencies for a fieldwork educator. *American Journal of Occupational Therapy, 60*(6), 650-651.

American Occupational Therapy Association. (2007). AOTA's American Centennial Vision and executive summary. *American Journal of Occupational Therapy, 61*(6), 613-614.

American Occupational Therapy Association. (2009a). Occupational therapy fieldwork education: Value and purpose. *American Journal of Occupational Therapy, 63*(6), 821-822.

American Occupational Therapy Association. (2009b). Specialized knowledge and skills of occupational therapy educators of the future. *American Journal of Occupational Therapy, 63*(6), 804-818.

American Occupational Therapy Association. (2012). Fieldwork Level II and occupational therapy students: A position paper. *American Journal of Occupational Therapy, 66*(Suppl. 1), S75-S77.

American Occupational Therapy Association. (2013a). COE guidelines for an occupational therapy fieldwork experience—Level II. Retrieved from http://www.aota.org/-/media/corporate/files/educationcareers/educators/fieldwork/levelii/coe%20guidelines%20for%20an%20occupational%20therapy%20fieldwork%20experience%20—%20level%20ii—final.pdf

American Occupational Therapy Association. (2013b). OT/OTA student supervision & Medicare requirements. Retrieved from http://www.aota.org/-/media/Corporate/Files/Secure/Advocacy/Reimb/Coverage/ot-ota-student-medicare-requirements.pdf

American Occupational Therapy Association. (2015). Occupational therapy code of ethics. Retrieved from http://www.aota.org/-/media/corporate/files/practice/ethics/code-of-ethics.pdf

Brandenburger-Shasby, S., Hills, L., Huie, C., Jansen, K., Johnson, L., & Josey-Lamont, A. (1998). Fieldwork: The critical link. *Education Special Interest Section Quarterly, 8*(3), 1-3.

Cara, E. (1998). Fieldwork supervision in a mental health setting. In E. Cara, & A. MacRae (Eds.), *Psychosocial occupational therapy: A clinical practice* (pp. 609-640). Albany, NY: Delmar Publishers.

Christie, B. A., Joyce, P. C., & Moeller, P. L. (1985). Fieldwork experience, part II: The supervisor's dilemma. *American Journal of Occupational Therapy, 39*(10), 675-681.

Costa, D. M. (2007). *Clinical supervision in occupational therapy: A guide for fieldwork and practice.* Bethesda, MD: AOTA Press.

Costa, D. M. (2011). Management of fieldwork education. In K. J. Jacobs & G. L. McCormack (Eds.), *The occupational therapy manager* (5th ed., pp. 591-605). Bethesda, MD: AOTA Press

Costa, D. M., Molinsky, R., & Sauerwald, C. (2012). Collaborative intraprofessional education with occupational therapy and occupational assistant students. *OT Practice, 17*(21), CE1-CE7.

Dillon, T. H. (2001). Practitioner perspectives: Effective intraprofessional relationships in occupational therapy. *Occupational Therapy in Healthcare, 14*(3-4), 1-15.

Gat, S., & Ratzon N. Z. (2014). Comparison of occupational therapy students' perceived skills after traditional and nontraditional fieldwork. *American Journal of Occupational Therapy, 68*(2), e47-e54.

Grenier, M. (2015). Facilitators and barriers to learning in occupational therapy fieldwork education: Student perspectives. *American Journal of Occupational Therapy, 69*(Suppl. 2), 6912185070.

Hanson, D. J., & DeIuliis, E. D. (2015). The collaborative model to fieldwork education: A blueprint for group supervision of students. *Occupational Therapy in Healthcare, 29*(2), 223-239.

Koski K. J., Simon, R. L., & Dooley, N. R. (2013). Valuable occupational therapy fieldwork educator behaviors. *Work, 44*, 307-315.

Martin, M., Morris, J., Moore, A., Saldo, G., & Crouch, V. (2004). Evaluating practice education models in occupational therapy: Comparing 1:1, 2:1 and 3:1 placement. *British Journal of Occupational Therapy, 67*(5), 192-200.

Mason, L. (1998). Fieldwork education: Collaborative group learning in community settings. *Australian Occupational Therapy Journal, 45*(4), 124-130.

Mulholland, S., & Derdall, M. (2005). A strategy for supervising occupational therapy students at community sites. *Occupational Therapy International, 12*, 28-43.

Neher, J., Gordon, K., Meyer, B., & Stevens, N. (1992). A five-step "microskills" model of clinical teaching. *Journal of the American Board of Family Practice, 5*, 419-424.

Scheerer, C. (2001). The partnering model: Occupational therapy assistant and occupational therapy students working together. *Occupational Therapy in Health Care, 15*(1-2), 193-208.

Schell, B. A., Gillen, G., Scaffa, M., & Cohn, E. S. (2009). *Willard and Spackman's occupational therapy* (12th ed.). Philadelphia, PA: Lippincott Williams & Wilkins.

Supervision. (2016, April 4). In Merriam-Webster dictionary. Retrieved from http://www.merriam-webster.com/dictionary/supervision

Vogel, K. A., Grice, K. O., Hill, S., & Moody, J. (2004). Supervisor and student expectations of level II fieldwork. *Occupational Therapy in Health Care, 18*(1-2), 5-19.

World Health Organization. (2010). Framework for action on interprofessional education & collaborative practice. Geneva, Switzerland: World Health Organization. Retrieved from http://whqlibdoc.who.int/hq/2010/WHO_HRH_HPN_10.3_eng.pdf

APPENDIX A: DUQUESNE UNIVERSITY DEPARTMENT OF OCCUPATIONAL THERAPY EVALUATION OF LEVEL I FIELDWORK STUDENT PERFORMANCE

☐ Level I A   ☐ Level I C

Student Name:

Name of Clinical Site:

Type of Site: (check primary)
Fieldwork Educator Name and Credentials (PRINT): _____

☐ Gerontology – SNF/ LTC	☐ Work Hardening	☐ Peds – Hospital	☐ Peds - Other
☐ Gerontology – Other	☐ Mental Health – Community	☐ Peds – School	☐ Phys Dys- Acute Care
☐ Home health	☐ Mental Health – Hospital	☐ Peds – Outpatient	☐ Phys Dys- Rehab
☐ Hand Therapy	☐ Mental Health – Other	☐ Peds – EI	☐ Phys Dys – Outpatient

☐ Other: _____

The purpose of this performance report is to identify the level of growth of the student' professional behaviors and clinical reasoning in preparation for level II FW and entry-level practice. Level I FW provides the student exposure to the role of occupational therapy and the opportunity to apply/observe newly learned theories, frames of reference, techniques and applications in practice arenas. *Please note that students have completed many of their occupational therapy intervention courses thus far in the curriculum, and are prepared for hands-on clinical practice! We encourage as much "hands-on" experience as possible and appropriate.*

Please complete this form in entirety, indicating the student's level of performance using the scale below. Please do not indicate any items as N/A. We are aware that not all behaviors may be observed or demonstrated during their level I FW experience. If an item on this evaluation is not applicable at your site, please attempt in assisting the student to achieve competency via discussion, role play, etc. Comments are appreciated.

0 = Below Standards: Opportunities for improvement exist. Student has not demonstrated adequate response to feedback. Work/performance/behaviors are occasionally unacceptable.

1= Meets Standards: Carries our required tasks and activities. This rating represents good, solid performance and should be used more than all the others

2 = Exceeds Standards: Frequently carries out tasks and activities that surpass requirements. Performance is exceptional

Thank you for your service, dedication and assistance in the educational process or our occupational therapy students. We deeply appreciate the unique learning opportunities you provide and the time and energy extended by you and other staff in creating a stimulating and successful experience.

NOTE: This evaluation must be completed by the fieldwork educator, reviewed by the student, signed by both the student and the FWED, and returned to the Course Instructor before the student will receive a grade for this fieldwork experience.

PROFESSIONAL BEHAVIORS		
DOES THE STUDENT DEMONSTRATE:	**SCORE**	**COMMENTS**
Time management skills • the ability to be prompt, arrives on time, completes assignments on time, meets deadlines, and if unable to meet deadlines informs necessary parties?	0 1 2	
Organization Skills • the ability to set priorities, be dependable, be organized, follow through with responsibilities?	0 1 2	
Engagement in Fieldwork Experience • an apparent level of interest, level of participation while on site; investment in individuals and treatment outcomes?	0 1 2	
Self-Directed Learning • the ability to take responsibility for own learning, demonstrate motivation, exhibits an enthusiasm for inquiry and discovery willingness to 'go the extra mile', volunteers or takes on additional responsibilities?	0 1 2	*continued*

PROFESSIONAL BEHAVIORS (CONTINUED)			
DOES THE STUDENT DEMONSTRATE:	**SCORE**		**COMMENTS**
Written Communication • appropriate grammar, spelling, legibility, successful completion of written assignments, documentation skills?	0	1 2	
Initiative • the ability to seek and acquire information from a variety of sources, uses downtime efficiently/productively?	0	1 2	
Verbal Communication/ Interpersonal Skills • the ability to interact appropriately with patients, families and staff, such as eye contact, empathy, limit setting, respectfulness, use of authority etc., degree/quality of verbal interactions, use of body language and nonverbal communication, exhibits confidence, handles conflict constructively?	0	1 2	
Professional and Personal Boundaries • the ability to recognize/handle personal/ professional frustration, balance personal/professional obligations, handle responsibilities, work with others cooperatively, considerately, effectively; responsive to social cues?	0	1 2	*continued*

PROFESSIONAL BEHAVIORS (CONTINUED)		
DOES THE STUDENT DEMONSTRATE:	**SCORE**	**COMMENTS**
Flexibility • Adapts, adjusts and copes with change well, (time schedule, assignments etc.), manages stressors in a positive and constructive manner, modifies own behavior accordingly to manage a variety of simultaneous clinical demands?	0 1 2	
Responsiveness to constructive feedback • the ability to modify performance after feedback, demonstrates ability to profit from constructive feedback, attentive learning, clarification of problem areas and appropriate attempts to change behavior	0 1 2	
Team Building and Interprofessional Skills • Strive to achieve team goals, is proactive in meeting needs of others, assists with problem solving, works efficiently in a group or with other disciplines	0 1 2	

OCCUPATIONAL THERAPY CLINICAL REASONING SKILLS			
DOES THE STUDENT DEMONSTRATE:	**SCORE**		**COMMENTS**
Clinical Observation Skills • the ability to actively observe relevant behaviors for performance areas and performance components, and to verbalize perceptions and observations?	0	1 2	
Clinical Problem Solving Skills • the ability to use self-reflection, willingness to ask questions, ability to analyze, synthesize and interpret information, and understand the OT Process?	0	1 2	
Use of professional terminology • the ability to respect confidentiality, appropriately apply professional terminology such as OTPF vocabulary, acronyms, abbreviations etc.) in written and oral communication	0	1 2	
Evaluation Skills • an understanding of the various evaluation tools and methods used, evidence of expanding clinical observations, can obtain appropriate data via interview (i.e. occupational profile)?	0	1 2	*continued*

OCCUPATIONAL THERAPY CLINICAL REASONING SKILLS (CONTINUED)			
DOES THE STUDENT DEMONSTRATE:	**SCORE**		**COMMENTS**
Treatment Planning Skills • the ability to analyze an activity to demonstrate which goals can be addressed through patient participation in such an activity, strives to use occupation-based interventions?	0 1 2		
Treatment Implementation • the use of more than one activity to address patient goals demonstrates an ability to grade activities, is able to modify activities based upon client's response/needs, adheres to safety/diagnostic precautions during treatment?	0 1 2		
Treatment Termination • an understanding of quality of care, ability to decipher appropriateness of discontinuing/discharging services, provides appropriate recommendations for next level of care, disposition needs, suggests appropriate adaptations in environment and activities to accommodate to client's functional level?	0 1 2		

Please mark the following items as satisfactory (S) or unsatisfactory (U). If unsatisfactory, please give example(s)

CRITERIA	SCORE		COMMENTS
Complies with dress code of facility	S	U	
Observes and adheres to safety precautions	S	U	
Demonstrates a positive attitude	S	U	
Complies with policies, procedures and rules of your facility	S	U	

Student Areas of Strength:

Student Areas of Growth/Improvement:

_____   _____
Occupational Therapy Student's Signature   Date

_____   _____
Fieldwork Educator's Signature   Date

APPENDIX B: STUDENT
EVALUATION OF FIELDWORK EXPERIENCE

The American Occupational Therapy Association, INC.

Purpose: This form is important feedback for your fieldwork experience supervisor, your faculty and other students at your school.

Directions: Complete this Student Evaluation of Fieldwork Experience (SEFWE) form in ink prior to your final meeting with your fieldwork supervisor. Your supervisor, too, will have completed your student performance evaluation for review at this meeting. Share the completed SEFWE with your supervisor, and the form should be co-signed. One copy remains with the fieldwork site and one copy is returned to your educational program.

Part I: IDENTIFYING INFORMATION

Academic Program_____

Facility Name_____

Address_____

Placement Dates: from_____ to _____

Order of Placement: 1   2   3   4   out of   1   2   3   4

Type of Fieldwork:_____
                                             Specialty/ Practice Area

Living Accommodations: *(include type, cost, location, condition)*

Part II: STRUCTURE OF FIELDWORK EDUCATION PROGRAM

A. Student Orientation

    1. Was a formal orientation provided?   Yes_____   No_____

    2. If yes, indicate your view of the orientation by *checking* "satisfactory" (S) or "Needs Improvement" (I) regarding the three factors of adequacy, organization, and timeliness.

Topic	Adequate		Organized		Timely	
	S	I	S	I	S	I
a. Staff introductions						
b. Physical facilities						
c. Organizational structure						
d. Facility/Department philosophy						
e. Facility services						
f. Facility/Department						
g. Occupational Therapy services						
h. Departmental documentation						
i. Safety/Emergency procedures						
j. Confidentiality						
k. Fieldwork objectives/requirements						
l. Student supervision						
m. Community resources						
n. Department frame(s) of reference						
o. Quality Improvement Program						
p. Requirements/Assignments						
q. Other						

    3. Comments or suggestions regarding your orientation to this fieldwork placement:

B. Written and Oral Assignments

1. Indicate whether the following assignments were required by *checking* "Yes" or "No".

   If required, indicate the number you did; also, indicate their value to your learning experience by *circling* the appropriate number with #1 being least valuable and #5 being the most valuable.

	Required Yes	Required No	How Many	Educational Value
a. Client/patient screening				1 2 3 4 5
b. Client/patient evaluations *(use specific names of evaluations)*				
				1 2 3 4 5
				1 2 3 4 5
				1 2 3 4 5
				1 2 3 4 5
				1 2 3 4 5
				1 2 3 4 5
				1 2 3 4 5
				1 2 3 4 5
				1 2 3 4 5
c. Written treatment/care plans				1 2 3 4 5
d. Discharge summary				1 2 3 4 5
e. Team meeting presentation				1 2 3 4 5
f. Inservice presentation				1 2 3 4 5
g. Case study				1 2 3 4 5
h. QI/Outcome/Efficacy study				1 2 3 4 5
i. Activity analysis				1 2 3 4 5
j. Other				1 2 3 4 5
k. Other				1 2 3 4 5

2. Comments or suggestions regarding assignments:

C. Caseload Description

1. List approximate number of each age category in your caseload.

Age	Number
0-5 years old	
6-12 years old	
13-21 years old	
Adult	
Older adult	

2. List diagnostic categories in your caseload and approximate number of each diagnosis.

Diagnosis	Number

3. List major therapeutic interventions frequently used and indicate whether it was provided in group or individually.

Therapeutic Interventions	Group	Individual

4. Suggestions for changes in caseload assignment that would improve your learning experience.

Part III: SUPERVISION

A. List all your supervisors

	Name	Title	Frequency	Individual	Group
1.					
2.					
3.					
4.					
5.					
6.					
7.					
8.					
9.					
10.					

B. Check categories which seem descriptive of your supervision.
   (You may wish to complete one chart for each clinical supervisor.)

	1= Rarely 2= Occasionally 3= Frequently 4= Consistently			
	1	2	3	4
Taught knowledge and skills as required				
Presented clear explanations and expectations				
Provided supervision as needed				
Used constructive feedback methods to address weaknesses				
Provided positive reinforcement for strengths				
Encouraged student to provide feedback to supervisor				
Facilitated student's problem-solving skills				
Encouraged self-directed learning				
Approachable and interested in students				
Adjusted workload to facilitate student's growth				
Reviewed written work in timely manner				
Made me feel comfortable and part of the department				
Demonstrated interest and commitment to job				
Provided a positive role model of professional behavior				
Provided a positive attitude towards other staff and students				
Provided feedback in timely manner				

C. General comments on supervision:

Part IV: PROFESSIONAL RELATIONSHIPS

A. Check categories which seem descriptive of your experience, referring to the code.

	1= Rarely 2= Occasionally 3= Frequently 4= Consistently			
	1	2	3	4
Provided with exposure to OTR/COTA/ Service Extender roles				
Provided with opportunities to network with other professionals				
Experienced interdisciplinary approach to care				
Observed OT staff modeling therapeutic relationships				
Informed of additional educational opportunities				
Participated in additional educational opportunities				
Provided chance to network with related agencies				
Provided with opportunity to expand interdisciplinary knowledge				
Expanded knowledge of community resources				

B. Which professionals were role models for you in your professional growth?

Please describe:

C. List the schools, disciplines and academic levels of students present during your fieldwork experience.

D. Describe how this affected your learning experience.

E. Comments or suggestions regarding professional relationships.

Part V: ACADEMIC PREPARATION

A. Rate the relevance and adequacy of your academic coursework relative to the needs of **THIS** fieldwork placement, *circling* the appropriate number.

Course	Preparation Minimal Excellent	COMMENTS
Foundations & Concepts of OT	1 2 3 4 5	
Lifespan Occupational Perf.		
Anatomy		
Human Motion and Movement		
Neuroscience		
Occ. Perf. Perspectives		
Fundamentals of Practice		
Occupational Perf. Evaluation		
Medical Conditions in OT		
Clinical Reasoning and FW 1A		
Humans, Groups & Occupations		
Psychosocial Function		
Biomechanical Function		
Sociocultural Systems & Networks		
Clinical Reasoning & FW 1B		
Neurosensorimotor I		
Principles of Research		
Qualitative Research		
Neurosensorimotor II		
Evidence Based Practice		
OT Administration		
Com. & World Healthcare Issues		
Env. Adapt. & Rehab. Technology		
Intervention Seminar		
Fieldwork Proposal		

B. What are the strongest aspects of your academic program relative to the needs of **THIS** Level II Fieldwork Experience? Be specific and include course references as appropriate.

C. Did you find correlation between theories and concepts and skills learned at school and their practical application at this center. Give examples of this type of correlation.

D. What changes would you recommend in your academic program relative to the needs of **THIS** Level II Fieldwork Experience?

Part VI: SUMMARY

A. What particular qualities or personal performance skills do you feel a
   student should have to function successfully on this fieldwork placement?

B. Overall, what changes would you recommend in this Level II Fieldwork
   Experience?

C. Would you recommend this center as a student Fieldwork Experience?
   YES_____No_____Why?

Part VII: ADDITIONAL COMMENTS

Please feel free to add any further comments, descriptions or information
concerning your fieldwork at this center. Please use another sheet if necessary.

We have mutually shared and clarified this Student Evaluation of Fieldwork
Experience report.

_____   _____
Student Signature   FW Supervisor Signature

_____   _____
Educational Program   Date

APPENDIX C: STUDENT/FIELDWORK EDUCATOR WEEKLY REVIEW

Week #: _____ Student: _____ Fieldwork Educator: _____

Strengths:

Growth Areas:

Goals for Next Week:

Meetings, Assignments Due, Etc.:

8

Professionalism and Fieldwork Education

Elizabeth D. DeIuliis, OTD, OTR/L

INTRODUCTION

Fieldwork education is one of the key academic experiences where occupational therapy students have the opportunity to carry out professionalism under the supervision of an occupational therapy practitioner. According to Delany and Bragge (2009), fieldwork education is essential to learning in the health professions, since it facilitates socializing in the practice community, develops professional identity and commitment to lifelong learning, promotes adaptability, and provides skills in collaboration with other professions—which is essential in the current health care environment. Therefore, fieldwork education directly influences professionalism by socializing occupational therapy students in the profession through the development of their attitudes and values to form their personal professional identity (Conner-Kerr, Wittman, & Muzzarelli, 1998; Nolinske, 1995; Sabari, 1985). When occupational therapy professionals have the tools needed for educating and socializing others, the field of occupational therapy becomes stronger.

KEY WORD

Rasch Analysis: A mathematical model of psychometric analysis that allows for distinctions to be made between the varying difficulties of items on an assessment or questionnaire

DeIuliis, E.D.
Professionalism Across Occupational Therapy Practice (pp 201-221).
© 2017 Taylor & Francis Group.

Box 8-1

It is important for occupational therapy fieldwork educators to view the fieldwork experience as a course, and to view the fieldwork student as a learner, not a worker.

Objectives

By the end of reading this chapter and completing the learning activities, the reader should be able to:

1. Identify how professionalism is formally evaluated during level II fieldwork

2. Compare and contract qualities of successful and unsuccessful fieldwork students

3. Compare and contrast qualities of effective and ineffective fieldwork educators

4. Evaluate generational considerations in fieldwork supervision

Fieldwork (FW) education is essential for the process of professional socialization (Argyris and Schon, 1974). FW education provides students with the opportunity to learn professional responsibilities by having them modeled by qualified and experienced personnel, and to then practice these responsibilities under supervision. This supervised learning experience is intended to promote students' development into competent, professional, entry-level practitioners. Once an occupational therapy practitioner agrees to supervise (teach) students for FW, he or she undertakes several responsibilities in training occupational therapy students to become professionals (Box 8-1) (Vogel, Grice, Oxford, Hill, & Moody, 2004).

Professional Behaviors and the American Occupational Therapy Association Fieldwork Performance Evaluation of the Level II Student

The purpose of the American Occupational Therapy Association (AOTA) Fieldwork Performance Evaluation of the Level II FW student (FWPE) is to measure entry-level competence. The AOTA FWPE was designed to measure occupational therapy student's performance of occupational therapy process across multiple settings. Forty-two items have been identified as key skills and behaviors which entry-level practitioners should exhibit. The Rasch Measurement Model was used to develop and analyze the AOTA FWPE, which indicated that not all of these 42 items are equal in level of difficulty. The 42 items range from simple to evaluate and measure, to more difficult and complex. Professionalism and professional behaviors are typical components on level I and II fieldwork evaluations. On the AOTA FWPE, items 28 through 42 pertain to professional behaviors. These items include basic work skills and specific competencies related to management of occupational therapy services, such as: meeting productivity requirements and organization of caseload; communication, including written, oral and nonverbal; and professional behaviors, which includes the qualities of being self-directed, response to constructive feedback, time management, and cultural sensitivity. Atler (2003) provides a helpful Rasch analysis of all 42 items on the FWPE, which indicated that these competencies related to professionalism tend to be "easier" for the fieldwork educator to score. Competencies such as positive interpersonal skills (item 41), responding to feedback (item 38), and adherence to ethics (item 2) were identified as easier items to score for the fieldwork educator.

ATTRIBUTES OF FIELDWORK STUDENTS AND FIELDWORK EDUCATORS THAT INFLUENCE PROFESSIONALISM

Similar to occupational therapy theories and practice models, there needs to be a synergy and complementary interaction between characteristics of both fieldwork students and fieldwork educators to foster the development of professionalism and the occurrence of successful fieldwork experiences. Since the fieldwork educator at the clinical practice site is responsible for the on-site supervision of the fieldwork student, variability exists in the delivery of occupational therapy education at different fieldwork sites. The fieldwork educator is given the autonomy to provide the fieldwork education in a manner that is safe, suitable, and appropriate for the student and for the practice site. The type, frequency, and amount of supervision may be affected by multiple factors including reimbursement issues, staffing concerns, and reimbursement for student-led services.

Fieldwork education, specifically the supervision provided, has the greatest influences on an occupational therapy student's professional development (Christie, Joyce, & Moeller, 1985; Hanson, 2011). "Supervision is the most critical aspect of the fieldwork experience … specifically the attitudinal and interpersonal variables" of the fieldwork educator (Christie et al., 1985, p. 10). In occupational therapy literature, as well as other allied health professional scholarly work, the fieldwork educator (preceptor, or clinical instructor) is cited as the principal influence on a student's learning in clinical education (Grenier, 2015; Hoover et al., 2014; Thomas et al., 2007). Numerous research studies have investigated the perceptions of fieldwork educators and fieldwork students on qualities that are considered effective and ineffective in fieldwork education. The summary Tables 8-1 to 8-4 provide an overview of the themes presented in not just occupational therapy literature, but in other allied health professions as well. Themes surrounding supervision, communication, teaching characteristics, and qualities of professionalism are prominent throughout all literature summarized (see Tables 8-1 to 8-4).

In summary, the literature on clinical education in allied health identifies many attributes of professionalism that both the student and clinical educators feel are important and beneficial in providing a positive learning experience (Boxes 8-2 to 8-5; Table 8-5). "What do I need to put into place in my own life that will enable me to reap the most out of having the privilege to participate in such a noble profession, and in turn, experience a more meaningful personal life in the process?" (Wicks, 2008)

RESOURCES FOR FIELDWORK EDUCATORS TO ENHANCE THEIR EFFECTIVENESS DURING THE FIELDWORK EXPERIENCE

Although many of the attributes listed as effective qualities of fieldwork educators may be inherent intrinsic or extrinsic qualities of professionals, some of these skills can be developed and refined through learning such as independent learning, workshops, or other resources (Hanson, 2011). The lifelong learning aspect of being a professional does not only pertain to clinical skill development. The outline below indicates several strategies and resources geared towards enhancing the effectiveness of fieldwork education.

- Develop and implement a professional development plan for mastery in the fieldwork educator role

- Review and Use Fieldwork Resources provided by the AOTA

	TABLE 8-1 **TRAITS OF EFFECTIVE FIELDWORK EDUCATORS**
An effective fieldwork educator has ...	• Strong interpersonal communication skills • A quality, professional relationship with students
An effective fieldwork educator is ...	• Flexible • Friendly • Welcoming • Encouraging • Organized • Caring • Empathetic • A competent, knowledgeable practitioner • Authoritative, yet supportive • Passionate about the profession • Committed to teaching • Interested in the student as an occupational being • A role model
An effective fieldwork educator does ...	• Communicate in a clear, specific, consistent manner • Provide a detailed orientation • Provide constructive feedback • Provide validation • Provide structured supervision • Provide positive reinforcement • Provide variety in patient caseload and other experiences • Demonstrate legal and ethical behavior • Demonstrate professional attitudes and actions • Demonstrate consistent work behaviors • Build the student's confidence • Model the use of reflection • Stimulate clinical reasoning • Use shared problem-solving • Utilize active learning • Ask probing or provoking questions: "Tell me why?" • Make the student feel like a member of the team <div align="right">*continued*</div>

TABLE 8-1 (CONTINUED)
TRAITS OF EFFECTIVE FIELDWORK EDUCATORS

	• Create a positive space for student learning
	• Create a supportive learning environment
	• Create clear and realistic entry-level expectations
	• Adapt teaching style to the needs of the student
	• Match teaching to the student's learning style
	• Act as a facilitator and a guider

Adapted from: Christie, B. A., Joyce, P. C., & Moeller, P. L. (1985). Fieldwork experience, part II: The supervisor's dilemma. *American Journal of Occupational Therapy, 39*(10), 675-681; Cohn, E., & Crist, P. (1995). Back to the future: New approaches to fieldwork education. *American Journal of Occupational Therapy, 49*(2), 103-106; Curtis, N., Helion, J. G., & Domsohn, M. (1998). Student athletic trainer perceptions of clinical supervisor behaviors: A critical incident study. *Journal of Athletic Training, 33*(3), 249-253; De Beer, M., & Vorster, C. (2012). Fieldwork education: Putting supervisors' interpersonal communication to the test. *South African Journal of Occupational Therapy, 42*(1), 21-26; Deluliis, E. (2011). Using the occupational profile for student-centered fieldwork. *OT Practice, 16*(14), 13; Doherty, G., Stagnitti, K., & Schoo, A. (2009). From student to therapist: A follow up of a first cohort of Bachelor of occupational therapy students. *Australian Occupational Therapy Journal, 56*(5), 341-349; Dunn, S. V., & Hansford, B. (1997). Undergraduate nursing students' perceptions of their clinical learning environment. *Journal of Advanced Nursing, 25*(6), 1299-1306; Grant, J., Kilminster, S., Jolly, B., & Cottrell, D. (2003). Clinical supervision of SpRs: Where does it happen, when does it happen and is it effective? *Medical Education, 37*(2), 140-148; Grenier, M. (2015). Facilitators and barriers to learning in occupational therapy fieldwork education: Student perspectives. *American Journal of Occupational Therapy, 69*(Suppl. 2), 6912185070; Hansford, D. (2002, June). Insights into managing an age-diverse workforce. *Workspan, 45*(6), 48-54; Hanson, D. (2011). The perspectives of fieldwork educators regarding level II fieldwork students. *Occupational Therapy in Healthcare, 25*(2-3), 164-167; Hanson, D. (2014). Level II fieldwork success: A cooperative effort. *OT Practice, 19*(12), 18-19; Hoover, K. D., Podvey, M. C., Carrico, N., Gochuico, M. J., Griffin, K., Lipnick, M., ... & Vongsoasup, P. (2014). Successful fieldwork experiences: A clinical educators' perspective. Retrieved from http://files.abstractsonline.com/CTRL/04/6/F75/982/ 192/4BE/989/186/78A/1BF/45E/80/a1481_1.pdf; Hummel, J. (1997). Effective fieldwork supervision: Occupational therapy student perspectives. *Australian Occupational Therapy Journal, 44*, 147-157; Landa-Gonzalez, B., Velis, E., & Greg, K. (2015). Learning styles as predictors of fieldwork performance and learning adaptability of graduate nontraditional occupational therapy students. *Journal of Allied Health, 44*(3), 145-151; Laurent, T., & Weidner, T. G. (2001). Clinical instructors' and student athletic trainers' perceptions of helpful clinical instructor characteristics. *Journal of Athletic Training, 36*(1), 56-61; Levy, L. S., Sexton, P., Willeford, K. S., Barnum, M. G., Guyer, M. S., Gardner, G., & Fincher, A. L. (2009). Clinical instructor characteristics, behaviors and skills in allied health care settings: A literature review. *Athletic Training Education Journal, 4*(1), 8-13; Mackenzie, L. (2002). Briefing and debriefing of student fieldwork experiences: Exploring concerns and reflecting on practice. *Australian Occupational Therapy Journal, 49*, 82-92; McGovern, M. A., & Dean, E. D. (1991). Clinical education: The supervisory process. *International Journal of Language & Communication Disorders, 26*(3), 373-381; Platt, L. S. (2000). Leadership skills and abilities, professional attributes, and teaching effectiveness in athletic training clinical instructors. *Dissertation Abstracts International, 61*(10), 5220B; Platt Meyer, L. S. (2002) Leadership characteristics as significant predictors of clinical-teaching effectiveness. *Athletic Therapy Today, 7*(5), 34-39; Provident, I., Leibold, M. L., Dolhi, C., & Jeffcoat, J. (2009, October 26). Becoming a fieldwork educator: Enhancing your teaching skills. *OT Practice, 14*(19) CE1–CE8; Richard, L. (2008). Exploring connections between theory and practice: Stories from fieldwork supervisors. *OT in Mental Health, 24*(2), 154-175; Stafford, E. M. (1986). Relationship between occupational therapy student learning styles and clinic performance. *American Journal of Occupational Therapy, 40*(1), 34-39; Stormont, D. A. (2001). The significance of the interpersonal relationship in practicum supervision: What is it about Fleur? Retrieved from www.aare.ed.au/98pap/sto98234.htm; Swann E. (2002). Communicating effectively as a clinical instructor. *Athletic Therapy Today, 7*(5), 28-33; Weidner, T. G., & Henning, J. M. (2002). Being an effective athletic training clinical instructor. *Athletic Therapy Today, 7*(5), 6-11; Weidner, T.G., Trethewey, J., & August, J.A. (1997). Learning clinical skills in athletic therapy. *Athletic Therapy Today, 2*(5), 43-49; Williams, P. L., & Webb, C. (1994). Clinical supervision skills: A Delphi and critical incident technique study. *Medical Teacher, 16*(2-3), 139-157; Wilson, R. (1996). Clinical preceptor conferences as a venue for total quality education. *Optometric Education, 21*(3), 85-89; Winstanley, J., & White, E. (2003). Clinical supervision: Models, measures and best practice. *Nurse Researcher, 10*(4), 7-38.

TABLE 8-2
TRAITS OF INEFFECTIVE FIELDWORK EDUCATORS

An ineffective fieldwork educator has ...	• Poor administrative skills • Poor communication skills • A high need for control • A lack of trust
An ineffective fieldwork educator is ...	• Unprofessional • Intimidating • Close-minded • A micro-manager

continued

TABLE 8-2 (CONTINUED)	
TRAITS OF INEFFECTIVE FIELDWORK EDUCATORS	
An ineffective fieldwork educator is ...	• Not evidence-based • Not enthusiastic • Not supportive • Burnt out • Unapproachable • Unethical • Unavailable to teach • Disorganized • Disengaged • Inflexible
An ineffective fieldwork educator does not ...	• Actively include the student • Make the student feel like a part of the team • Introduce the student to other team and staff members • Respect confidentiality of clients and students • Clearly explain complex concepts • Provide the student a workspace in the clinic • Provide student-centered learning • Provide sufficient supervision • Provide an adequate model • Provide constructive feedback • Advocate for the profession

Adapted from: Christie, B. A., Joyce, P. C., & Moeller, P. L. (1985). Fieldwork experience, part II: The supervisor's dilemma. *American Journal of Occupational Therapy, 39*(10), 675-681; Curtis, N., Helion, J. G., & Domsohn, M. (1998). Student athletic trainer perceptions of clinical supervisor behaviors: A critical incident study. *Journal of Athletic Training, 33*(3), 249-253; Grenier, M. (2015). Facilitators and barriers to learning in occupational therapy fieldwork education: Student perspectives. *American Journal of Occupational Therapy, 69*(Suppl. 2), 6912185070; Hanson, D. (2011). The perspectives of fieldwork educators regarding level II fieldwork students. *Occupational Therapy in Healthcare, 25*(2-3), 164-167; Kinsella, E. A., Park, A. J., Appiagyei, J., Chang, E., & Chow, D. (2008). Through the eyes of students: Ethical tensions in occupational therapy practice. *Canadian Journal of Occupational Therapy, 75*(3), 176-183; Lew, N., Cara, E., & Richardson, P. (2007). When fieldwork takes a detour. *Occupational Therapy in Healthcare, 21*, 105-122; Li, C. Y., Chung, L., Chen, T. J., Shih, M. J., Yang, N. T., & Pan, A. W. (2006). Investigation of the professional identity among occupational therapists: viewpoints of national college students. *Medical Education, 10*, 197e208; Mackenzie, L. (2002). Briefing and debriefing of student fieldwork experiences: Exploring concerns and reflecting on practice. *Australian Occupational Therapy Journal, 49*, 82-92; Williams, P. L., & Webb, C. (1994). Clinical supervision skills: A Delphi and critical incident technique study. *Medical Teacher, 16*(2-3), 139-157.

TABLE 8-3
TRAITS OF SUCCESSFUL FIELDWORK STUDENTS

A successful fieldwork student has ...	• Self-awareness • Emotional intelligence • Emotional maturity • Strong communication skills • Strong organization skills • Strong problem-solving skills • Initiative • Drive • Autonomy • Honesty • Integrity • Good common sense • Clinical competency • Strong work ethic
A successful fieldwork student is ...	• Able to build therapeutic relationships • Self-directed • Self-motivating • Solutions-oriented • Eager to learn • Assertive • Professional • Ethical • Accountable • Empathetic • Flexible • Adaptable • Hands-on • Social • Understanding of boundaries

continued

TABLE 8-3 (CONTINUED)
TRAITS OF SUCCESSFUL FIELDWORK STUDENTS

A successful fieldwork student does …	<ul><li>Seek out feedback</li><li>Respond well to feedback</li><li>Demonstrate conflict-resolution skills</li><li>Take risks</li><li>Ask questions</li><li>Make eye contact</li><li>Present self well</li><li>Follow through</li><li>Engage actively</li><li>Collaborate effectively</li><li>Demonstrate good safety and judgement</li><li>Accept supervision</li><li>Know when to ask for help</li><li>Balance productivity, leisure, and rest</li><li>Demonstrate commitment and dedication to the profession</li></ul>

Adapted from Campbell, M. K., & Corpus, K. (2015). Fieldwork educators' perspectives: Professional behavior attributes of Level II fieldwork students. *Open Journal of Occupational Therapy, 3*(4), Article 7; Cohn, E., & Crist, P. (1995). Back to the future: New approaches to fieldwork education. *American Journal of Occupational Therapy, 49*(2), 103-106; Grenier, M. (2015). Facilitators and barriers to learning in occupational therapy fieldwork education: Student perspectives. *American Journal of Occupational Therapy, 69*(Suppl. 2), 6912185070; Gutman, S. A., McGreedy, P., & Heisler, P. (1998). Student level II fieldwork failure: Strategies for intervention. *American Journal of Occupational Therapy, 52*(2), 143-149; Hammer, D. (2000). Professional attitudes and behaviors: The "A's and B's" of professionalism. *American Journal of Pharmaceutical Education, 64*, 455-464; Hanson, D. (2011). The perspectives of fieldwork educators regarding level II fieldwork students. *Occupational Therapy in Healthcare, 25*(2-3), 164-167; Hoover, K. D., Podvey, M. C., Carrico, N., Gochuico, M. J., Griffin, K., Lipnick, M., … & Vongsoasup, P. (2014). Successful fieldwork experiences: A clinical educators' perspective. Retrieved from http://files.abstractsonline.com/CTRL/04/6/F75/982/ 192/4BE/989/186/78A/1BF/45E/80/a1481_1.pdf; Krusen, N. E. (2015). Student voices following fieldwork failure: A phenomenological inquiry. *International Journal of Practice-based Learning in Health and Social Care, 3*(1), 16-29; Landa-Gonzalez, B., Velis, E., & Greg, K. (2015). Learning styles as predictors of fieldwork performance and learning adaptability of graduate nontraditional occupational therapy students. *Journal of Allied Health, 44*(3), 145-151; Richard, L. (2008). Exploring connections between theory and practice: Stories from fieldwork supervisors. *OT in Mental Health, 24*(2), 154-175; Werther, K., & Schmitz, C. (2014). Valued qualities exhibited by occupational therapy students: An exploration of preceptor perspectives [PowerPoint presentation]. Retrieved from http://enothe.eu/Wordpress%20Documents/2014%20Powerpoints/Valued%20qualities%20exhibited%20by%20occupational%20therpay%20students%3B%20an%20exploration%20of%20preceptor%20perspectives.pdf

TABLE 8-4
TRAITS OF UNSUCCESSFUL FIELDWORK STUDENTS

An unsuccessful fieldwork student has …	<ul><li>Poor communication skills</li><li>Poor organization skills</li><li>Difficulty relating to other professionals</li><li>Difficulty responding to feedback</li><li>Difficulty making decisions; hesitates excessively</li><li>Difficulty engaging in the supervisory process</li><li>Limited personal awareness</li></ul>

continued

	TABLE 8-4 (CONTINUED) **TRAITS OF UNSUCCESSFUL FIELDWORK STUDENTS**
An unsuccessful fieldwork student has ...	• Lack of insight into their learning style • Lack of emotional intelligence • Reduced flexibility • Preference for passive reflection
An unsuccessful fieldwork student is ...	• Unenthusiastic • Disinterested • Outwardly overwhelmed • Resistive • Defensive • Not confident enough or overly confident • Uncomfortable in handling clients
An unsuccessful fieldwork student does not ...	• Regularly initiate engagement • Ask questions • Multi-task • Demonstrate progress with efficacy and independence • Demonstrate good safety and judgement

Adapted from Grenier, M. (2015). Facilitators and barriers to learning in occupational therapy fieldwork education: Student perspectives. *American Journal of Occupational Therapy, 69*(Suppl. 2), 6912185070; Gutman, S. A., McGreedy, P., & Heisler, P. (1998). Student level II fieldwork failure: Strategies for intervention. *American Journal of Occupational Therapy, 52*(2), 143-149; Hanson, D. (2011). The perspectives of fieldwork educators regarding level II fieldwork students. *Occupational Therapy in Healthcare, 25*(2-3), 164-167; Hummel, J. (1997). Effective fieldwork supervision: Occupational therapy student perspectives. *Australian Occupational Therapy Journal, 44*, 147-157; James, K., & Mussleman, L. (2006). Commonalities in level II fieldwork students. *Occupational Therapy in Healthcare, 21*, 105-122; Jarski, R. W., Kulig, K., & Olson, R. E. (1990). Clinical teaching in physical therapy: Student and teacher perceptions. *Physical Therapy, 70*(3), 173-178; Kramer, P., & Stern, K. (1995). Case report: Approaches to improve student performance on fieldwork. *American Journal of Occupational Therapy, 49*, 156-159; Landa-Gonzalez, B., Velis, E., & Greg, K. (2015). Learning styles as predictors of fieldwork performance and learning adaptability of graduate nontraditional occupational therapy students. *Journal of Allied Health, 44*(3), 145-151; Mackenzie, L. (2002). Briefing and debriefing of student fieldwork experiences: Exploring concerns and reflecting on practice. *Australian Occupational Therapy Journal, 49*, 82-92; Richard, L. (2008). Exploring connections between theory and practice: Stories from fieldwork supervisors. *OT in Mental Health, 24*(2), 154-175.

BOX 8-2

WHAT CAN UNPROFESSIONALISM DURING FIELDWORK LOOK LIKE?

Unprofessionalism during fieldwork can be a result of poor intrinsic qualities, extrinsic qualities, or a combination of both types of qualities of professionalism.

Extrinsic:

• Sloppy, unkempt appearance

• Failure to be prepared

• Requires continual reminders about responsibilities or patient care assignments

• Poor interpersonal interaction with fellow students, instructors, patients, and families

• Chronic fatigue and sleep deprivation   *continued*

Box 8-2 (CONTINUED)

WHAT CAN UNPROFESSIONALISM DURING FIELDWORK LOOK LIKE?

Extrinsic (continued):

- Arrogant and demeaning behaviors
- Excessive tardiness or absenteeism

Intrinsic:

- Lack of conscientiousness or failure to fulfill responsibilities at an acceptable level

Both:

- Lack of effort and enthusiasm towards developing and improving clinical skills
- Failure to accept responsibility for errors and learn from mistakes
- Unethical behavior such as failure to abide by confidentiality and privacy regulations

Box 8-3

CONSEQUENCES OF UNPROFESSIONALISM ON FIELDWORK

- Academic Consequences: Failure of FW course(s)
  - Extend FW course
  - Repeat FW, which may include re-register for credits (financial implications)
- Potential legal/civil consequences: such as fine, imprisonment
  - i.e., HIPAA violation
  - Revocation of AOTA membership
  - Inability to take National Board for Certification in Occupational Therapy exam

Box 8-4

TIPS FOR FIELDWORK STUDENTS TO INCREASE ORGANIZATION AND TIME MANAGEMENT

- Use a clipboard and take notes
- Write to-do lists, use post-it notes, have a planner/schedule
- Set deadlines
- Learn to multi-task
- Use down-time productively
- Engage in point-of-contact documentation
- Put equipment/supplies back after use

continued

Box 8-4 (CONTINUED)

TIPS FOR FIELDWORK STUDENTS TO INCREASE ORGANIZATION AND TIME MANAGEMENT

- Learn to delegate nonclinical tasks to other team members such as aides or technicians
- Observe others who are good time managers

Adapted from Napier, B. (2011). *Occupational therapy student fieldwork survival guide* (2nd ed.). Bethesda, MD: AOTA.

Box 8-5

TIPS TO MANAGING AND/OR REDUCING STRESS ON FIELDWORK

- Engage in regular relaxation, exercise, solid nutrition, and sleep
- Partake in nonfieldwork related activities or hobbies
- Be proactive
- Ask for help when needed
- Journal
- Spend time with your family and friends outside of fieldwork
- Practice fieldwork-life-balance

Adapted from American Occupational Therapy Association. (2006). Level II fieldwork survival guide. Retrieved from https://intraweb.stockton.edu/eyos/gradstudies/content/docs/msot/Level%20II%20Fieldwork%20Survival%20Guide%20for%20Students.pdf.

TABLE 8-5

SUGGESTIONS TO PROMOTE A SUCCESSFUL FIELDWORK EXPERIENCE

PHASE	ACTION
Pre-FW	<ul><li>Provide student a learning style inventory (see Chapter 5)</li><li>Use a teaching style inventory (see Chapter 5)</li><li>Seek to understand your student as an occupational being (Deluliis, 2011)</li><li>Establish SMART site-specific objectives (remember the novice-to-expert continuum)</li><li>Create weekly schedule for skill progression (patient caseload, responsibilities, projects etc.); see Appendix A</li><li>Plan for structured time for feedback (weekly review forms) see Appendix B</li><li>Create a fieldwork manual specifying clear expectations for your fieldwork students. Suggested policies: dress code, time/attendance, use of technology and social media, confidentiality, and privacy</li></ul>

continued

PHASE	ACTION
During	<ul><li>Provide student with fieldwork manual</li><li>Provide a detailed orientation for student to staff, space and environment</li><li>Incorporate time and space for feedback sessions</li><li>Share your time management strategies with the student</li><li>Use teachable moments: one minute preceptors (Grenier, 2015)</li><li>Identify learning activities outside of patient care: i.e. staffing meetings, supervision of volunteers, etc., observe a surgery, shadow/interview other health care providers</li><li>Ask for help! Use academic fieldwork coordinators or site supervisor as a resource</li><li>Learning contract; see Appendix C</li><li>Document! Document! Document! Document! Keep organized fieldwork files, and track feedback sessions and evaluations</li></ul>
After	<ul><li>Seek out feedback from the student on your role as the fieldwork educator</li><li>Reflect</li><li>Seek out resources to enhance your effectiveness</li></ul>

TABLE 8-5 (CONTINUED)
SUGGESTIONS TO PROMOTE A SUCCESSFUL FIELDWORK EXPERIENCE

The AOTA offers many resources to support Fieldwork Educators. The AOTA website (www.aota.org) provides many useful documents that can be downloaded, including:

- Resources for establishing a new fieldwork program
- Sample weekly learning schedules for fieldwork students
- Suggestions for an onsite fieldwork manual
- Sample site-specific objectives

AOTA Self-Assessment Tool for Fieldwork Educator Competency

The AOTA Self-Assessment Tool for Fieldwork Educator Competency identifies the competencies a fieldwork educator should have: professional practice, education, supervision, evaluation, and administration (AOTA, 2009). The AOTA's Fieldwork Experience Assessment Tool was designed to promote discussions between students and fieldwork educators, facilitate reflection and problem solving, encourage observation and modeling, and allow fieldwork educators to provide graded learning experiences as a teaching strategy (AOTA, 2001).

The Fieldwork Experience Assessment Tool

The Fieldwork Experience Assessment Tool, which can be completed by both the fieldwork educator and fieldwork student, was designed to enhance the learning experience during level II FW.

The tool consists of a form that evaluates three key components of the fieldwork experience including the environment, fieldwork educator, and the fieldwork student. Each of these three components are further broken down; for example, the fieldwork educator section includes a deep dive into the fieldwork educator's attitude, professional attributes and teaching style, and the fieldwork student section looks at the student's attitude and learning behaviors. This tool can be an excellent strategy to identify concerns with professional behaviors and create an opportunity to discuss the common and different perspectives of the fieldwork educator and the student.

Self-Assessment for Fieldwork Educator Competency

A tool designed to help fieldwork educators "evaluate their degree of competency in supervising students, while also identifying areas for enhancement of development of necessary skills" (Geraci & Hanson, 2014, p. 7). The five main areas of competence are: professional practice, education, supervision, and evaluation of fieldwork student performance. The tool also includes a fieldwork educator professional development plan, encouraging the fieldwork educator to identify goals to enhance their supervisory skills.

SEEK OUT TRAINING AND CONTINUING EDUCATION

- The AOTA Fieldwork Educators Certificate Program
  - This hands-on workshop is designed for both novice and experienced fieldwork educators, and is geared towards deepening participants' understanding of the fieldwork educator role. This two day workshop includes learning modules such as administration, education, supervision, and evaluation, which are key aspects of the fieldwork educator role. Participants can obtain up to 15 contact hours for licensure renewal and/or National Board for Certification in Occupational Therapy recertification.
- Become a member of Education Special Interest Section
  - Members of the AOTA are able to select up to two areas of interest and receive quarterly supplements. The Education Special Interest Section focuses on academic and clinical education topics.
- Network with other fieldwork educators and academic fieldwork coordinators
  - AOTA.org provides information about fieldwork councils and consortia across the country. Fieldwork consortia are typically made up of academic professionals represented from occupational therapy and occupational therapy assistant programs and fieldwork educators who are dedicated to enhancing the quality of occupational therapy fieldwork. These consortia may have meetings, workshops, or continuing education opportunities specifically focused on fieldwork education.

SUMMARY

A synthesis of the literature presented in this chapter indicates that while clinical competency and skill mastery are obvious critical requirements for success during fieldwork, there is an equal or arguably heavier emphasis on the many intrinsic and extrinsic qualities of professionalism. Professionalism is expected and required of both a successful fieldwork student and an effective fieldwork educator. Fieldwork education is vital in shaping and enhancing not only the clinical and professional reasoning of occupational therapy students, but propelling the occupational therapy profession forward as a whole.

LEARNING ACTIVITIES

1. A learning contract is not used just for remediation. Using the format presented in Appendix C, create three SMART goals for yourself as you prepare for upcoming fieldwork experiences. Outline specific strategies to accomplish these goals.

2. Reflect on fieldwork educators you have had during your occupational therapy education. Identify strategies that helped to promote your learning

3. Write a letter to your future self describing the type of fieldwork educator you aspire to be. List a few things you remember that most helped you be successful in fieldwork. List a few things you swear you will never do as a fieldwork educator.

4. Metaphors provide means of understanding and experiencing one thing in relationship to another. For example, "fieldwork is like a box of chocolates, you never know what you are going to get." Use the following prompts to create metaphors about your fieldwork experiences:

   a. Collaborating with other professionals on fieldwork is like …

   b. Fieldwork supervision is like …

   c. Dealing with challenging clients on fieldwork is like …

   d. Getting feedback from my fieldwork educator is like …

REFERENCES

American Occupational Therapy Association. (2001). Fieldwork experience assessment tool (FEAT). Retrieved from https://www.aota.org/-/media/Corporate/Files/EducationCareers/ Accredit/FEATCHARTMidterm.pdf

American Occupational Therapy Association. (2006). Level II fieldwork survival guide. Retrieved from https://intraweb.stockton.edu/eyos/gradstudies/content/docs/msot/Level%20II%20Fieldwork%20Survival%20Guide%20for%20Students.pdf

American Occupational Therapy Association. (2009). The American Occupational Therapy Association self-assessment tool for fieldwork educator competency. Retrieved from https://www.aota.org/-/media/Corporate/Files/EducationCareers/Educators/Fieldwork/Supervisor/Forms/Self-Assessment%20Tool%20FW%20Ed%20Competency%20%282009%29.pdf

Argyris, C., & Schon, D. (1974). *Theory and practice: Increasing professional effectiveness.* San Francisco, CA: Jossey Bass.

Atler, K. (2003). *The complete guide: Using the fieldwork performance evaluation forms.* State College, PA: AOTA Press.

Campbell, M. K., & Corpus, K. (2015). Fieldwork educators' perspectives: Professional behavior attributes of Level II fieldwork students. *Open Journal of Occupational Therapy, 3*(4), Article 7.

Christie, B. A., Joyce, P. C., & Moeller, P. L. (1985). Fieldwork experience, part II: The supervisor's dilemma. *American Journal of Occupational Therapy, 39*(10), 675-681.

Cohn, E., & Crist, P. (1995). Back to the future: New approaches to fieldwork education. *American Journal of Occupational Therapy, 49*(2), 103-106.

Conner-Kerr, T. A., Wittman, P., & Muzzarelli, R. (1998). Analysis of practice-role perceptions of physical therapy, occupational therapy and speech-language pathology students. *Journal of Allied Health, 27*(3), 128-131.

Curtis, N., Helion, J. G., & Domsohn, M. (1998). Student athletic trainer perceptions of clinical supervisor behaviors: A critical incident study. *Journal of Athletic Training, 33*(3), 249-253.

De Beer, M., & Vorster, C. (2012). Fieldwork education: Putting supervisors' interpersonal communication to the test. *South African Journal of Occupational Therapy, 42*(1), 21-26.

DeIuliis, E. (2011). Using the occupational profile for student-centered fieldwork. *OT Practice, 16*(14), 13.

Delany, C., & Bragge, P. (2009). A study of physiotherapy students' and clinical educators' perceptions of learning and teaching. *Medical Teacher, 31*(9), e402-e411.

Doherty, G., Stagnitti, K., & Schoo, A. (2009). From student to therapist: A follow up of a first cohort of Bachelor of occupational therapy students. *Australian Occupational Therapy Journal, 56*(5), 341-349.

Dunn, S. V., & Hansford, B. (1997). Undergraduate nursing students' perceptions of their clinical learning environment. *Journal of Advanced Nursing, 25*(6), 1299-1306.

Geraci, J., & Hanson, D. (2014, January 20). Resources for fieldwork education. *OT Practice, 19*(1), 7-8.

Grant, J., Kilminster, S., Jolly, B., & Cottrell, D. (2003). Clinical supervision of SpRs: Where does it happen, when does it happen and is it effective? *Medical Education, 37*(2), 140-148.

Grenier, M. (2015). Facilitators and barriers to learning in occupational therapy fieldwork education: Student perspectives. *American Journal of Occupational Therapy, 69*(Suppl. 2), 6912185070.

Gutman, S. A., McGreedy, P., & Heisler, P. (1998). Student level II fieldwork failure: Strategies for intervention. *American Journal of Occupational Therapy, 52*(2), 143-149.

Hammer, D. (2000). Professional attitudes and behaviors: The "A's and B's" of professionalism. *American Journal of Pharmaceutical Education, 64*, 455-464.

Hansford, D. (2002, June). Insights into managing an age-diverse workforce. *Workspan, 45*(6), 48-54.

Hanson, D. (2011). The perspectives of fieldwork educators regarding level II fieldwork students. *Occupational Therapy in Healthcare, 25*(2-3), 164-167.

Hanson, D. (2014). Level II fieldwork success: A cooperative effort. *OT Practice, 19*(12), 18-19.

Hoover, K. D., Podvey, M. C., Carrico, N., Gochuico, M. J., Griffin, K., Lipnick, M., ... & Vongsoasup, P. (2014). Successful fieldwork experiences: A clinical educators' perspective. Retrieved from http://files.abstractsonline.com/CTRL/04/6/F75/982/ 192/4BE/989/186/78A/1BF/45E/80/a1481_1.pdf

Hummel, J. (1997). Effective fieldwork supervision: Occupational therapy student perspectives. *Australian Occupational Therapy Journal, 44*, 147-157.

James, K., & Mussleman, L. (2006). Commonalities in level II fieldwork students. *Occupational Therapy in Healthcare, 21*, 105-122.

Jarski, R. W., Kulig, K., & Olson, R. E. (1990). Clinical teaching in physical therapy: Student and teacher perceptions. *Physical Therapy, 70*(3), 173-178.

Kinsella, E. A., Park, A. J., Appiagyei, J., Chang, E., & Chow, D. (2008). Through the eyes of students: Ethical tensions in occupational therapy practice. *Canadian Journal of Occupational Therapy, 75*(3), 176-183.

Kramer, P., & Stern, K. (1995). Case report: Approaches to improve student performance on fieldwork. *American Journal of Occupational Therapy, 49*, 156-159.

Krusen, N. E. (2015). Student voices following fieldwork failure: A phenomenological inquiry. *International Journal of Practice-based Learning in Health and Social Care, 3*(1), 16-29.

Landa-Gonzalez, B., Velis, E., & Greg, K. (2015). Learning styles as predictors of fieldwork performance and learning adaptability of graduate nontraditional occupational therapy students. *Journal of Allied Health, 44*(3), 145-151.

Laurent, T., & Weidner, T. G. (2001). Clinical instructors' and student athletic trainers' perceptions of helpful clinical instructor characteristics. *Journal of Athletic Training, 36*(1), 56-61.

Levy, L. S., Sexton, P., Willeford, K. S., Barnum, M. G., Guyer, M. S., Gardner, G., & Fincher, A. L. (2009). Clinical instructor characteristics, behaviors and skills in allied health care settings: A literature review. *Athletic Training Education Journal, 4*(1), 8-13.

Lew, N., Cara, E., & Richardson, P. (2007). When fieldwork takes a detour. *Occupational Therapy in Healthcare, 21*, 105-122.

Li, C. Y., Chung, L., Chen, T. J., Shih, M. J., Yang, N. T., & Pan, A. W. (2006). Investigation of the professional identity among occupational therapists: viewpoints of national college students. *Medical Education, 10*, 197e208.

Mackenzie, L. (2002). Briefing and debriefing of student fieldwork experiences: Exploring concerns and reflecting on practice. *Australian Occupational Therapy Journal, 49*, 82-92.

McGovern, M. A., & Dean, E. D. (1991). Clinical education: The supervisory process. *International Journal of Language & Communication Disorders, 26*(3), 373-381.

Napier, B. (2011). *Occupational therapy student fieldwork survival guide* (2nd ed.). Bethesda, MD: AOTA.

Nolinske, T. (1995). Multiple mentoring relationships facilitate learning during fieldwork. *American Journal of Occupational Therapy, 49*(1), 39-43.

Platt, L. S. (2000). Leadership skills and abilities, professional attributes, and teaching effectiveness in athletic training clinical instructors. *Dissertation Abstracts International, 61*(10), 5220B.

Platt Meyer, L. S. (2002) Leadership characteristics as significant predictors of clinical-teaching effectiveness. *Athletic Therapy Today, 7*(5), 34-39.

Provident, I., Leibold, M. L., Dolhi, C., & Jeffcoat, J. (2009, October 26). Becoming a fieldwork educator: Enhancing your teaching skills. *OT Practice, 14*(19) CE1–CE8.

Richard, L. (2008). Exploring connections between theory and practice: Stories from fieldwork supervisors. *OT in Mental Health, 24*(2), 154-175.

Sabari, J. S. (1985). Professional socialization: Implications for occupational therapy education. *American Journal of Occupational Therapy, 39*(2), 96-102.

Stafford, E. M. (1986). Relationship between occupational therapy student learning styles and clinic performance. *American Journal of Occupational Therapy, 40*(1), 34-39.

Stormont, D. A. (2001). The significance of the interpersonal relationship in practicum supervision: What is it about Fleur? Retrieved from www.aare.ed.au/98pap/sto98234.htm

Swann E. (2002). Communicating effectively as a clinical instructor. *Athletic Therapy Today, 7*(5), 28-33.

Thomas, Y., Dickson, D., Broadbridge, J., Hopper, L., Hawkins, R., Edwards, A., & McBryde, C. (2007). Benefits and challenges of supervising occupational therapy fieldwork students: Supervisors' perspectives. *Australian Occupational Therapy Journal, 54*, S2-S12.

Vogel, K. A., Grice, K. O., Hill, S., & Moody, J. (2004). Supervisor and student expectations of level II fieldwork. *Occupational Therapy in Health Care, 18*(1-2), 5-19.

Weidner, T. G., & Henning, J. M. (2002). Being an effective athletic training clinical instructor. *Athletic Therapy Today, 7*(5), 6-11.

Weidner, T.G., Trethewey, J., & August, J.A. (1997). Learning clinical skills in athletic therapy. *Athletic Therapy Today, 2*(5), 43-49.

Werther, K., & Schmitz, C. (2014). Valued qualities exhibited by occupational therapy students: An exploration of preceptor perspectives [PowerPoint presentation]. Retrieved from http://enothe.eu/Wordpress%20 Documents/2014%20Powerpoints/Valued%20qualities%20exhibited%20by%20occupational%20therpay%20 students%3B%20an%20exploration%20of%20preceptor%20perspectives.pdf

Wicks, R. J. (2008). *The resilient clinician.* Oxford, United Kingdom: Oxford University Press.

Williams, P. L., & Webb, C. (1994). Clinical supervision skills: A Delphi and critical incident technique study. *Medical Teacher, 16*(2-3), 139-157.

Wilson, R. (1996). Clinical preceptor conferences as a venue for total quality education. *Optometric Education, 21*(3), 85-89

Winstanley, J., & White, E. (2003). Clinical supervision: Models, measures and best practice. *Nurse Researcher, 10*(4), 7-38.

APPENDIX A: LEVEL II FIELDWORK EDUCATION OCCUPATIONAL THERAPY STUDENT WEEKLY BEHAVORIAL OJECTIVES TEMPLATE

LEVEL II FIELDWORK EDUCATION
OCCUPATIONAL THERAPY STUDENT WEEKLY BEHAVIORAL OBJECTIVES TEMPLATE

WEEK	RESPONSIBILITIES	CASELOAD	ASSIGNMENTS
1			
2			
3			
4			
5			
6			

continued

Level II Fieldwork Education

Occupational Therapy Student Weekly Behavioral Objectives Template (Continued)

WEEK	RESPONSIBILITIES	CASELOAD	ASSIGNMENTS
7			
8			
9			
10			
11			
12			

APPENDIX B: STUDENT/ FIELDWORK EDUCATOR WEEKLY REVIEW

Week #: _____ Student: _____ Fieldwork Educator: _____

Strengths:

Growth Areas:

Goals for Next Week:

Meetings, Assignments Due, Etc.:

APPENDIX C: SAMPLE LEARNING CONTRACT

PERFORMANCE ISSUE/ CONCERN (BE SPECIFIC)	EXPECTED PERFORMANCE GOAL (BEHAVIORAL GOAL- SMART)	STRATEGIES, ACTIONS AND RESOURCE(S) REQUIRED TO MEET THE GOAL	PLAN FOR FOLLOW-UP/ TIMELINE (ESTABLISH DATE/TIME FOR PERFORMANCE TO BE RE-EVAL- UATED)	CONSEQUENCES IF PERFOR- MANCE NOT IMPROVED

By providing a signature, both parties are acknowledging the above performance issues, and agree to participate in the performance improvement plan as outlined above. It is the student's responsibility to access resources, carry out these and/or other strategies to improve his or her performance and implement feedback in the identified problem areas. Failure to meet expected performance in established timeline may indicate disciplinary action and/or failed fieldwork experience.

Student signature: _____ Date: _____

Fieldwork Educator(s) signature(s): _____ Date: _____

For use at follow-up meeting

Learning Contract/Action Plan REVIEW OUTCOME

Evidence to demonstrate change in performance/outcome:

_____Review met expectations
_____Review did not meet expectations* Disciplinary action may be necessary.

Student signature:_____ Date: _____

Fieldwork Educator(s) signature(s): _____ Date: _____

*encourage all parties involved to keep copy for their records

9

Clinical Vignettes
Common Fieldwork Professional Behavior Scenarios

Elizabeth D. DeIuliis, OTD, OTR/L

INTRODUCTION

Fieldwork tests a student's resolve. The transition from classroom to clinic can be one of the most stressful and challenging experiences a student will encounter. This transition involves leaving a familiar environment—campus, classes, friends, and faculty—and challenges occupational therapy students to adapt to a new environment and new expectations, which requires an emotional adjustment. This can be a time of personal growth and maturation, as well as a time of increased stress, which may challenge students to rise to the professional expectations of the real world and the profession. This chapter will provide examples of common unprofessional scenarios that could occur during fieldwork, as well as identify strategies in how to handle them. Although there is no one "right" way to handle any of these scenarios, strategies are presented to guide professional behavior, attitude, and conduct.

UNPROFESSIONAL FIELDWORK STUDENT SCENARIOS

Scenario 1: Fieldwork Student Has Difficulty Accepting Constructive Feedback

A fieldwork (FW) educator provides constructive feedback to a FW student about how to perform a stand-pivot-transfer with better body mechanics. The FW student tells the FW educator that she was taught a different way to transfer in school, and prefers to transfer the way she was taught rather than considering the FW educator's advice.

DeIuliis, E.D.
Professionalism Across Occupational Therapy Practice (pp 223-227).
© 2017 Taylor & Francis Group.

How to Prevent the Situation

Fieldwork education provides plenty of opportunities for occupational therapy students to be provided with constructive feedback, which is a crucial part of their learning and development in becoming an entry-level practitioner. To prevent having a difficult time accepting constructive feedback, the student should understand that FW is a learning process that will inevitably include receiving feedback.

How to Handle the Situation

The student should acknowledge the FW educator's experience and knowledge, and should make an effort in the future to be open to new techniques and different perspectives. Instead of challenging the FW educator's expertise, the student may use a phrase such as "Can you help me understand the clinical rationale of this technique?" as means to gather additional information to support their learning. The FW educator should continue to provide the student with feedback that will be beneficial to sharpening and broadening the student's clinical skills.

Scenario 2: Overly Confident Fieldwork Student

An occupational therapy assistant student is beginning week four of an eight week Level II FW experience on an inpatient psychiatric unit. The student received a satisfactory midterm score, yet several areas were noted as progressing and needing improvement. The student is ultimately pleased with the midterm evaluation and takes initiative in beginning the morning group therapy session with individuals with schizophrenia, even though the FW educator instructed the student to wait until they were present to begin.

How to Prevent the Situation

Fieldwork students should be knowledgeable about their role, supervisor expectations and overall responsibilities during fieldwork experiences. The FW student should acknowledge that ultimately the FW educator is responsible for the FW student and should comply with their instructions.

How to Handle the Situation

Fieldwork students need to remember that they are developing practitioners. Their FW educators, who are more experienced, may have a different viewpoint and perspective, especially in regards to safety. In this scenario, without the counsel of the FW educator, the student may not be aware of key safety information such as a client with new symptoms of suicide ideation, or self-injurious behavior. Occupational therapy FW students should initiate conversation with their fieldwork educator and know their boundaries with their role.

Scenario 3: Fieldwork Student Chooses to "Coast" After Receiving a Passing Midterm Score

During his or her final Level II experience, a FW student receives a passing score on the AOTA fieldwork performance evaluation form. The student then chooses to "coast" through the second half of the rotation.

How to Prevent the Situation

To prevent this situation, the student should set professional development goals for herself in the beginning of the FW experience. The student should work consistently throughout the entire FW experience to not only meet their professional development goals, but to exceed them. Occupational therapy fieldwork educators should establish site-specific behavioral objectives to guide the FW experience, demonstrating a realistic progression of student learning and responsibilities.

How to Handle the Situation

The FW student needs to find motivation in other aspects of the FW experience apart from grades. The student should focus on other motivating factors and continue to try her best throughout the second half of the rotation.

Scenario 4: Being Unaware of Unprofessional Behaviors

A FW student with an outgoing personality is very social with clients, often asking them personal and unrelated questions. The FW student thinks she is being friendly, but the FW educator finds the conversations to be inappropriate.

How to Prevent the Situation

The student should be aware of appropriate conversation topics and be educated on how to use the therapeutic modes to create a professional and trusting relationship with the client. Fieldwork educators should model professional interaction with clients and colleagues. The use of role play may be a helpful strategy to simulate appropriate clinical encounters.

How to Handle the Situation

The FW educator should immediately address the situation with the fieldwork student, and identify clear examples of unprofessional behavior. The FW educator can provide the student with appropriate conversation topics and related questions the student can use when speaking with clients.

UNPROFESSIONAL FIELDWORK EDUCATOR SCENARIOS

Scenario 1: Crossing Professional Boundaries

A FW educator asks their current FW student (or a patient) to be their "friend" on a social media site.

How to Prevent the Situation

The FW educator is responsible for demonstrating and role modeling professional relationships for the FW student. The FW educator is also responsible for complying with all employer policies related to use of social media. Integrating social media with the student FW educator relationship or practitioner patient relationship crosses a boundary that can lead to unethical practice.

How to Handle the Situation

As a student professional, an occupational therapy student is required to maintain a professional relationship with their FW educator. The student should comply with their academic program policies and not accept the request. The student should also notify the academic FW coordinators. The student can respectfully ignore the "friend" request until after the FW placement is finished, and accept the "friend" request after. The student can ask the FW educator what the facility's policies and regulations are on adding patients on social media websites to determine if any policies are being violated.

Scenario 2: Degrading the Student as "Just a Student"

During treatment sessions, the FW educator frequently refers to the FW student as "just a student" in front of the patient and other health care team members.

How to Prevent the Situation

The FW educator and site clinical coordinator for fieldwork are responsible for being knowledgeable about the role, expectations, and responsibilities of occupational therapy fieldwork students. The student should take the initiative and introduce themselves to the client by stating "Hi, my name is _____ and I am an occupational therapy student from _____ University."

How to Handle the Situation

The student can have a conversation with the FW educator about how the student is more than "just a student", and by telling other health care professionals that could hurt the amount of participation they allow the student with clients. In addition, the student can explain his or her experience and education, and the supervision being provided by the FW educator. The student can ask the FW educator what the difference is between a FW student and a student observing to clarify an understanding that the two positions are different.

Scenario 3: Poor Modeling of Confidentiality

During the lunch hour in the cafeteria, the FW student observes their fieldwork educator talking about patient-protected health information of one of their clients with a clinician who is not providing care to this particular client, and who is not on a need-to-know basis.

How to Prevent the Situation

All health care providers, including students, are responsible for complying with HIPAA regulations. Competencies and trainings can be used to teach and verify understanding for both employees, students, and volunteers. Fieldwork educators are responsible for being professional and ethical role models for fieldwork students.

How to Handle the Situation

The student can approach the fieldwork educator and inform them that they overheard the conversation and did not want to make assumptions. However, they were under the impression that the other clinician was not part of the client's current health care team. The student can also ask the FW educator about rules on patient confidentially and what the consequences are if a clinician breaks these rules.

Scenario 4: Unethical Scoring of Fieldwork Performance Evaluation

During the formal midterm review of the AOTA fieldwork performance evaluation, the fieldwork educator reports that they give every Level II student a "2" at midterm, regardless of their performance, and never assign a score of a "3."

How to Prevent the Situation

The FW educator is responsible for being knowledgeable and competent in using and scoring the AOTA fieldwork performance evaluation. If unsure, the FW educator can counsel with the academic fieldwork coordinators.

How to Handle the Situation

The student can have a conversation with the FW educator after receiving a "2" and request more specific feedback from the educator on his or her performance. If the FW educator does not provide a rationale for scoring a "2" on the performance evaluation, the student should talk with their academic fieldwork coordinators to discuss the issue.

SUMMARY

The transition from the classroom to the clinic can be a challenging experience for both the occupational therapy student and the fieldwork educator. Fieldwork education provides an opportunity and a context for occupational therapy students and fieldwork educators to apply and refine both clinical and professional skill sets. Having clear expectations, policies, and procedures to enforce professional behaviors are necessary measures for fieldwork sites and academic programs. As professionals, FW educators and fieldwork students have an obligation to enforce professional behavior policies and report misconduct to the appropriate individual(s), which may include Academic Fieldwork Coordinator, Compliance Officer, or Administrator. Maintaining neat and detailed documentation of unprofessional scenarios is essential. Increasing the emphasis of professionalism during FW education will assist the profession in embodying the Centennial Vision.

Part IV

Professionalism in Clinical Practice

Professionalism isn't just something expected by faculty and fieldwork educators. Employers, patients, and other health care providers are also concerned with an occupational therapy practitioner's knowledge, attitudes, behaviors, and actions surrounding professionalism. The final section of this textbook is intended to discuss the importance of professionalism throughout clinical practice as an occupational therapy practitioner, including navigating the credentialing process after graduation, job searching, interviewing, and the importance of continued competence and engagement in professional service and other scholarly activities.

10

The Credentialing Process

Elizabeth D. DeIuliis, OTD, OTR/L

INTRODUCTION

Congratulations, you did it! After completing the requirements for graduation from an accredited occupational therapy education program, the next step is to secure the credentials of certified or registered and licensed practitioner. Registration and certification is obtained by passing the National Board Certification Exam (NBCOT). Licensure is granted by the state. It is the occupational therapy graduate's professional responsibility to be knowledgeable about the process and requirements for each of these important tasks. This chapter will discuss the occupational therapy practitioner's professional responsibilities throughout the credentialing process.

KEY WORDS

Certification: Refers to the confirmation of certain characteristics of an person

Competency: The ability to do something successfully or meet necessary standards

Continuing Education Unit: A unit of credit equal to ten hours of participation in a learning program, designed for professionals with certificates or licenses to practice in various professions, to secure credentials

Credential: A qualification, achievement, or aspect of an individual's background, typically awarded through a document or certificate, indicating they are competent to practice in their field; can apply to a variety of levels, such as state and national

Professional Development Unit: A unit of measure for professional learning and development to meet professional body requirements, such as the National Board for Certification in Occupational Therapy

DeIuliis, E.D.
Professionalism Across Occupational Therapy Practice (pp 231-237).
© 2017 Taylor & Francis Group.

OBJECTIVES

By the end of reading this chapter and completing the learning activities, the reader should be able to:

1. Describe the credentialing process for a new graduate
2. Understand the professional responsibility required to obtain initial licensure/certification and/or registration
3. Explain the importance and professional responsibility required to seek renewal of licensure/certification and/or registration

A credential is a qualification, achievement, or aspect of an individual's background typically used to indicate they are suitable to perform a job. In many occasions, it is awarded in the form of a document or certificate proving a person's identity or qualifications. Most health care providers are required to seek and maintain various credentials throughout their professional career indicating they are legitimate, fit, and competent to practice in their field. To enter practice after successful completion of their educational program, occupational therapy graduates must seek credentials from the National Board for Certification in Occupational Therapy (NBCOT), as well as through the state(s) in which they desire to practice.

STATE LICENSURE

Occupational therapy practice is regulated in all 50 states, the District of Columbia, Puerto Rico, and Guam. Different states have various types of regulation that range from licensure, the strongest form of regulation, to title protection or trademark law, the weakest form of regulation. To obtain a license, a practitioner needs to:

- Graduate from an accredited Occupational Therapy or Occupational Therapy Assistant educational program
- Complete all fieldwork requirements
- Apply for and pass the NBCOT Certification Examination (more about the NBCOT exam will be discussed later in this chapter)
- Apply for a license and pay a fee for each state/jurisdiction in which you wish to practice or hold a license (if applying for a travel/contract position, you may be required to obtain licensure in multiple states)

Many, but not all, states allow practitioners to practice on a temporary license or limited permit while waiting to take or receive the results of the certification exam. If you do not pass the exam on your first attempt, you may not be able to continue to practice on a temporary license. Each state occupational therapy regulatory agency should be consulted for specific requirements. Many times there is a waiting period between the time an individual submits a completed application with all requirements met until they receive their license and are able to practice. Some states also require first-time license applicants to take a test on the rules and regulations specific to that state. Likewise, maintenance of one's license varies according to the state. Most states require the practitioner to renew his or her license every two years. It is a professional's responsibility to be knowledgeable about the credentialing process and to know what resources are available when questions arise. You can visit www.aota.org for further details regarding state occupational therapy practice acts and regulations.

CERTIFICATION AND REGISTRATION

The purpose of the NBCOT certification exam is to protect the public interest by certifying only those candidates who have the necessary knowledge of occupational therapy to practice (NBCOT, 2016a). The registered occupational therapist (OTR) and certified occupational therapy assistant (COTA) examinations are constructed to measure entry-level competence of candidates who have met eligibility requirements for certification of their respective credential. Initial certification by the NBCOT is a requisite for licensure in all 50 U.S. states and the District of Columbia. The certification process for U.S. candidates consists of three main phases, each with its own set of requirements, forms, and/or fees.

Determine Your Eligibility

To be deemed eligible to sit for the NBCOT certification examination, U.S. candidates must have graduated (including completion of fieldwork requirements) with one of the following accredited/approved entry-level occupational therapy degrees:

- Associate degree in occupational therapy (COTA Exam)
- Entry-level master's degree in occupational therapy (OTR Exam)
- Entry-level doctoral degree in occupational therapy (OTR Exam)

Apply for the Exam

After applying for the NBCOT Certification examination through MyNBCOT, a candidate must submit an official final college or university transcript that indicates the degree date and title, or an academic credential verification form within six months of the candidate receiving his or her final degree. The pass/fail status of candidates who submit an academic credential verification form will not be released until the NBCOT receives an official final transcript.

Agree to Abide by the NBCOT Practice Standards/Code of Conduct

The Standards of Practice in Occupational Therapy are the baseline for quality occupational therapy care, holding OTR and COTA certificants accountable for delivering consistent, high quality health care services (NBCOT, 2016b). The Standards provide guidelines that can be used to determine what the OTR or COTA should and should not do when providing services to clients. These Standards represent the expectations of the NBCOT and may be used to evaluate performance for ongoing professional development and/or disciplinary action.

The NBCOT Standards of Practice consist of four sections:

- Practice domains
- Code of professional conduct
- Supervision
- Documentation

National Board for Certification in Occupational Therapy expects both certificants—those who are already certified and/or registered—and applicants to uphold the organization's Code of Conduct Principles. There are eight principles which deal with honesty, integrity, accountability, responsibility, professional behavior, and ethical behavior, paralleling many of the values of the occupational therapy Code of Ethics (Boxes 10-1 and 10-2) (NBCOT, 2016c).

Box 10-1

BEING PROFESSIONAL IN YOUR PREPARATION FOR THE NBCOT EXAM

Preparing for the NBCOT exam requires more than just studying. Adequate preparation requires an individual to display professionalism through demonstrating strong time management skills in developing a study plan, organizational skills in preparing study materials, and proactivity in completing the process to apply for the exam. According to data collected by the NBCOT, candidates are most likely to pass the certification exam on the first attempt when taken within the first 60 days post-graduation (Grace, 2015).

Box 10-2

HELPFUL STUDY RESOURCES FOR THE NBCOT EXAM

- DiZazzo-Miller and Pellerito (2009) in their text, "Preparing for the OT National Board Exam: 45 Days and Counting", provide a detailed schedule for 45 days of study.

- TherapyEd (2016) provides preparatory classes and study guides, which include information on test taking strategies, realistic practice questions, and outlines.

- AOTA's NBCOT Exam Prep includes retired COTA and OTR Exam questions, which are copyrighted 2013 by the National Board for Certification in Occupational Therapy, Inc. This study resource provides the option of a realistic test experience, including timed questions.

The NBCOT completes periodic surveys to identify textbooks and peer-reviewed journals commonly used in occupational therapy and occupational therapy assistant educational programs. These surveys result in an updated reference list of publications used in entry-level occupational therapy academic programs which will be used by NBCOT item writers to reference items developed for the OTR and COTA certification examinations. The references will also be available to the Certification Examination Validation Committee (CEVC) to verify and validate items appearing on the certification examinations. You can access the registered occupational therapy and occupational therapy assistant curriculum text and peer-reviewed journal report at www.nbcot.org (NBCOT, 2016d).

How to Apply for NBCOT Exam

Once you have prepared yourself for the exam content, the next step is to apply to take the exam. Please note, you must complete the exam application in one sitting. You cannot exit the screen, login, and start where you left off.

1. Be sure to read the exam handbook

2. Register for your account through MyNBCOT using a valid email address—make sure you check whether your occupational therapy school email address remains valid after graduation

3. Complete and submit the exam application and pay using a major credit card

4. Have your school registrar submit an official final transcript or academic credential verification form

5. Schedule the exam through Prometric (see Box 10-3 for more information)

6. Take the exam

Box 10-3

PREPARATION FOR PROMETRICS TESTING CENTER

On the day of the test, candidates must arrive at least 30 minutes prior to the start of the exam, and are required to present two pieces of official identification at the Prometric Test Center. Both forms of identification must match the first and last names as they appear on the authorization to test letter. If the identification does not match the authorization to test letter, you will not be able to test, and your exam fee will be forfeited. A currently valid government issued photo ID with legal name and legible signature is acceptable as a primary form of identification. Acceptable secondary identification include a current major credit card with expiration date (i.e. Visa, MasterCard, American Express, or Discover), ATM card, Employee ID card, voter registration card or letter, or Student ID card. Social Security cards are not acceptable forms of identification. More FAQs regarding how to best prepare for the day of the exam can be found at www. nbcot.org.

For additional information regarding the examination, including ordering score transfers and/or state confirmation notices, refer to www. nbcot.org (Box 10-3).

Certification/Registration Renewal

Being knowledgeable about the certification and registration process is not only important for new graduates, but also for practicing occupational therapists. Whereas completion of the NBCOT certification exam is mandatory to obtain initial credentials and state licensure, the certification itself is technically voluntary. Despite being voluntary, many occupational therapists choose to maintain certification to stay competitive and current in this field. Continuing education and professional development is required to maintain the OTR or COTA designation. It is also important to ensure that certification is renewed on time. Late renewals may result in a penalty fee, delayed renewal, or suspension of credentials.

NBCOT certification is granted for a three-year period. Certificants who complete all certification renewal requirements by their scheduled renewal date will be granted Active in Good Standing certification status for another three-year period. The certification renewal season occurs between January and March annually, regardless of the month indicated on the certificant's initial certification document. During the renewal process, certificants must complete an attestation stating that they have complied with the professional development unit requirements, as well as remain compliant with the certificant code of conduct. A minimum of 36 professional development units are required to renew certification and/or registration. The NBCOT offers a professional development unit log as a method for certificants to track their professional development unit accrual as well as store documentation of completion. Certificants who do not submit their certification renewal application by the scheduled renewal date will have their certification status changed to Noncompliant-Inactive. An individual who has Noncompliant-Inactive certification cannot use the OTR or COTA certification marks (Boxes 10-4 and 10-5).

Box 10-4

PROFESSIONAL DEVELOPMENT UNITS

There are 33 different ways to earn professional development units for NBCOT. The six main categories of types of units are:

- Workshops/Courses/Independent Learning: Employer-sponsored continuing education, attendance to professional conferences, independent learning, etc.

- Fieldwork Supervision: Formal supervision of Level I or II fieldwork students, or occupational therapy department students

- Presenting: Serving as an adjunct faculty member or guest lecturer, or presenting at a conference

- Publishing: Developing instructional materials or publications

- Professional Service: Volunteering, or mentoring as discussed in Chapter 6

- NBCOT Navigator: This is the newest method to accrue professional development units, occurring through interactive learning tools and games

---

Box 10-5

TIPS ON BEING PROFESSIONAL IN THE CREDENTIALING PROCESS

- Be organized: Use a professional portfolio to maintain and organize documentation of professional development unit and Continuing Education Unit activities

- Be proactive: Know your recertification period; have the necessary forms, paperwork and signatures needed ahead of time

- New graduates, communicate with your occupational therapy faculty. Many state forms needs to be signed off by the Program Director and/or Registrar, or academic fieldwork coordinators regarding proof of fieldwork experiences

- Be thorough and detail oriented

- Be ethical and honest: Application for the certification examination includes some questions that relate to felony convictions

- Maintain a professional portfolio: Suggestions for what to include and showcase are discussed in Chapter 11

SUMMARY

Being knowledgeable about the process and expectations for initial and recredentialing is a responsibility of being an occupational therapy professional. Occupational therapy practitioners are able to validate their entry-level competence, as well as mastery of skills, knowledge, and abilities through the (re)credentialing process. It is evident that our clients, colleagues, and peers all benefit from credentialing.

LEARNING ACTIVITIES

1. Find and review the occupational therapy practice act or state licensure board website for your state. Discuss what it lists regarding continuing competence credits, malpractice insurance, working on a temporary license, occurrence of failing the NBCOT exam when operating with a temporary license, supervision of COTA/Ls, and delegation of tasks to non-occupational therapy personnel such as aides or technicians. If you are completing fieldwork in a different state, find and review the practice act for this state as well.

2. Create two SMART goals for yourself that you will accomplish in regards to the NBCOT study prep process

3. Determine the licensure process in your home state. Provide information regarding renewal requirement, including continuing competence if required.

REFERENCES

DiZazzo-Miller, R., & Pellerito, J. (2009). *Preparing for the OT National Board exam: 45 days and counting.* Burlington, MA: Jones & Bartlett Learning.

Grace, P. (2015, October). *NBCOT report.* Presentation presented at AOTA/OTCAS Education Summit, Denver, CO.

National Board for Certification in Occupational Therapy. (2016a). About NBCOT. Retrieved from http://www.nbcot.org/about-us

National Board for Certification in Occupational Therapy. (2016b). Practice standards. Retrieved from http://www.nbcot.org/practice-standards-regulators

National Board for Certification in Occupational Therapy. (2016c). Practice standards/code of conduct. Retrieved from http://www.nbcot.org/certificant-code-of-conduct

National Board for Certification in Occupational Therapy. (2016d). Curriculum textbook and peer-reviewed journal reports: OTR & COTA. Retrieved from http://www.nbcot.org/textbook-journal-reports

TherapyEd. (2016). Prepare for the NBCOT exam. Retrieved from https://www.therapyed.com/occupational-therapy

Marketing Yourself as a Professional

Elizabeth D. DeIuliis, OTD, OTR/L

INTRODUCTION

Whether you are a new graduate or an experienced practitioner, the current job market is intense. Regardless of our backgrounds, we all want to make great first impressions with potential employers. Your cover letter and résumé or curriculum vitae (CV) are typically the first impressionable part of the job search process. This chapter will cover best practices and strategies for successfully presenting yourself to a potential employer, both on paper through a competitive and professional cover letter, résumé, and/or CV, as well as in person during an interview.

According to research, employers and recruiters tend to follow a consistent visual path when removing cover letters and résumés from consideration. Therefore, layout and organization of these documents is crucial. In fact, a study by TheLadders.com showed that recruiters spend about six seconds scanning a résumé before sending it into the "yes" or "no" pile (Evans, 2012). Whereas employers read through résumés to determine experience and qualifications, review of these documents also showcases elements of the individual's professional identity. They may not win you the job by themselves, but it is all too true that a poorly crafted cover letter and résumé can squash your chances of ever getting to the next level in the job search process. So, if it's a job interview you're after, it's worth the extra time and effort to make sure your cover letter and résumé sparkle accordingly. After all, they are representing you!

KEY WORDS

Cover Letter: A document sent with a résumé to provide additional information on the prospective employee's skills and experience

DeIuliis, E.D.
Professionalism Across Occupational Therapy Practice (pp 239-281).
© 2017 Taylor & Francis Group.

Curriculum Vitae: A detailed document which contains information on a person's academic background, including teaching experiences, degrees, research, awards, publications, presentations, service, and other achievements

Résumé: A document that contains a person's education, qualifications, and previous experience, typically sent with a job application or provided during a job interview

Teaching Philosophy Statement: A self-reflective statement of an educator's beliefs about teaching and learning

OBJECTIVES

By the end of reading this chapter and completing the learning activities, the reader should be able to:

1. Describe the professional intent of a cover letter, résumé, and CV

2. Understand the benefits of a professional portfolio

3. Demonstrate the ability to design a professional cover letter and résumé

COVER LETTER

A cover letter is an application or introductory letter of interest for a particular job, whether solicited from advertisement or unsolicited (Lasovich, 2009). A professional should always submit a cover letter with a résumé. It introduces the job hunter to an employer and indicates a desire for an interview with that employer. A cover letter is typically a one-page document (Appendices A and B).

Three Components to a Cover Letter

First Paragraph

States why you are writing, how you learned about the desired position, and basic information about yourself.

Second Paragraph

Includes the body of the letter and explains why you should be hired by describing how your work experience qualifies you for the job. Demonstrate that you know enough about the employer or position to relate your background to what is being sought out. Mention specific qualifications which make you a good fit for the employer's needs. Focus on what you can do for the employer, not what the employer can do for you. This is an opportunity to explain in more detail relevant items in your résumé. Refer to the fact that your résumé is enclosed. Mention other enclosures if such are required to apply for a position. Indicate why you are interested in the company. Use a third paragraph to further explain your qualifications and interests if necessary.

Final Paragraph

Indicates a desire for an interview. Include contact information and indicate the type of response that you anticipate from the letter. Always detail how you will follow up on your application. Indicate that you would like the opportunity to interview for a position or to talk with the employer to learn more about their opportunities or hiring plans. State what you will do to follow

---

Box 11-1

TIPS ON DRAFTING A PROFESSIONAL COVER LETTER

- Use the same format and style (i.e. font, heading, paper quality, etc.) as your résumé.

- Always address the cover letter to a specific person, usually the individual responsible for filling the position. Never address the cover letter to "Sir or Madam" or "To Whom It May Concern." This is a letter to a real person, so it should be addressed to that person's name. A "Dear Mr. Smith" greeting comes across more friendly and knowledgeable than a "To Whom It May Concern" one. Also, using the name within the body of the letter creates a warm yet professional atmosphere for the reader. Call or research the company at the library or over the Internet to get the name and title of the person responsible for hiring new employees. If you cannot find a particular person's name, use the person's specific title—such as "Human Resource Manager."

- Be concise, enthusiastic, and natural when writing the cover letter. Write the letter similar to the way you normally speak. You want this letter to be a representation of your authentic professional self.

- Omit any personal information. Remember that this is a formal letter.

- Do not use clichés such as "I've taken the liberty of enclosing my résumé," or "I'm a people person." A cover letter should be unique to your talents and capabilities. The more unique the letter, the higher your chance of securing an interview. Avoid sending standard cover letters to employers. You never know if one hiring manager at one company knows a hiring manager at another company. You would not want both individuals to discover that they each received the same letter!

- Always proofread the letter for grammatical and spelling mistakes.

---

up, such as telephone the employer within two weeks. If you will be in the employer's location and could offer to schedule a visit, indicate when this could occur. State that you would be glad to provide the employer with any additional information needed. Thank the employer for her or his consideration.

Sincerely,

Your handwritten signature (on hard copy) (Box 11-1).

RÉSUMÉ

A résumé is a professional document that summarizes your education, experiences, and competencies. It's designed to introduce you to an employer and highlight your qualifications for a specific job or type of work. The art of crafting a professional résumé is an important quality for both students and practitioners at any level of experience. You may not think of it this way, but your résumé is a personal marketing tool, and can certainly help to land a job, secure a fieldwork opportunity, or assist in the admissions process for a graduate or advanced certificate program.

Process to Develop Your Professional Résumé

Drafting your first professional résumé may be something you are asked to do as a student, and can be a difficult task. Here are a few tips to start the process:

Box 11-2

PROFESSIONAL TIP

Tip: It may be beneficial to have more than one version of your résumé. For example, as a new graduate, if you are unsure whether you are interested in working in pediatrics or in an adult physical disability setting, it may be beneficial to have one résumé highlighting your pediatric skill set and a different résumé for working with adults.

Brainstorm and begin with a self-assessment. To put together an effective résumé, it is important to know your abilities, what skills you have developed, what values are important to you in a career, and what you can offer to an employer. The first step in preparing your résumé is to think about yourself, your experiences, and your accomplishments. Ask yourself these kinds of questions:

- What skills have I developed?
- What are my strengths?
- What have I accomplished
- Why should someone hire me?
- Who is my target audience?

Make a list of your present and past experiences, accomplishments, and skills. Often, employers look for applicants with two skill sets: hard skills and soft skills (Box 11-2). Hard skills are the technical skills and typically the knowledge gained from your occupational therapy education, continuing education, or advanced training. For example, hard skills would pertain to clinical populations you have experience with, evaluation tools or assessments you are competent in administering, intervention skills you are familiar with, advanced training such as being a certified lymphedema therapist, etc.

Soft skills can be harder to quantify and more often relate to those intrinsic and extrinsic qualities of professionalism such as interpersonal skills, teamwork, problem solving, leadership abilities, etc. The National Association of Colleges and Employers (2014) conducted a study on 260 employers and found the following five soft skills to be the most valuable in employees, in order of importance:

1. Ability to work in a team structure
2. Ability to make decisions and solve problems
3. Ability to communicate verbally with people inside and outside an organization
4. Ability to plan, organize, and prioritize work
5. Ability to obtain and process information

Although you need the hard skills to get your foot in the door for a position, it is often the soft skills that make you stand out and ultimately get hired. Therefore, it is imperative to highlight both of these types of skills in your résumé and during the interview process (Box 11-3).

Select from this list the information that will be pertinent for your résumé and the job for which you are applying. Draw from academic work and honors, clubs and activities, volunteer experiences, and prior work experiences. You may have developed many basic skills in diverse contexts that can be transferred to a variety of work environments, such as organizational, communication, and interpersonal skills, as well as learning to meet deadlines and communicate ideas to a variety of people. Getting together basic ideas about your set of skills will make writing your résumé an easier task (Box 11-4).

Box 11-3

SOFT SKILLS THAT EXEMPLIFY QUALITIES OF PROFESSIONALISM

- Flexibility: Adapts to changing conditions
- Teamwork skills: Ability to work interprofessionally, cooperative attitude
- Time management: Ability to effectively manage multiple tasks, set priorities, and meet deadlines
- Interpersonal skills: Effective communicator
- Leadership: Ability to motivate others
- Generational competence: Ability to build rapport with a diverse workforce
- Organization: Attention to detail
- Critical thinking skills: Ability to problem solve and make decisions
- Self-management: Conscientious, go-getter

Box 11-4

APPLICABLE SKILL SETS FROM WORK EXPERIENCE

Part-time job as a waiter

- Skill sets: Customer service (communication), multi-tasking, teamwork

Part-time job in the library

- Skill sets: Organization, attention to detail, time management

Part-time job as a lifeguard

- Skill sets: Discipline, focus, responsibility, judgment

Box 11-5

EXAMPLES OF POWER VERBS

Demonstrated, accomplished, executed, performed, initiated, participated, completed, created, fulfilled, developed, employed, established, led, managed, achieved, etc.

Elaborate on your list by writing a short, concise description of each experience, accomplishment or skill. Try to have at least two to three bullets for each accomplishment or skill. Begin each phrase with a unique action or power verb. For example, instead of writing that you worked with clients who have neurological injuries, instead state that you demonstrated competency with clinical evaluation and intervention within the acute neurological population (Box 11-5).

With each experience you list on your résumé, highlight a different skill set you gained or refined. Try not to repeat or overuse the same professional skill word, action verb, or other characterizing words in describing your background and experiences.

Organize your résumé in an effective format by placing the most critical and current information first. Use a reverse chronological order to list your accomplishments. Whereas most

---

Box 11-6

BASIC COMPONENTS TO A PROFESSIONAL RÉSUMÉ

- Your name and contact information; be sure that your contact information includes a professional email address—not coolestOT@email.com
- Objective of résumé submission
- Educational experience
- Achievements, honors, awards, and scholarships
- Scholarship such as presentations, publications, and research projects
- Relevant experience, such as clinical positions held, fieldwork placements, service learning, etc.
- Other related experience, such as other jobs, or roles
- Service such as volunteerism and leadership positions in organizations
- Memberships and qualifications with the AOTA, state occupational therapy association, etc.
- Continuing education, with a list of professional development units/continuing education units received, unique trainings, etc.

---

careers recommend a one-page résumé (short and sweet), in service careers such as health care, you are starting off with valid, relevant experience (i.e. fieldwork experience, service learning, etc.) Therefore, a two to three page résumé is both recommended and okay for an occupational therapy practitioner. The best way to market yourself as a professional and practitioner is to list and describe your experiences. However, you must be sure to choose elements that are necessary and relevant to the job you are seeking. Therefore, you may have more than one résumé at any given time. As a new graduate, if you are looking into various different practice settings, you may have one résumé geared toward pediatric practice which highlights a certain skill set, and another résumé geared toward physical disability practice, each showcasing different abilities and experiences (Box 11-6).

Format your résumé using a professional style and font. Keep your résumé easy to read by being cognizant of the type and size of your font, ensuring that these remain consistent throughout. It is recommended to use a simple classic font such as Times New Roman, Arial, Helvetica, or Courier.

Read and review your résumé. Be sure to use spell check, and have a friend or colleague review your cover letter and résumé as well. According to the Recruitment and Employment Commission, around 50% of all résumés received by recruitment consultants contain spelling or grammatical errors (Jones & Ashton, 2009). Spelling and grammar mistakes can indicate that the individual did not take the time to proofread, or lacks important written communication skills. Make sure that your résumé is not one of those 50%! (Boxes 11-7 to 11-9)

Professional References

Employers usually ask for professional references, individuals who can vouch for your skills and qualifications, before making a hiring choice. Some jobs require a list of individuals who can speak with the employer. Other jobs require formal written letters of recommendation. In either case, it is beneficial to have a combination of individuals who can serve as professional references that can

---

Box 11-7

WHAT NOT TO INCLUDE IN YOUR RÉSUMÉ

- Irrelevant personal information such as sex, religious beliefs, political affiliation, or date of birth
- Irrelevant work experience
- Salary expectations
- Photograph
- Inaccurate information

Box 11-8

RÉSUMÉ TIPS

- Invest in high-quality paper! If you are submitting via U.S. postal service or in person during an interview, the use of formal résumé paper is recommended. Résumé paper is slightly thicker paper than standard printer paper. It is a subtle way to make a great professional impression. Many argue that having a color that is slightly different than white helps a résumé to stand out in a large stack of papers, as well. For this purpose, use soft, nonoffensive colors such as cream, ivory, and grey.

- Attend to the spacing and margins. Your résumé should look "clean," not cluttered.

- Demonstrate correct spelling and grammar—this is critical. Stellar written communication skills show competence and professionalism.

- Use power verbs! (See Box 11-5 for examples.)

- Avoid use of abbreviations.

- Pay attention to the verb tenses you use—be consistent.

- Showcase your abilities and skills! Detailing your experiences can be difficult, especially since societal norms often prevent us from boasting about our success and talents. Your résumé and interview are one of the only socially acceptable opportunities to toot your own horn!

- Update frequently. Once you have the foundation set for your professional résumé, it is easy to update and maintain. Make it an effort to revise and add in pertinent information to your résumé at least twice a year.

Box 11-9

METHODS TO DELIVER YOUR RÉSUMÉ AND COVER LETTER

Electronic: In today's age of technology, it is common to apply and submit application materials including your cover letter and résumé electronically, either via email or an online database system. You may be prompted to upload your cover letter and résumé documents, or manually input information. Sometimes formatting can be altered, so be sure to preview all versions prior to submission. *continued*

Box 11-9 (CONTINUED)

METHODS TO DELIVER YOUR RÉSUMÉ AND COVER LETTER

Electronic (continued): If sending an email, be sure that you have the correct email address, and include an appropriate subject line, perhaps referencing the job ID you are applying for, or the department.

Fax: Double check that you have the correct fax number, and use a cover sheet for confidentiality purposes. Be sure to get a confirmation that your fax was received.

U. S. Postal Service: Use nice quality paper as previously indicated. Be sure that any information that is handwritten, such as the address, is legible and easy to read.

In person: In addition to using good quality résumé paper, be sure that you are professionally dressed and polite when delivering your résumé materials.

Box 11-10

STEPS TO BUILD YOUR PROFESSIONAL REFERENCE LIST

- Always ask for permission from your references before using them as a reference.
- Be sure to get the correct spelling of their name, position title, credentials, and current contact information.
- Typically seek out at least three individuals to serve as your professional references. They may be a former fieldwork educator, faculty member, Academic Fieldwork Coordinator, boss, mentor, or another respected person from your personal life (other than family members), etc.
- Do not choose people who are not well versed on your background and accomplishments.
- Prepare your references in advance by sharing your current résumé or CV and cover letter, and the position description you may be applying for.

---

speak to both your technical, clinical, or hard skills, as well as personal attributes or soft skills such as professionalism. Examples of professional behaviors your references should be able to speak to are time management, punctuality, ability to work in a team, integrity, leadership, interpersonal skills, and more (Box 11-10).

Examples of sample résumés and reference lists are provided to you as appendices to this chapter (Appendices C to E).

PROFESSIONAL PORTFOLIO

The use of a portfolio is common to many careers and professions. For example, a photographer, architect, or interior designer may use a "pitch book" to showcase his or her talents to potential customers. Like cover letters and résumés, a professional portfolio can be an effective way to provide a highly focused profile of one's skills, abilities, and professional accomplishments. Although occupational therapy students may be instructed to create a portfolio during their educational journey, even a more experienced occupational therapy practitioner can benefit from maintaining a professional portfolio. A portfolio is a collection of evidence or "artifacts," which demonstrate the continuing acquisition of skills, knowledge, attitudes, understanding, and achievements (Brown, 1992; Wilcox,1997).

According to Nagayda, Schindehette, and Richardson (2005), "a portfolio is a visual representation of personal and professional goals and accomplishments" (p. 7). A common job interview question is to "Describe an experience when…" What better way for a job candidate to do so than with a tangible, physical artifact from their portfolio? Since occupational therapy personnel can move across a variety of roles and settings, the portfolio, as a historical and working record, can be used to facilitate reflection on one's various roles and functions. Occupational therapy literature regarding the maintenance of portfolios advocates for their use to record and verify skill acquisition and learning experiences in career development, and to document learning outcomes. A professional's portfolio is expected to be more than just a collection of accomplishments, as they show in detail how the individual grew through a reflective process, documenting what and how something was learned. Thus, the portfolios serve not only as a basis for a retrospective review of accomplishments, but also become a prospective guide for future professional development planning.

The purpose of a professional portfolio is to:

1. Provide concrete examples of your professional and technical skill set

2. Show your career path and growth as a professional

3. Prepare for recertification process, serving as a means to track and organize all professional development and continuing education materials

Your portfolio can be kept in hard copy, such as a 3-ring binder or leather portfolio with plastic sheet protectors and dividers to stay organized. You can also develop an electronic portfolio instead. Adobe Acrobat has a portfolio option, or you can alternatively scan important documents and pictures into PDFs and load them onto a disc or jump drive. This may be a good option when you would like to leave information after an interview ends with a potential employer. Funk (2007) investigated the use of portfolios in occupational therapy education and found that they assisted students to develop the professional skills of organization, motivation, and higher-order thinking. While your résumé may list specific accomplishments and accolades of your professional career, your portfolio is a way to elaborate and show tangible and authentic evidence of your achieved performance and success (Miller & Tuekam, 2011). Using your portfolio during the interview process is a great way to "wow" your interviewer. It could be "the thing" that separates you from the other candidates (Box 11-11).

Steps to Building Your Professional Portfolio

Regardless of where you are in your career as an occupational therapy practitioner—start to build your portfolio now! A portfolio only begins to take shape as you select and arrange the artifacts contained in your collection with a particular audience or purpose in mind. Then, when you go on to compose reflections exploring the meaning of the artifacts, your work folder is transformed into a potentially powerful document representing a self-aware professional. The key to the portfolio process is in understanding the relationship between collection, selection, and reflection (Box 11-12).

The first step in portfolio preparation is collection. You may well want to become a "pack rat," collecting everything related to your career as an occupational therapy practitioner—beginning with your educational path. Once you have collected and selected the artifacts to use in your portfolio, you need to reflect on the significance and meaning of major events in your professional

---

Box 11-11

CASE EXAMPLE OF USING A PROFESSIONAL PORTFOLIO DURING AN INTERVIEW

Two new graduates are interviewing for the same position at a skilled nursing facility. Both students graduated at the top of their class, and excelled during Level II fieldwork. Both students demonstrated professionalism during the interview. However, only one student brought and showcased a professional portfolio during the interview. During the course of the interview, the student effectively referred to accomplishments and activities displayed in the portfolio. For example, during their professional coursework, a student created an exceptional piece of adaptive equipment for an elderly adult client. The student photographed the equipment and created a brief narrative describing the assignment, product created, and a brief reflection of skills learned. In another class, this student generated an exceptional evidence-based review of effective treatments addressing social participation in elderly persons who were depressed, and added this to their portfolio. Finally, in a research class, the student chose to focus on designing a pilot study that looked at reducing falls in a geriatric setting. When she interviewed for her first job in a rehabilitation hospital specializing in geriatric clients, she took these items from the showcase section of her portfolio with her as evidence of her abilities.

Box 11-12

SUGGESTIONS FOR PROFESSIONAL PORTFOLIO

- Cover page including your contact information and current résumé or CV
- Credentials; important documents such as transcripts, background and security clearances, health history or immunization report, licensure and/or registration/certification
- Journal reflections or personal vision statement regarding your identity as an occupational therapy practitioner
- Professional development plan(s)
- Evaluations by faculty, peers, and fieldwork educators
- Photographs of meaningful projects, copies of exemplary assignments
- Papers and/or reviews of professional literature
- Letters of recommendation and appreciation
- Awards and/or recognitions such as thank you notes or letters from clients, families, or colleagues
- Activities in part with or recognitions from professional organizations
- Proof of attendance and/or presentations at conferences, as well as documentation of continuing education

---

Box 11-13

PROFESSIONAL TIP

Tip: As with any professional documents, updates and maintenance to your professional portfolio should occur at least twice a year.

A great resource for building your professional portfolio is:

Nagayda, J., Schindehette, S., & Richardson, J. (2005). *The professional portfolio in occupational therapy: Career development and continuing competence.* Thorofare, NJ: SLACK Incorporated.

---

development, as well as the relevancy of the curriculum and requirements of your major program of study. You should insert narratives when appropriate to describe and explain the contents of your portfolio. For example, in the case example in Box 11-11, the student was applying for a job with the geriatric population. This student would do well to select accomplishments and activities that showcase experiences relevant to geriatric practice. Your portfolio should provide evidence of growth and change in your philosophy as well as connecting your education to your career goals and needs.

It is important to emphasize that a portfolio should be used throughout your professional career. Therefore, the content of your portfolio will change as you grow in your career as an occupational therapy professional. You will want to continue to develop your portfolio as you navigate through your career. The Commission on Continuing Competence and Professional Development, a part of AOTA, has created the Professional Development Tool, which is available free as an AOTA member benefit (AOTA, 2003). The Professional Development Tool is designed to help you assess your individual learning needs and interests, create a professional development plan, and document your professional development activities (Box 11-13).

How to Use Your Professional Portfolio

It is one thing to create a professional portfolio; however, it is another thing to learn to use your portfolio successfully. As stated, the use of a portfolio can be an effective strategy during the interview process to make yourself stand out. But knowing how and when to use it during the interview is important. Don't wait until the interview is over to show your portfolio. Most likely, the interviewer won't have time to read it at that point. It will serve you best when you can use it as part of the interview. Common interview questions that may prompt the use and discussion of the portfolio could be:

1. "Tell me a bit about yourself."
2. "Can you give me an example of a project you completed that would be similar to what we do here?"
3. "Where do you see yourself in 5 years?"
4. "What is your proudest accomplishment?"

The best way to use your portfolio is to provide concrete and tangible examples that back up your résumé and your response to the interviewer's questions. Also, it is common for an interviewer, during closure of the interview process, to ask something such as "Is there anything else you would like to share about yourself that I haven't asked?" This would be an excellent opportunity to showcase specific artifacts from your portfolio that showcase the skill set that the employer is looking for.

Box 11-14

TYPICAL INFORMATION INCLUDED IN A CV

- Name and Contact Information: Providing contact information for your current institution or place of employment may work best for this, unless you do not want your colleagues to know that you are job hunting.

- Areas of Interest: A listing of your varied academic and/or scholarly interests.

- Education: A list of your degrees earned or in progress, the institutions of your education, and years of graduation. You may also include the titles of your dissertation or thesis here.

- Grants, Honors, and Awards: A list of grants received, honors bestowed upon you for your work, and awards you may have received for teaching or service.

- Publications and Presentations: A list of your published articles and books, as well as presentations given at conferences. If there are many of both, you might consider having one section for publications and another for presentations.

- Employment and Experience: This section may include separate lists of teaching experiences, laboratory experiences, field experiences, volunteer work, leadership, or other relevant experiences.

- Scholarly or Professional Memberships: A listing of the professional organizations of which you are a member. If you have held an office or position in a particular organization, you can either say so here or leave this information for the experience section.

- Service: A list of service responsibilities within academia, the profession, or the community.

- Professional Licenses/Certifications: A list of licenses or certifications that you hold, such as specialty certifications.

CURRICULUM VITAE

The terms résumé and CV are often used interchangeably. However, a résumé is typically used for the search of a job or employment, whereas a CV is used when applying for research or post-secondary teaching positions in higher education. The phrase curriculum vitae translates to "course of life" in Latin ("Curriculum Vitae," 2017). It is a comprehensive document that details all of an individual's educational background, as well as related positions including teaching and research experience. It is the standard representation of credentials and experience in academia. One of the primary differences between a résumé and a CV is the audience. A résumé is typically read by hiring managers in a non-academic organization who hire for a wide variety of positions. A CV is read by an academic audience. When applying for a scholarly position, such as a role in academia or research, the CV serves as the means to demonstrate academic achievement and scholarly potential including research funding, teaching, and service. Due to the level of detail required, it is common for a CV to be 15 pages or longer in length. See Appendix F for a sample CV (Box 11-14).

BOX 11-15

TYPICAL COMPONENTS OF A TEACHING PHILOSOPHY

- Content mastery
- Education pedagogy (i.e., active learning, experiential learning, service learning, etc.)
  - Refer to Chapter 5 for more details
- Approach to critical thinking
- Perspective on discovery of knowledge
- Design of learning environment

Teaching Philosophy Statement

When applying or interviewing for an academic position, the inclusion or description of a teaching philosophy is common practice. A teaching philosophy is a narrative statement that conveys the educator's values, beliefs, and goals regarding teaching and learning. A teaching philosophy statement is often written within a cover letter or letter of interest when applying to an academic institution (Box 11-15).

The following prompts may be useful for those that desire to create a teaching philosophy statement.

- The purpose of education is to _____.
- Why do you want to teach your subject/content area?
- Students learn best by _____.
- When you are teaching your subject, what are your goals?
- The most effective methods for teaching are _____.
- I know this because _____.
- The most important aspects of my teaching are _____.

A sample teaching philosophy statement is provided in Appendix G.

SUMMARY

Professional documents such as a cover letter, résumé, CV, and/or teaching philosophy statement play a critical role in giving an employer, colleague, or your clients a positive first impression regarding your skill set and professionalism. As you craft each of these documents, keep in mind that you are creating and selling a personal brand for yourself that will precede face-to-face interaction. Remember to accentuate your strengths and unique features that may diversify you from the competition. Sell your brand, and toot your horn with confidence! Each of these documents should be flawless in spelling and grammar, consistent in content and message, and tailored specifically to the employer and position you are applying for. Always keep the reader and audience in mind! The reader should be able to put your experience into context. These documents not only show off your writing skills, but are also good measures of your communication abilities, organization, and use of technology (if you are submitting forms electronically). Chapter 12 will build upon this with a direct focus on the job search, interview, and negotiation process.

LEARNING ACTIVITIES

1. Create a list of your educational, work, and leadership experiences. Describe each using a power verb to highlight an intrinsic or extrinsic quality of professionalism.

2. Identify two individuals you would ask to be a professional reference. Write a sample reference letter. What professional qualities would they highlight of you?

3. Write a cover letter as if you were applying for a full-time position at one of your fieldwork sites.

4. Students or future educators, use the prompts provided in this chapter and create your teaching philosophy:

    a. The purpose of education is to _____.

    b. Why do you want to teach your subject?

    c. Students learn best by _____.

    d. When you are teaching your subject, what are your goals?

    e. The most effective methods for teaching are _____.

    f. I know this because _____.

    g. The most important aspects of my teaching are _____.

REFERENCES

American Occupational Therapy Association. (2003). *Professional development tool.* Retrieved from http://www.aota.org/education-careers/advance-career/pdt.aspx.\

Brown, R. A. (1992). *Portfolio development and profiling for nurses.* Lancaster, CA: Quay Books.

Curriculum Vitae. (2017). In Dictionary.com. Retrieved from http://www.dictionary.com/browse/curriculum-vitae?s=t

Evans, W. (2012). Eye tracking online metacognition: Cognitive complexity and recruiter decision making. Retrieved from http://info.theladders.com/inside-theladders/You-only-get-6-seconds-of-fame-make-it-count

Funk, K. P. (2007). Student experiences of learning portfolios in occupational therapy education. *Occupational Therapy in Health Care, 21*(1-2), 175-184.

Jones, E., & Ashton, R. (2009, April 21). Spell it out. Retrieved from http://www.theguardian.com/careers/cv-mistakes

Lasovich, S. (2009). Professional resumes: The purpose and importance of a good resume. Retrieved from https://my.usa.edu/ICS/icsfs/Resume_for_jobs_portlet.pdf?target=0dedee05-abd3-4c91-a40f-1b681a2eef93

Miller, P. A., & Tuekam, R. (2011). The feasibility and acceptability of using a portfolio to assess professional competence. *Physiotherapy Canada, 63*(1), 78–85.

Nagayda, J., Schindehette, S., & Richardson, J. (2005). *The professional portfolio in occupational therapy: Career development and continuing competence.* Thorofare, NJ: SLACK Incorporated.

National Association of Colleagues and Employers. (2014). NACE job outlook 2015. Retrieved from https://www.umuc.edu/upload/NACE-Job-Outlook-2015.pdf

Wilcox, B. L. (1997). The teacher's portfolio: An essential tool for professional development. *The Reading Teacher, 51*(2), 170-173.

APPENDIX A: SAMPLE COVER LETTER FOR A NEW GRADUATE

YOUR NAME
CONTACT INFO HERE

(DATE)

Suzie Smith, OTR/L
Lead Occupational Therapist
Best Hospital
1000 OT Way, Suite 120
Pittsburgh, PA 15317

Dear Suzie Smith,

This letter is to express my interest in an Occupational Therapy position within your company because of the reputation for quality services that your staff provides. I recently graduated Magna Cum Laude from Duquesne University with a Bachelors Degree in Health Sciences and anticipate graduation in January of 2017 with a Masters of Science Degree in Occupational Therapy. My academic schoolwork and fieldwork evaluations have been consistently superior, demonstrating my skill and ability to provide above standards work.

I have completed fieldwork at an acute rehabilitation hospital, and am finishing my final fieldwork placement at an outpatient children's therapy center. Additionally, I have volunteer experience on the stroke and traumatic brain injury floors at Mercy Hospital. Through my fieldwork and professional experience I have had the opportunity to work with a variety of diagnoses. I have evaluated patients with physical and mental disabilities; established goals based on patient's specific needs, developed and implemented treatment plans, conducted group therapy, utilized therapeutic modalities, and participated in interdisciplinary team meetings. Through these experiences I have addressed comprehensive health and wellness needs of both adult and pediatric populations. Based upon my fieldwork experiences, I am confident that working within the pediatric patient population is _____ and believe I can contribute greatly to the success of your company.

Enclosed, I have included a résumé that summarizes my education, experiences, and accomplishments that you may find helpful in assisting your interviewing process. I am eager to continue to contribute to this valuable profession and would welcome a personal interview to more accurately reveal my qualifications. I am confident that my skills, personal attributes and work ethic will be an asset to The Best Hospital.

Thank you for your time and consideration, and please do not hesitate to contact me if you have any questions.

I look forward to hearing from you soon.

Respectfully,
YOUR NAME, OTS

APPENDIX B: SAMPLE COVER LETTER FOR AN EXPERIENCED OCCUPATIONAL THERAPY PRACTITIONER

Attention Ms. Jesse Smith – Occupational Therapy manager
Re: Occupational therapy Assistant Position Job ID # 5555

I am writing to apply for the position of occupational therapy assistant at Viva Hospital, as advertised recently in *OT Practice*.

I am a motivated and passionate occupational therapy assistant, with a Bachelor of Business Management, and over eight years of experience in working in skilled nursing and long-term care practice settings, as both a clinician and a supervisor.

In my current role, I am responsible for managing a large case load, working with a wide range of clients in both assistive living, skilled nursing, and long-term care. I am currently responsible for supervising three COTA/L's and the recreation therapist, which includes their annual performance reviews and program development. I am also responsible for the delivery of moving and handling training and consulting with the nursing staff, focusing on the minimization of workplace injury risk, body mechanics and workplace wellness

I am a self-motivated professional who is passionate about caring for clients and getting the best results for their recovery. I possess very strong communication skills and pride myself on my highly developed interpersonal skills, which have allowed me to achieve great results both individually and when working as part of a team.

I am a self-directed, life-long learner, and have sought out advanced training to further my clinical and professional knowledge. I currently hold specialty certification in Environmental Modication through The American Occupational Therapy Association, and certified by NBCOT.

I am confident that my unique background, training and experiences, along with my extensive training in environmental modifications makes me a good contender for this position within your facility.

My professional résumé is attached and I look forward to being able to discuss the position with you further.

Yours sincerely,

Jane Jones, COTA/L, BA

APPENDIX C: RÉSUMÉ TEMPLATE

Jane Doe, OTD, OTR/L
600 Smith Road
Pittsburgh, PA 14512
doej@duq.edu
555-555-5555

Objective:

-state your intent, be specific to position applying for.

Ex: To obtain an occupational therapy position that allows the utilization of my educational and clinical training, in addition to providing opportunities for personal growth and professional development

Education:

- Include Full Title of Degree, institution received from, expected/anticipated graduation/completion dates
- Include any relevant educational accomplishments, awards, scholarships, honor societies, etc.
- Graduate students: add any info related to research or capstone project

> Ex: ***OTD School University, Pittsburgh, Pennsylvania***
> ***Doctor of Occupational Therapy, December 2016***
> <u>Scholar Capstone/Dissertation</u>
> *"An Occupational Therapy Initiative": A Post-Operative Breast Cancer In-patient Rehabilitation Program*
> <u>Curriculum</u>
> *Occupational Science, Administration/Management, Education and Theory, Leadership, Methods of Evaluation and Evidenced-Based Practice*

> ***Duquesne University, Pittsburgh, Pennsylvania***
> ***Master's of Occupational Therapy, May 7, 2015***
> ***Bachelor's of Health Science, May 3, 2014***
> - *Golden Key International Honor Society 2013Inductee*
> - *Dean's List 1999-2003,*
> - *Presidential Scholarship 2010-2014*

Scholarship (if did Faculty research, presented at undergraduate research symposium, etc.)

Research Apprentice, Dates

- Faculty Advisor
- Roles/responsibilities
  Presentations/Papers (indicate whether it was peer-reviewed, referred, invited)

  List Authorship, Title of Presentation, Type of presentation (poster, workshop, institute, etc.) Name of conference, Location and Dates

Ex: Sexuality in Occupational Therapy Research Project

Advisor: Dr. John Smith, PhD, OTR/L

-submerged into literature, and completed evidence-based literature review on Sexuality in Occupational Therapy education, assisted with analyzing and coding data, completed in-person interviews with participants regarding their spiritual practices
Presentation:

Smith, J., **Doe, J.,** Guzak, G., & Frank, L. Evidence and Techniques Integrating Sexuality Into Occupational Therapy Practice. Poster Presentation at the 94th Annual AOTA Conference & Expo, Baltimore, MD, April 4, 2014.

Clinical Experience:

- Include fieldwork, service learning experience, most recent experiences should be on top
- Include facilitate/site, dates, and brief description of your responsibilities/experiences
- Be sure each fieldwork experience highlights different skills/responsibilities

Ex: Level II Fieldwork Affiliation – UPMC Mercy Hospital, Pittsburgh, Pennsylvania September – December 2011

- *Performed evaluations and interventions on adult patient population including spinal cord injury, traumatic brain injury, orthopedic surgeries, etc.*
- *Demonstrated competency in transferring/moving and handling a variety of clients*
- *Achieved full caseload requirements and met monthly productivity*

Level II Fieldwork Affiliation – Health South Harmerville, Pittsburgh, Pennsylvania, June – September 2011

- *Participated in multidisciplinary team meetings and demonstrated excellent communication skills with physical therapists, social workers, physicians, nurses, etc.*

Level I c Fieldwork Affiliation-etc.

Level I b Fieldwork Affiliation (Service Learning or Community Engaged Learning)

Level 1a Fieldwork Affiliation

Supplemental Experience

Include any other relevant paid/unpaid experiences (i.e. volunteering, shadowing, etc.)

Ex:
Waitress, #1 Restaurant, (Pittsburgh, PA)
Developed skills to deliver quality service to customers such as: teamwork,
handled a high volume of customers, interpersonal skills, time management, adaptability, strong communication skills, high energy, listening skills, and problem solving.

Volunteer, Vincentian Nursing Home: September 2014-November 2014

-Implemented occupational leisure activities with the residents,
-Assisted recreation therapist in set-up and clean-up of group activites
- Achieved 87 volunteer hours

Leadership

SOTA leadership, student ambassador, officer position in sorority/fraternity, etc.

Service

Volunteering, service organizations, best buddies, etc.

Memberships/Certifications

AOTA Member – ID # 4949494
State OT Association Member – ID # 34343
Date of Background Check: 4-26-2012
Date of CPR Expiration: 5-25-2015

Continuing Education (If have any relevant continuing education that you want to include)
List Date, Name of Course, Provider/Location, Date, # of CEU's/PDU's

Ex:

4/18/16: Lymphedema and Complete Decongestive Therapy, Cross Country Education, Pittsburgh, PA, 8 CEU's

APPENDIX D: SAMPLE RÉSUMÉ

Ann S. Ewing, OTD, OTR/L
4942 Dolly Rd
Pittsfield, PA 15400
(412) 555-2819
astuart1@email.com

Education

OTD, Chatham University	2009-2010
MOT, Western Michigan University	1978-1980
B.S. in Psychology, St Lawrence University	1971-1975

Professional Experience

Director of Rehab Almond Ridge Memory Care Pittsfield, Pennsylvania	2011-current
Homecare Occupational Therapist HomeCare OT services, LLC Pittsfield, Pennsylvania	1987-2011
Director of Occupational Therapy HealthSouth Rehab of Centuryville Pittsfield, Pennsylvania	1985-1987
OTR/Head Injury Specialist Rehabilitation Institute of Pittsburgh Pittsfield, Pennsylvania	1983-1985
Director of Occupational Therapy Wightman Health Care Center Pittsfield, Pennsylvania	1980-1983
OTR/Team Leader Harmarville Rehab Center Pittsfield, Pennsylvania	1975-1983

Advanced Clinical Training

AOTA Fieldwork Certificate Workshop	2011
Certified Lymphedema Therapist	1997
Certified Brain Injury Specialist	1991
NDT/Bobath Certificate Course in the Management of Adults with Stroke and Brain Injury	1984

Academic Appointments

Adjunct Instructor Department of OT OTR University Pittsfield, PA	1980-August 2015

Certification and Licensure

NBCOT (#AA2130462 expires 3/31/2017)
PA Licensure (#OC0003749L expires 6/30/2017)
CPR (expires 6/2016)

Honors and Awards

POTA President's Award for Leadership Innovation POTA Master Clinician Award

Memberships

AOTA (#43072 expires 11I30/2016)

POTA (#0677 expires 3/31/17)

Professional Service

AOTA Emerging Leaders Development Committee	2014-2015
PA Alternate Rep to AOTA Representative Assembly	2 terms
POTA Commission on Conference	1980-present
POTA Ad Hoc Committee on Leadership Development-Chair	2010-2013
POTA Local Conference Committee (Special Events, Conference Co-Chair roles)	2008-2010
	1990-2013
District II Delegate to POTA Board	
District II Board (including appointed Legislative, OT Administrators Committee,	2 terms
Conference, Leadership Development roles)	1985-2013

APPENDIX E: SAMPLE PROFESSIONAL REFERENCE LIST

Jane Doe, OTD, OTR/L

600 Smith Road

Pittsburgh, PA 14512

doej@duq.edu

555-555-5555

Davey Crocket, DPT
Director of Rehabilitation Services
Pittsburgh Hospital
444 Hospital Drive
Pittsburgh, PA 14494
555-456-7895
crocketd@pghhosp.org

Sherry Waters, MOT, OTR/L
Level II FW Educator
Pittsburgh Hospital
444 Hospital Drive
Pittsburgh, PA 14494
555-456-3215
Waterss@pghhosp.org

Elizabeth D. DeIuliis, OTD, OTR/L
Academic Fieldwork Coordinator, Faculty Mentor
Duquesne University
Department of Occupational Therapy
600 Forbes Avenue
Pittsburgh, PA 15282
deiuliise@duq.edu
555-555-5555

APPENDIX F: SAMPLE CV

Elizabeth Dwyer DeIuliis

Duquesne University
John G. Rangos Sr. School of Health Sciences
Department of Occupational Therapy
221 Health Sciences Building
600 Forbes Ave
Pittsburgh, Pennsylvania 15282
deiuliise@duq.edu
412.396.5411 office
412.952.6358 mobile

Education

OTD   Doctorate of Occupational Therapy, Chatham University, 2009

             Scholar Capstone: *"An Occupational Therapy Initiative": A Post-Operative Breast Cancer In-Patient Rehabilitation Program*

MOT   Occupational Therapy, Duquesne University, 2004

BS   Health Sciences, Duquesne University, 2003

             Awards/Achievements: Golden Key International Honor Society Inductee 2002, Dean's List 1999-2003, Presidential Scholarship 1999-2003

Academic Appointments

2015   **Assistant Department Chairperson,Director of Community & Clinical Education, Academic Fieldwork Coordinator**
             Department of Occupational Therapy
             John G. Rangos, Sr., School of Health Sciences
             Duquesne University, Pittsburgh, PA

2010-2015   **Assistant Professor/Academic Fieldwork Coordinator/Curriculum Coordinator**
             Department of Occupational Therapy
             John G. Rangos, Sr., School of Health Sciences
             Duquesne University, Pittsburgh, PA

2005- 2010   **Adjunct Clinical Instructor**
             Department of Occupational Therapy

John G. Rangos, Sr., School of Health Sciences
Duquesne University, Pittsburgh, PA

2005-2008   **Adjunct Clinical Instructor**
Department of Occupational Therapy
School of Health & Rehabilitation Sciences
University of Pittsburgh, Pittsburgh, PA

Teaching Responsibilities

Current Teaching Responsibilities:
OCCT 530 Biomechanical Function/Lab
Role: Primary Instructor 2010-2011
Role: Co-Instructor 2012 - present
4 credit course/14-week semester/8.8 Contact hours/9 lectures
Description of Course: This course examines evaluation and intervention strategies related to the biomechanical and rehabilitation frames of reference across the human lifespan via lecture, class discussion, self-directed and experiential/ lab learning activities.

REHS Biomechanical Intervention & Treatment/Lab
Role: Course Developer & Co-instructor 2014-present
4 credit course/14-week semester/8.8 contact hours/10 lectures
Description of Course: This course and curriculum was created for students from Shanghai University in China. This course examines evaluation and intervention strategies related to the U.S. biomechanical and rehabilitation frames of reference across the human lifespan via lecture, class discussion, self-directed and experiential/ lab learning activities. Additional self-study modules were developed to further introduce International students to U.S. models and scope of OT Practice.

OCT 520 Neurosensorimotor Function II/Lab
Role: Primary Instructor 2011-present
4 credit course/6.4 contact hours /14-week semester/ 20 lectures
Description of Course: This course examines neuromotor learning and sensory theories with a focus on the application of neuro-physiological principles, and specific evaluation and intervention strategies related to young adult through geriatric clients. The influence of cognitive, perceptual rehabilitation and motor learning theories and approaches on evaluation and treatment is discussed as related to their influence on recovery of the client via lecture, class discussion, self-directed and experiential/ lab learning activities. An interprofessional grand rounds seminar also occurs in this class, as an IPE event between the Schools of Health sciences, nursing & pharmacy.

OCCT 555 – 558 Level II Fieldwork
Role: Primary Instructor
16 credit course
Description of Course: The purpose of the fieldwork experience is to provide students with the opportunities to integrate the theory and skills learned in the classroom within the clinical setting. I developed and implemented online discussion reflection sessions for students during Level II fieldwork, to discuss relevant trends and issues occurring in their practice sites. This instructional strategy allows me to provide guidance to promote continued learning while they are in the course, as well as meet relevant ACOTE standards. The online discussion enables me to remain in good communication with the students and allows for monitoring potential attitudinal or performance concerns. Upon completion of the fieldwork experiences, the student is expected to perform at or above the minimum skill level of the entry-level occupational therapy professional. Level II FW is a total of 16 credits. *online education component

OCCT 552 Clinical Seminar A
Role: Primary Instructor
2 credit course
Description of Course: This graduate seminar uses online class discussion and reflection over the course of level II FW to integrate the relationship between graduate students' clinical experiences and essential curriculum concepts. *online education component

OCCT 553 Clinical Seminar B/Lab
Role: Primary Instructor
0 credits/12 Contact hours/3-week semester
Description of Course: This graduate seminar uses in-class discussion to integrate the relationship between graduate students' clinical experiences and essential curriculum concepts. Reflection questions completed online in OCCT 552 Clinical Seminar A are revisited and seminar discussion of advanced topics connect occupation-based practice to a variety of settings with particular attention to the impact of contextual factors on the management and delivery of occupational therapy services and students continued professional development as practice scholars and future fieldwork educators. Students organize and deliver a continuing education symposium for undergraduate students, fieldwork educators, and practitioners in the community focused on state of the art practice learned throughout the curriculum and in fieldwork.

OCCT 574 Fieldwork Proposal
Role: Co-Instructor
1 credit course
Description of Course: This course is the final component of the student research sequence in the curriculum. Following the qualitative and quantitative research courses and the evidence-based practice course, this course encourages students to think as clinician-researchers, asking questions of interest based on clinical observations, and designing studies to address those questions. The student's project for the course is to

write a fieldwork proposal, similar in structure to a research grant proposal. The proposed research study must address a question of interest within occupational therapy, and the study must be one that could realistically be carried out at the student's Fieldwork IIA site. Faculty serve as advisors to this scholarly capstone project. # of MSOT Students personally mentored from 2011-present: 14

Past Teaching Responsibilities

OT Overview
Role: Primary Instructor 2010-present
0-3 credits
Description of Course: This course is designed to be an introduction to occupational therapy as a profession and practice. Transfer, Post-Bachelor and articulation students are required to take this course online to meet ACOTE standards. Content includes the history, philosophies, organizations, roles and functions, standards of practice, ethics and future directions. Basic professional information literacy and retrieval skills will be developed. In addition, fundamental practice skills will be obtained in readiness for fieldwork and experiential learning. The course establishes a foundation for higher levels of learning. *online education component

OCCT 535 Occupational Performance Evaluation/Lab
Role: Primary Instructor 2010-2012
3 credits
Description of Course: This course provides an introduction to evaluation, assessment and screening processes in occupational therapy practice across the human lifespan. This includes learning the basics regarding, observation, interviewing, psychometrics (test and measurement theories, methods, scales, procedures, statistics and test interpretation), ethics and assessment administration. This is a foundational course that supports learning of specific assessments in future intervention courses. A primary goal for the student is to develop fundamental concepts and initial skills as an evaluator to engage in the critical review and professional administration of assessments and evaluation program development as an entry-level practitioner.

OCCT 522 Intervention Seminar/Lab
Role: Co-Instructor 2010-2013
3 credit course
Description of Course: This course uses a guided analysis of case studies with an emphasis on application of theories and principles of evaluation & intervention across the lifespan. The focus of this course is on understanding the comprehensive needs of various populations and how to achieve occupational performance outcomes prior to level II FW experiences.

OCCT 610 Research Project I: Prospectus
Role: Primary Instructor

1 credit course

Description of Course: This is the first course in the elective 3-course research project sequence. Working with a faculty research mentor, the graduate student designs a research proposal using quantitative and/or qualitative research methods, and submits the proposal to the University's Institution Review Board.

OCCT 611W Research Project II: Engagement
Role: Primary Instructor
1 credit course

Description of Course: This is the second course in the elective 3-course research project sequence. Under the guidance of a faculty mentor, the student collects data for the research project approved by the University Institution Review Board.

OCCT 612W Research Project III: Dissemination
Role: Primary Instructor
1 credit course

Description of Course: This is the final course in the elective research project sequence. Under the guidance of a faculty mentor, the student analyzes the data and completes a dissemination project, including presentation and/or publication at regional, state or national level.

OCCT 561 OT Administration
Role: Primary Instructor: 2011-2013
Role Co-Instructor: 2014
3 credit course/15 contact hours/7-week semester/lectures

Description of Course: This course addresses the entrepreneur, managerial and consultant roles of the occupational therapist. The content focuses on health care trends, reimbursement regulations, legislative policies, practice environments, strategies for maintaining continued competence, and emerging professional issues. Supervision, planning, budgeting, quality management, staffing, program development and standards of professional practice are presented via lecture, class discussion, self-directed and experiential/lab learning activities.

Course/Curriculum Development:

OCCT 640 Doctoral Experiential Component
12 credits

Description of Course:

Students pursuing a doctoral degree (OTD) are required to complete one additional sixteen-week Doctoral Experiential Component (DEC) following level II FW. The goal of this experiential component is to develop occupational therapists with advanced skills (those beyond a generalist level), and it is integral to acquiring deeper practice-scholar competencies as reflected in the program's curriculum design

This 12 credit course provides an in-depth, customized experience specific to the doctoral pursuit of the occupational therapy student, and the opportunity to extend and refine knowledge & skills acquired in the curriculum. Students may participate in learning experiences that include a focus on theory development, research, policy, advanced clinical practice, advocacy, teaching, administration, leadership, etc. Each OTD student must successfully complete a minimum of 16 weeks (640) hours of the DEC. I was responsible for developing the objectives, curriculum, and evaluation methods associated with this course.

OCCT 635, 645 & 655 Practice Scholar Doctoral Capstone Project Sequence
1 credit for each course (3) total
Description of Course: DU OTD students' complete a series of courses to prepare and deliver a practice scholar capstone project as the culminating product of their doctoral studies. The capstone project reflects the OTD student's transformative journey into becoming an advanced Practice Scholar. The capstone project reflects the student's synthesis of knowledge, reflective practice and application of occupational therapy concepts and analytic and leadership skills developed throughout the OTD program. The doctoral project is evidence that the student can *serve, do, question and lead* as a practice scholar at the doctoral level. The primary purpose of the capstone project is to focus the student on the development, implementation, and evaluation of a scholarly project related to their area of practice, current job site, specialty area or within the community. All projects will be evidence driven and consist of project development, implementation, and evaluation. I was responsible in developing the objectives, curriculum and sequence for these 3 courses.

Advanced Teaching to Professionals

"Best Practice in Item Writing", Presented to Department of Occupational Therapy Faculty, April 1st, 2016

Guest Lectures

Duquesne University Doctor of Physical Therapy Program
PHYT 421: Principles of Practice 3: Ethical, Moral and Legal Issues
"Interprofessional Lecture on Stroke Care – OT"
January 31, 2014

Non-Teaching Responsibilities

- Co-led department in completing ACOTE self-study initial and annual reports for MS and OTD programs

- Coordinates curriculum in the pre-professional and professional phases to assure compliance with all ACOTE accreditation standards for these phases, including writing self-study document with Program Director
- Coordinates implementation of department strategic planning including monitoring outcomes of key departmental committees and projects
- Coordinates reporting of all program and learning outcomes including FW and exit surveys, alumni and employer surveys, student learning outcomes and teaching evaluations of clinical and adjunct faculty
- Oversees and manages all experiential community education including level I FW, level II FW and doctoral experiential component including responsibilities and processes including adhering to Accreditation standards, monitoring of program evaluation outcomes for continuous quality improvement and annual reports, recruitment of clinical sites, reservation management, communication, conflict resolution, site visits, student placement and procurement of students' pre-clinical health and security requirements
- Directly supervises 3 Non-Tenure Clinical Faculty positions and an Administrative Assistant I position including performance review process
- Co-manages occupational therapy curriculum content and delivery
- Coordinates with admission team regarding articulation agreements and student recruitment
- Directs and facilitates department admissions for post-baccalaureate MS program and OTD programs via OTCAS online centralized application service
- Assists with OTD curriculum development
- Assists with curriculum development for Shanghai University students
- Faculty advisor to the Student Occupational Therapy Association
- Ensures the maintenance of health records, background checks and drug screens for students through certifiedbackground.com.
- Mentoring/advising of about 25 Occupational Therapy Students each academic year
- Advisor to graduate students for fieldwork proposal
- Mentors clinical faculty
- Chair, RSHS Clinical Coordinator Committee
- Chair & Member, OT Faculty Search Committee
- Duties as assigned by Department Chair

Summary of National & Local Level I, II Fieldwork and DEC Placements Secured for MSOT & OTD Students

Graduation Year	2011	2012	2013	2014	2015	2016	2017*
Students (n)	29	27	27	27	33	28	

Placements (n)	116	108	108	135	165	140	

*includes newly developed OCCT 640 Doctoral Experiential Component

# of fieldwork site visits from 2011-present - 150 +

# of new fieldwork affiliation agreements initiated – 35 +

Clinical Appointments

Areas of Clinical Expertise: acute care, hospital, intensive care and skilled nursing setting; orthopedic, neurology, cardiothoriacs, musculoskeletal, oncology conditions.

2010–present **Casual Occupational Therapist**
Centers for Rehab Services at UPMC Shadyside Hospital, Pittsburgh, PA

2008–2010   **Assistant Facility Director/Clinical Coordinator of Education**
Centers for Rehab Services at UPMC Shadyside Hospital, Pittsburgh, PA

2007–2008   **Team Leader/Clinical Coordinator of Education**
Centers for Rehab Services at UPMC Braddock Hospital, Pittsburgh, PA

2005–2007   **Senior Occupational Therapist/Clinical Coordinator of Education**
Centers for Rehab Services at UPMC Braddock Hospital, Pittsburgh, PA

2004–2005   **Staff Occupational Therapist**
Centers for Rehab Services at UPMC Braddock Hospital, Pittsburgh, PA

Professional Certifications & Licensure

2010   American Occupational Therapy Fieldwork Educator Workshop Certificate

2004–present Occupational Therapy Board Certified & Registered OTR
Certification #: 1071173

2004–present Licensed Occupational Therapist by the State of Pennsylvania
License #: OC009437

Professional Awards

2015   **Dedication Service Award**
        Awarded by POTA President Mary Muhlenhaupt, OTD, OTR/L, FAOTA
        Pennsylvania Occupational Therapy Association

2015   **Dean's Award for Excellence in Teaching**
        John G. Rangos, Sr., School of Health Sciences
        Duquesne University, Pittsburgh, PA

2015   **Outstanding Organization Advisor of the Year Nomination**
        Student Organization Leadership & Service Awards
        Duquesne University, Pittsburgh, PA

2014   **Creative Teaching Award**
        "Interprofessional Grand Rounds"
        Center for Teaching Excellence
        Duquesne University, Pittsburgh, PA

2010   **Quality Improvement Award**
        UPMC Community Providers Services Quality Fair

2007   **Health Ranger Mentor Award**
        UPMC Braddock Health Rangers Program

Professional Associations

Member: The American Occupational Therapy Association   Member ID: 000004264193

Member: The Pennsylvania Occupational Therapy Association   Member ID: 11308

Member: Greater Pittsburgh Fieldwork Council

SCHOLARSHIP

Textbook (Sole Author)

Deluliis, E. Professionalism across Occupational Therapy Clinical Practice, {Provisional title}
        SLACK Incorporated; Thorofare, New Jersey. [In progress and under contract].

Online Continuing Education Course

Deluliis, E., & Hellstead, S. *The Role of Occupational Therapy with Individuals with Breast Cancer,* 3 hour distance learning course, Western Schools; {In progress and under contract}.

Referred Publications

Wallace, S.E., Turocy, P., DiBartola, L., **Deluliis, E.**, Weideman, Y., Morgan, A., Astle, J., Cousino, S., O'Neil, C., & Simko, L. (in press). Interprofessional education outcome study: Learning and understanding professional roles in stroke care. *Journal of Physical Therapy Education* (expected publication in late 2016)

Hanson, D. & **Deluliis, E.** (2015) "The Collaborative Model to Fieldwork Education: A blueprint for group supervision of students", *OT in Healthcare: Special Issue in Education,* (29) 2, 223-239.

Peer Reviewed Publications

Deluliis, E. (2013). Answering questions about level I fieldwork, *OT Practice, 18 (12), p. 8-9.*

Deluliis, E, Cohen, S., Campell, C. & Slowman, L. (2012). Connecting through OT connections: an occupational therapy breast cancer initiative, *OT Practice, 17 (*16), 15-17.

Deluliis, E. (2011). Using the occupational profile for student-centered fieldwork. *OT Practice, 16 (14), p. 13.*

Deluliis, E. & Hughes, J. (2012). Occupational Therapy's Role in the Rehabilitation of Breast Cancer. *American Occupational Therapy Association.*

Published Abstracts

Benson, J.D., Szucs, K.A, & **Deluliis, E.** *Impact of Student Response Systems on Student Retention of Course Content*
International Lily Conference on College Teaching Oxford, Ohio, November, 2014
Conference Theme: Evidenced-based learning and Teaching

Grants

Funded

Benson, J.D., Szucs, K., **Deluliis, E**. (2013) Duquesne University Academic Learning Outcome

Assessment Grant. To support research on student retention of content introduced utilizing a Student Response System. $1000.

Professional Presentations/Papers

2016 Peer Reviewed Accepted
Donoso Brown, E., & Deluliis, E.
> *Navigating the Transition from the Clinic to Academia: Identifying a Path and Creating a Plan*
> Poster Presentation, 2016 American Occupational Therapy Association Annual Conference
> Chicago, Illinois, April 2016

2016 Peer Review Accepted

Kane, A., **Deluliis, E.,** & Munoz, J.
> *"(Re)Discovering the Utility of the IRM in Professional Reasoning"*
> Poster Presentation, 2016 American Occupational Therapy Association Annual Conference
> Chicago, Illinois, April 2016

2015 Peer Review Accepted
Deluliis, E.D & Donoso Brown, E.
> *Academia as an OT Practice Setting?*
> Presentation, 2015 Pennsylvania Occupational Therapy Association Annual Conference
> Scranton, Pennsylvania, October 2015

2015 Peer Review Accepted
Donoso Brown, E., Kane, A., Witchger-Hansen, A., et al.
> Contributing Author: **Deluliis, E.**
> *Cultural Integration Program: Promoting Success of Foreign Students in and out of the Classroom*
> Presentation, 2015 American Occupational Therapy Association Annual Conference, Nashville, Tennessee, April, 2015.

2015 Peer Review Accepted
Benson, J.D., Szucs, K.A, & **Deluliis, E.** *Impact of Student Response Systems on Student Retention of Course Content*
> Poster Presentation, 2015 American Occupational Therapy Association Annual Conference, Nashville, Tennessee, April, 2015.

2014 Peer Review Accepted (International Conference)

Benson, J.D., Szucs, K.A, & **Deluliis, E.** *Impact of Student Response Systems on Student Retention of Course Content*
Platform Presentation, International Lily Conference on College Teaching, Oxford, Ohio, November, 2014

2014 Peer Review Accepted

Benson, J.D., Szucs, K.A, & **Deluliis, E.** *Impact of Student Response Systems on Student Retention of Course Content*
Poster Presentation, Pennsylvania Occupational Therapy Association Annual Conference, Valley Forge, Pennsylvania October 2014

2014 Peer Review Accepted (International Conference)

Dibartola, L., **Deluliis, E.** & Wallace, S. *Interprofessional Education Workshop in Stroke Rehabilitation*
Poster Presentation, All Together Better Health VII, Pittsburgh, Pennsylvania, June 7,2014

2014 Peer Review Accepted

Wallace S, Turocy P, DiBartola L, **Deluliis E**, Astle J, Cousino S, Morgan A, O'Neil C, Simko L, Weideman Y. *Interprofessional education workshop in stroke rehabilitation.*
Poster Presentation, Pennsylvania Speech-Language and Hearing Association Annual Conference, Pittsburgh, Pennsylvania. April 2014

2013   Peer Reviewed Accepted

Deluliis, E & McCann, M. *Perspectives on the Collaborative Student Supervision Model in Level 2 Fieldwork*
Workshop, Pennsylvania Occupational Therapy Association Annual Conference, Pittsburgh, Pennsylvania, November 9, 2013.

2013   Peer Reviewed Accepted

Dolhi,C., Leibold, M.& **Deluliis, E.** *Fieldwork Educators: Can We Talk?*
Workshop, Pennsylvania Occupational Therapy Association Annual Conference, Pittsburgh, Pennsylvania November 9, 2013

2013   Peer Reviewed Accepted

Fairman, A., Bateson, J. & **Deluliis, E.** *Ready for Change? Transitioning to new practice settings*
Workshop, Pennsylvania Occupational Therapy Association Annual Conference, Pittsburgh, Pennsylvania November 9, 2013

2013 Peer Reviewed Accepted

Deluliis, E., Wallace, S., DiBartola, L., & Turocy, P. *We are all in this together–An Interprofessional Education Collaboration.*
Workshop, Pennsylvania Occupational Therapy Association Annual Conference, Pittsburgh, Pennsylvania, November 9, 2013

2013 Peer Reviewed Accepted

Zimmerman, E., Syrko,S. & Hirynk, R. **Deluliis, E.** *Unwrapping the mysteries of level 1 fieldwork*
Poster Presentation, Pennsylvania Occupational Therapy Association Annual Conference, Pittsburgh, Pennsylvania, November 9, 2013

2013   Peer Reviewed Accepted

Dibartola,L. **Deluliis,E,** Wallace, S. & Turocy, P. *We are all in this together- An Interprofessional Education Collaboration*
Workshop, Association of Schools of Allied Health Professions, Orlando, Florida Oct 23-25, 2013

2013   Peer Reviewed Accepted

Wallace, S.E., Turocy, P., DiBartola, L., **Deluliis, E**., Astle, J., Cousino, S., Morgan, A., O'Neil, Simko, L., & Weideman, Y. Learning Outcomes from an 8-discipline Interprofessional Education Program
 Poster Presentation, Association of Schools of Allied Health Professions, Orlando, Florida, Oct 23-25, 2013

2012   Invited Presentation

Hughes, J., Cohen, S., Lyons, K., Munoz, L. & **Deluliis, E.** *Emerging area of occupational therapy practice: OT interventions across the treatment continuum for women with breast cancer*
Workshop, American Occupational Therapy Association Annual Conference, Indianapolis, Indiana 2012

2012   Invited Presentation (International Conference)

Crist, P., Munoz, J., Hansen, A.M., Benson, J.D, **Deluliis, E**, Szucs, K. *Developing Practice-Scholars: An Outcome Oriented Curriculum & Practice Models for Engagement in the Scholarship of Practice,* Presentation, The International Perspective Conference, Poland, 2012

2010   Peer Reviewed Accepted

Deluliis, E. *A Post-Operative Breast Cancer Inpatient Rehabilitation Program*
Poster Presentation, Pennsylvania Occupational Therapy Association Annual Conference, Scranton, Pennsylvania, October 31, 2010

2010   Peer Reviewed Accepted

Deluliis, E. *A Post-operative Breast Cancer Inpatient Rehab Program*

Platform Presentation, UPMC Community Services Providers Quality Fair, Pittsburgh, Pennsylvania, September, 2010

2007   Invited Presentation
Deluliis, E. *Addressing Psychosocial Issues in a Rehab/Hospital Setting*
Platform Presentation, AOTA/NBCOT Student Conclave, Pittsburgh, Pennsylvania, September, 2007

Faculty Mentored Research Project

2013-2015 Research Project Title: *Role Expectations of Academic Fieldwork Coordinators in Occupational Therapy Programs*
Graduate Student: Alyssa Hines, MSOT Class of 2015

SERVICE / LEADERSHIP

University

2016   Member, PA Department Search Commitee

2016   Co-Chair, OT Faculty Search Committee (3 searches)

2015   Member, 25th Anniversary Anna. L Rangos Rizakus Student Symposium Planning Committee

2015   Co-Chair, OT Faculty Search Committee (3 searches)

2015   Member, RSHS Dean's Advisory Committee

2014   Co-Chair, OT Faculty Search Committee (2 searches)

2013   Member, RSHS Academic Integrity Committee

2013   Member, OT Faculty Search Committee (2 searches)

2012–present Member, OTD Curriculum Development Committee

2012–present Chair, RSHS Clinical Coordinator Committee

2011–present Member, Inteprofessional Education Collaborative Committee

2009–2012   Member, Clinical Coordinator Committee

2010–present Faculty Advisor, Student Occupational Therapy Association

2009–present   Volunteer/Participant in Annual RSHS Recruitment Activities – Open House &
               DUQ Fest

Profession - National

2016   Invited Team Leader/Subject Matter Expert
               NBCOT Item Development Meeting, July 21 – July 23, 2016

2016   Appointed Member/Subject Matter Expert
               NBCOT OTR Examination Certification Development and Validation Committee –
               Multiple Choice (OTRCE – MC), March 18-19, 2016 & September 23-24, 2016

2015   Appointed Member/Subject Matter Expert
               NBCOT Certification Examination Development & Validation Committee
               September 10-September 12, 2015

2015   Invited Team Leader/Subject Matter Expert
               NBCOT Item Development Meeting, July 30 – August 1, 2015

2015   Appointed Member
               NBCOT Certification Validation Examination Committee, March 14-16, 2015

2015   Invited Member/Subject Matter Expert
               NBCOT Item Development Pilot Meeting, January 8 – 10, 2015

2014   Manuscript Reviewer
               F.A. Davis, *Health Professions Today*
               Chapter 19 Occupational Therapy

2014   Appointed Member
               NBCOT Certification Validation Examination Committee

2013   Appointed Member
               NBCOT Standard Setting Study

2013   Appointed Member
               NBCOT Certification Validation Examination Committee

2012   Appointed Member
               NBCOT Certification Validation Examination Committee

2012–present   Manuscript Reviewer
F. A. Davis, *Radomski & Trombly's text Occupational Therapy for Physical Dysfunction,* 7th *edition*

2012–present   Manuscript Reviewer
F.A Davis text, Braveman, B. *Leading & Managing OT Services*

2011   Invited Member
NBCOT Item Enhancement Team

2011–present   Proposal Reviewer
American Occupational Therapy Association Annual Conference

Professional - State/Regional

2016   Appointed Position
District II Delegate to the POTA Board of Directors

2013–2016   Appointed Chair
POTA, District II, Continuing Education Committee

2012–2013   Invited Program Co-Chair
POTA Local Conference Planning Committee – Program

2011–present Proposal Reviewer
Pennsylvania Occupational Therapy Annual Conference

2006–2008   Health Rangers Mentoring Program
UPMC Braddock Hospital

2009–present Member/Leader in Steering Committee
Greater Pittsburgh Area FW Council

2008–2009   Invited Member
CRS/UPMC Network OT committee

Community

2011–present Volunteer
Cystic Fibrosis Foundation- Local Chapter, Pittsburgh, Pennsylvania

Abbreviated Attended Continued Education (last 4 years)

3/18-3/19/2016 *"Certification Examination Development and Validation Committee,"* presented by The National Board for Certification in Occupational Therapy, Long Beach, California

2/17/2016   *"Working with ESL (English as a Second Language) Students,"* presented by Center for Teaching Excellence, Duquesne University, Pittsburgh, Pennsylvania

1/14 -1/15/16 *" ACOTE Self-Study Preparation Workshop"* presented by Accreditation Council for Occupational Therapy Education Council, Alexandria, Virginia.

10/24/15, *"Reiki Level I Training,"* Annual 2015 Pennsylvania Occupational Therapy Conference, Scranton, PA

10/23/15 *"Student Learning 2.0: Integrating New Technologies into the Classroom,"* Annual 2015 Pennsylvania Occupational Therapy Conference, Scranton, PA

10/23/15 *"An OT's Guide to Patient Reported Outcomes,"* Annual 2015 Pennsylvania Occupational Therapy Conference, Scranton, PA

9/11-9/12/2015 *"Certification Examination Development and Validation Committee,"* presented by The National Board for Certification in Occupational Therapy, Minneapolis, Minnesota

8/19/2015 *"Department Chairperson Orientation,"* presented by Associate Provost for Academic Affairs, Alexandra Gregory, Duquesne University, Pittsburgh, Pennsylvania

7/31 -8/2/2015 *"Item Development Meeting,"* presented by The National Board for Certification in Occupational Therapy, Orlando, Florida.

 1/10/2015 *"Item Development Pilot Program,"* presented by The National Board for Certification in Occupational Therapy, Scottsdale, Arizona.

1/5/2015 *"Recognizing and Reporting Child Abuse: Mandates and Permissive Reporting in Pennsylvania,"* presented by University of Pittsburgh School of Social Work, PA Child Welfare Resource Center

12/11/2014 *"Use of Intensive Therapy and the Universal Exercise Unit (UEU) to Change Function,"* POTA District II Event, presented by Mary Jo Smith, OTR/L & Kristen Bowman, OTR/L

9/12/2014 *"2014 OTR Certification Examination Validation Committee Meeting,"* presented by the National Board for Certification in Occupational Therapy

9/8/14 *"DU OT Department In-service: SafeAssign Feature on Blackboard (plagiarism detector),"* presented by Elena Donoso Brown, PhD, OTR/L

6/28/14 *"DU OT Department In-service-Rangos 240: Covered aspects of technology for use in face to face and online environments. (SMART monitor, doc cam, Bamboo pad),"* presented by Elena Donoso Brown, PhD, OTR/L

6/14/2014 *"Manual Treatment for Shoulder, Elbow, & Hand for Occupational Therapists: Introductory Course,"* POTA District II Event, presented by Pearl Clinical Education, LLC

6/5/2014 *"DU OT Department In-service -Rangos 240: Video Capture techniques including video capture methods for use in online mediums: Camtasia and Explain everything,"* presented by Elena Donoso Brown, PhD, OTR/L

5/15/2014 *"Tutorial on New Teaching Equipment in PBL Lab 233 – Short throw projector & whiteboard with capture features,"* presented by Lauren Turin, DU Media Services

4/4/14 *"SC 242 Vision to Fruition: Reflections on Applying the OT Model to Curriculum to an Entry-Level Doctoral Program,"* presented by 2014 AOTA Annual Conference and Expo

4/4/14 *"Presidential Address Attitude, Authenticity, and Action: Building Capacity got Occupational Therapy,"* presented by 2014 AOTA Annual Conference and Expo

4/4/14 *"Eleanor Clarke Slagle Lecture Education as Engine,"* presented by 2014 AOTA Annual Conference and Expo

4/3/14 *"WS108 (AOTA) Academic Fieldwork Coordinators Forum,"* presented by 2014 AOTA Annual Conference and Expo

12/14/2013 *"Getting a grip on G-Codes: Implications on OT Documentation and Reimbursement,"* POTA District II Event, presented Lynne Huber, OTD, OTR/L & Theresa Wubbens, PT, MPM

10/23/2013 *"2013 ASAHP ANNUAL MEETING"*, presented by Association of Schools of Alied Health Professions

9/2013 *"Collaborate Web Conferencing Workshop,"* presented by Duquesne University Rangos School of Health Sciences

8/21/13 *"Blackboard 9 Updates,"* presented by DU Center Technology Services

7/12/2013 *"2013 OTR Certification Examination Validation Committee Meeting,"* presented by the National Board for Certification in Occupational Therapy

6-8/2013 *"Creating a Powerful Online Learning Experience,"* Online Course, presented by DU Instructional Technology Department

4/18/2013 *"Lymphedema and Complete Decongestive Therapy,"* presented by Cross Country Education

3/15/2013 *"2013 OTR Standard Setting Meeting,"* presented by the National Board for Certification in Occupational Therapy

3/14/2013 *"2013 OTR Certification Examination Validation Committee Meeting,"* presented by the National Board for Certification in Occupational Therapy

11/2012 *"Tutorial on Turningpoint Software (SRS),"* presented by Lauren Turin, DU Media Services

10/5/2012 *"Combined Program Directors Academic Fieldwork Coordinators Meeting,"* presented by The American Occupational Therapy Association, Inc

9/21/2012 *"2012 OTR Certification Examination Validation Committee Meeting,"* presented by the National Board for Certification in Occupational Therapy

4/29/2012 *"Emerging Area of Occupational Therapy Practice: OT Interventions across the treatment Continuum for Woman with Breast Cancer,"* presented by the American Occupational Therapy Association.

Appendix G: Sample Teaching Philosophy

I whole-heartedly enjoy teaching and am committed to the education of future occupational therapy practitioners. As a teaching scholar, my philosophy is congruent with many of the foundational pillars of the occupational therapy profession. As an occupational therapist, I believe in the power of doing. I believe that the most effective learning takes place when students are actively engaged with the content. I believe that in order for students to learn, the learning experience must be personally relevant, so I view my ability to weave professional clinical examples with the content as essential in helping students learn, make connections, and prepare for contemporary practice. Different content calls for different teaching methodologies. Being flexible to teach using a vast array of methods that are best suited for particular content is the hallmark of an effective educator. I expect students to take responsibility for their own learning, and I will do whatever I can to facilitate it. For example, I expect students to have done the readings or complete self-study modules before class, and I teach as if they had. Most of my classes have discussions, role-play, simulation, use of student response systems ("clickers"), or case examples built into them. I believe that this helps shift the responsibility of learning onto the students who become their own architects of learning which helps lay the foundation for lifelong independent learning.

Both practice skills and professional behavior are essential to be an effective occupational therapist. Developing clinical/professional reasoning skills is as important as learning specific techniques. As a teaching-scholar, I understand that there is a responsibility to instill values of life-long learning, professionalism, compassion and ethics. I would like to think that my own personal and professional journey as an occupational therapy practitioner has emulated these values to my colleagues and students. These values help prepare the student to become a servant leader and practice-scholar with a vision and commitment to enhance practice and society. I have developed a teaching style that focuses not only on delivering content, but also on promoting clinical thinking and professionalism.

I am a firm believer that I am educating my future colleagues. I believe that the development of both practice skills and professional behavior are essential to be an effective occupational therapist and practice-scholar. Developing clinical /professional reasoning skills is as important as learning specific techniques. Many of my assignments offer opportunities to exercise initiative, leadership and organizational skills. Likewise, I try to enrich my teaching with as many case examples as possible, garnered from my more than 11 years of clinical practice. I aim to bring dedication and competence to my teaching. It helps that I really enjoy teaching, so working hard at it is not onerous. It also helps that I am so enthusiastic about occupational therapy. I try to infect my students with that enthusiasm, so that they will not find the hard work of learning onerous.

I believe in being frank and open with students about my expectations and philosophy. Students have said that they find my expectations high but reasonable. Other students, however, have indicated that they are not distressed by my high expectations, valuing a good mark from me as a real achievement and appreciating my concern for their future clients. I do not apologize for my high standards. I truly believe that a good education is not necessarily an easy one, and I am committed to providing a good education. That is what a professional teacher offers; that is what a professional student wants; that is what a professional occupational therapist needs; and that is what every future client of my students deserves!

As a fieldwork educator and academic fieldwork coordinator, I wholeheartedly embrace John Dewey's philosophy that learning occurs through experience, I strive to find and set-up students with unique, individually-tailored experiences in fieldwork, and in the health care arena based upon many variables such as the students' clinical interest, learning style and work ethic.

Not unlike the domain and process of the occupational therapy profession, teaching is a complex process involving the dynamic interaction between the students, educator, and the knowledge.

It is ever-changing affected by the individual values and life experiences of each student that enters the classroom. The power of teaching is found in the strength of the connections between the students, teacher, and knowledge.

12

The Job Search and Interview Process

Elizabeth D. DeIuliis, OTD, OTR/L

INTRODUCTION

Professionalism includes practicing basic etiquette and following the norms of acceptable workplace behavior. The way you dress, enter the interview room, shake hands, smile, and introduce yourself to the hiring manager are all essential elements of professionalism. Contrary to popular belief, interviewing is not just about answering questions. It is a series of steps and a sequence of events that allow the potential employer to determine if you are the best candidate for the job. Presenting a professional approach to your interview can affect the way you are perceived, and ultimately make or break the interview's outcome.

KEY WORDS

Behavioral Interview Questions: Interview questions that are geared to learning an interviewee's behavior in certain work situations

Hard Skills: Job skills that can be defined and taught

Soft Skills: Personality-driven skills or personal attributes

Technical Interview Questions: Interview questions that are geared toward the role or job you are interviewing for; they may be based around a patient population, setting, or group of intervention approaches

DeIuliis, E.D.
Professionalism Across Occupational Therapy Practice (pp 283-297).
© 2017 Taylor & Francis Group.

OBJECTIVES

By the end of reading this chapter and completing the learning activities, the reader should be able to:

1. Describe key elements of professionalism that are required during the job search process

2. Identify the importance of making a professional impression during job interviews

3. Define professional behaviors and attitudes which are essential to demonstrate during the job interview process

WHAT IS A JOB INTERVIEW?

An interview is a formal meeting between the candidate and the employer. The interview is a mutual process in which the candidate learns more about the job position, the employer or company, and allows the employer to learn about the candidate. A job interview typically precedes the hiring decision and is used to formally evaluate the candidate ("Job Interview," 2016). The interview allows candidates an opportunity to make an in-person impression. Even if you had a stellar cover letter and résumé, you will still have to make a positive impression in person. According to a survey by Monster.com, 33% of employers claimed that they knew within the first 90 seconds of an interview if they would hire someone or not (Sundberg, n.d.). What will you do to showcase your intrinsic and extrinsic skills as a professional within those 90 seconds?

GENERAL COMPONENTS OF A JOB INTERVIEW

Job interviews can take various forms; these will be discussed later in this chapter. However, the general format is typically the same (Boxes 12-1 to 12-3).

- Introductions
  - Clearly reiterate the purpose of the meeting and the position being interviewed for
  - Communicate the schedule and process of the interview
    - For example: who will you be meeting with? Possibility of a tour of the facility?
- Description of position in detail, as well as positive aspects of the job
- Discuss expectations for an individual in this role
- Explain needs of the department as they relate to the open position
- Questioning
  - The purpose of an interview is to identify and hire candidates who will perform well and want to remain with their employer. To achieve this purpose, the interview process should assess the candidate's technical skills and abilities, personal preferences, and behavior
    - Q & A by Interviewer: When asked questions, always listen carefully. If you don't understand any question, ask them to clarify the question. If you do not know the answer to the question, be honest and say so, but do offer to get back to them with the answer later. If this happens, do get back to them with your response. (Sample questions will be provided later in this chapter.)
    - Q & A by Interviewee: Remember, the job interview is for your benefit as well. Ask questions about the actual job requirements, benefits, and type of work that you will be expected to do. Determine if the job will fit in with your educational background and

Box 12-1

PROFESSIONAL TIP

Make sure your initial nonverbal communication is positive. For example, smile when you first see the person interviewing you. Have a firm handshake and establish good eye contact when talking. Be the one to start off the conversation.

Box 12-2

PROFESSIONAL TIP

Write down all the names and position titles of the people you meet or get business cards. This will helpful for writing your handwritten thank-you notes.

Box 12-3

PROFESSIONAL TIP

Be enthusiastic, engaging, smile, and show positive body language. Realize that everyone you encounter could be a person to provide feedback on your impression.

career goals. Be prepared to take notes during the interview. This demonstrates that you came prepared. (Sample interview questions will be provided later in this chapter.)

- Meet with potential pertinent co-workers or consumers
  - You may have the opportunity to observe, shadow, or meet with other staff members at the site
- Tour facility
- Regroup for final Q & A
  - Your interviewer may have a few remaining questions, or perhaps you do, after the tour or meeting with other individuals
- Closure
  - Perhaps discuss other candidates, timeline of recruitment, and how the decision will be communicated

PREPARING FOR A JOB INTERVIEW

1. Research the company and the job. Know the history of the organization, and the specifications and requirements of the job which you are applying for. For example, from the company website you may be able to find out that the site recently became re-certified by the Commission on Accreditation of Rehabilitation Facilities, won a prestigious award for disease-specific clinical care from The Joint Commission, or maintains a relatively high case mix index in their acute rehabilitation unit. Convince your interviewer that you know the company well, and be able to articulate what makes it special compared to its competitors.

Box 12-4

PROFESSIONAL TIP

Never respond with "I don't have any" when asked about your weaknesses. This can indicate a number of things to the interviewer:

1. That you haven't thought enough about your professional development and skill set

2. It can also provide insight that you may not respond well to critique or constructive feedback

3. If you are an individual who cannot see your own weakness, will you be able to accept it when others see it in you?

---

2. Know whom you are interviewing with and the general structure. Is it the human resources manager, recruiter, or department head? Is there a time limit for the interview? Will it be a group interview with multiple candidates, or an individual interview? Will there be time for a facility tour?

3. Review and update your résumé, cover letter, and portfolio. Be prepared to speak in detail about your experience, accomplishments, and how your own experience relates to the job you are applying for. For example, if the job description states that this position requires competence with splint fabrication, identify experiences in your career that demonstrate your knowledge and skill level with orthoses.

4. Practice! You will likely be asked questions about your technical skills, interpersonal relations, teamwork skills, and ability to work in a diverse environment. Do a mock interview with a friend and use the provided sample interview questions to practice your responses. Interview questions will likely be geared towards gaining information about those "hard and soft skills" you possess that were discussed previously.

Sample behavioral questions (regarding soft skills) which you may be asked:

- What are your strengths?

When you answer this question, you should answer it in terms of "what are the top two or three skills that I bring to this job?" Because of this, your strengths that you are willing to discuss will usually change from interview to interview, depending on the job and the organization you are meeting with. For example, you are not going to tell an interviewer that you throw a great fastball. Make sure the information you provide pertains to the position you are interviewing for (Box 12-4).

- What are your weaknesses?

Many people view this question as a way for an employer to find out your shortcomings as an employee. This is not the case. The typical reason why this question is asked during the interview process is to determine your level of awareness of your shortcomings. When answering this question, it is important for you to avoid weaknesses that may hinder your job performance or will disclose personal issues. You should choose a weakness before an interview, and only pick one! You should also be able to tell the interviewer steps that you took/are taking to overcome the weakness. The trick to this question is to spin it as a positive or reveal it is as a strength in disguise. Identify a real weakness that does not damage your potential for the position, but also does not come across as unprofessional, such as "lazy," "dishonest," or "immature."

New Graduate Example: "Some people would consider the fact that I have never worked in this field before as a weakness. However, being highly trainable and open minded, I have no preconceived notions on how to perform my job. Working with your organization will give me the

---

Box 12-5

THE STAR APPROACH

1. Situation: "Think about when you _____." The interviewer describes a specific situation which identifies a soft skill.
2. Task: What needed to be done about the situation?
3. Action: What did you do to resolve the situation?
4. Result: What was the result?

---

opportunity to learn the job the way you want it done, not the way I believe it is done. In addition, although I have no former on-the-job experience, I do bring with me extensive hands-on training and experience which can only enhance my ability to learn extremely quickly."

Example: Instead of saying that you have difficulty meeting deadlines or writing daily progress notes in a timely fashion, you could discuss how you are a very detail-oriented individual and take great pride in the quality of your work. With any stated weakness, be sure to indicate specific strategies that you are using to work on this area of development.

- What prompted you to pursue this position?
- Tell me about a time when you handled a difficult client or conflict.
- Tell me about a time when you had to meet a deadline.
- Tell me about a group project you worked on.
- Tell me about a time where you made a mistake. How did you find out you made this mistake, and what did you do to rectify it?
- Where do you see yourself in three or five years?
- How would a friend, colleague, or professor describe you?
- How did your fieldwork experiences prepare you for a position here?
- How did you get involved in the occupational therapy profession?
- What are you looking for in a job that would make you say—"that is a place I want to work"?
- Why do you think you are a good fit for this position?
- How do you handle criticism or negative feedback?
- Can you think of an experience or situation where you turned a negative situation into a positive one?
- How do you define doing a good job as an occupational therapy practitioner?

A popular method to use in answering behavioral questions is the STAR approach (Box 12-5). The acronym stands for Situation, Task, Action, and Result. The STAR approach provides a structured manner of responding to behavioral-based interview questions to gather all the relevant information about a specific capability that the job requires (Wayne State University, 2017).

Using the STAR approach allows you, as the interviewee, to answer a behavioral question in the form of a story (Box 12-6).

Some technical questions, meant to examine hard skills, which you may be asked include:

- What pediatric assessments are you familiar with?
- Describe an evaluation and treatment session with a client who had a total hip replacement surgery one day ago?

Box 12-6

EXAMPLE OF THE STAR APPROACH

Think about a time when you went above and beyond your expectations.

Interviewer Question: "Tell me about a time you demonstrated leadership skills."

Interviewee Answer

- Situation: "During my Level II B FW, I was the first Level II FW student at the site, and they decided they wanted to build a more structured fieldwork program."

- Task: "My fieldwork educator and the department head asked me to create and administer a training module for occupational therapy staff who would be supervising fieldwork students."

- Action: "To complete this task, first, I created a fieldwork manual, including an orientation checklist, site policies, and site procedures. I also initiated communication with each occupational therapy education program in the area to obtain their curriculum philosophy, fieldwork expectations, and school policies. Finally, I presented the information to the staff at my site."

- Result: "The training was a huge success. On a survey completed after the training, each occupational therapy practitioner rated the training a 10 out of 10 in the areas of usefulness and creativity. In addition, my communication and leadership styles were rated as 'excellent.'"

- Describe an example of how you implemented an occupation-based group intervention session for individuals with moderate Alzheimer disease?

- New graduate question, if allowed in state: When do you plan to take the National Board for Certification in Occupational Therapy exam? Are you planning to apply for temporary licensure?

- Describe your experience with rotating between multiple inpatient units. How do you react to dynamic, changing environments?

- Question aimed at interprofessional collaboration: Tell me about your experiences in working with other health care professionals.

QUESTIONS THE INTERVIEWER CANNOT ASK, AND THAT YOU DON'T HAVE TO ANSWER

According to the United States Equal Employment Opportunity Commission, federal law makes it illegal to discriminate against job applicants because of race, ethnicity, religion, sex, pregnancy, national origin, disability, or age (Equal Employment Opportunity Commission, n.d.). Handling these questions during an interview can be difficult. Legally, you are not obligated to answer any of the questions listed above. However, if you feel comfortable answering an illegal interview question, should it arise, you should not hesitate to answer the question. If you do feel uncomfortable answering such a question simply tell the interviewer that you do not feel comfortable answering that question.

+--+
| # Box 12-7 |
| |
| ## QUESTIONS AN INTERVIEWEE SHOULD NOT ASK |
+--+

- "What does this company do?" (Do your research ahead of time!)

- "If I get the job, when can I take time off for vacation?" (Wait until you get the offer to mention prior commitments).

- "Can I change my schedule if I get the job?" (If you need to figure out the logistics of getting to work, don't mention it now.)

- "Did I get the job?" (Don't be impatient. They'll let you know.)

When interviewing a job applicant, a good rule of thumb is to ask only questions that relate directly to the job (Box 12-7). To decide what questions to ask, keep in mind that the purpose of the interview, from the employer's perspective, is to discover which applicant is best qualified, most able, and most willing to do the job. Evaluating an applicant's qualifications and ability is fairly straightforward; ask specific questions about education, training, and work experience. But be sure that you don't ask an applicant to volunteer information that could potentially be used against them, such as "Are you recently engaged?" "Do you have small children at home?" or "Disclose something about your medical history."

Remember that there may be questions during the interview process that you did not anticipate. When this happens, breathe, and take a moment to think about your experience to find the best response. It is appropriate to say "That is a great question. Can I have a moment to think about my response?"

1. Do a dress rehearsal. During the preparatory mock interview indicated above, you should wear the same clothes, hairstyle, and jewelry that you plan to wear to the actual interview. Get feedback on your overall professional image.

2. Prepare a list of questions to ask of the employer/company (Box 12-8). In many situations, the questions you ask in an interview can be more revealing than the answers you give. Employers are looking for candidates who ask insightful questions throughout the recruitment process; they see candidates' questions for employers as clues about their analytical skills. Eliminate questions that can be answered by reading the website or marketing brochures.

3. Lastly, and most importantly, be yourself. While you want to be on your "A" game and present yourself as a professional, it is also important to be authentic.

TYPES OF INTERVIEWS

There are various types of interviews, each serving different purposes. For example, a phone interview may be used to screen initial applicants, while a face-to-face or panel interview may be used to distinguish final candidates.

Phone Interview

Phone interview etiquette is just as important as in-person job interview etiquette when it comes to seeking employment (Box 12-9). The goal of the phone interview is to convince the interviewer to bring you in for a face-to-face interview, which is the next step in the recruitment process.

Box 12-8

SAMPLE QUESTIONS FOR THE INTERVIEWEE TO ASK

- "Can you describe what a typical work day is like here?"
- "Describe the staffing, please. What is the experience level of the other employees? How long have they worked here?"
- "What are the department's short-term and long-term goals?"
  - Show that you did your research—ask questions that relate to the organization's mission/vision statement or value statements.
- "What is your favorite thing about working here?"
- "What would make someone really successful in this position?"
- "What is the company's stance on professional development and continuing education?"
- "Are there any opportunities for mentoring?"
- "When do you hope to make a decision regarding this position?"
- "Is there anything else that I can answer for you?"

Box 12-9

TIPS FOR A PROFESSIONAL PHONE INTERVIEW

- Set up your interview space. Eliminate background noise and the risk of interruptions; have interview materials at your fingertips such as your résumé, reference list, portfolio, or any notes you have prepared.
- Prepare your phone. Be sure your phone is charged and has a good signal; use a landline instead of a cellular phone if possible.
- Don't use speakerphone. It may be beneficial to use a headset with a microphone so that you are free to express yourself with your hands.
- Listen to yourself. Be aware of your pace, volume, tone, and clarity.
- Don't interrupt. Be a patient listener; hold your thoughts or write them down until there's a natural break in the dialogue.
- Dress for the part. Although you may be at home during your telephone interview, consider getting out of your pajamas and put on a professional business casual outfit. While you will not see the interviewer face to face, you will feel more composed, confident, aware, and ready to share your views.

Nonverbal Communication Skills to Be Aware of During a Phone Interview

- Sounds and expressions such as laughter, sighs, and gasps
- Mannerisms of talking such as pauses, stresses on words, "umms," "like," "you know"
- Facial expressions such as smiles and frowns; don't forget to smile!

Box 12-10

WHAT TO BRING TO A PROFESSIONAL INTERVIEW

- Bring and use a pen and paper to write down notes and questions.
- Bring your portfolio so all of your documents are readily accessible.
- Bring extra copies of your résumé, curriculum vitae, and professional reference list. Remember to provide them to the employer, you don't want to be asked for them!

Box 12-11

WHAT TO DO DURING A PROFESSIONAL INTERVIEW

- Arrive early. It is recommended to be 15 minutes early for an interview (Elkins, 2015). Allow yourself extra time to get lost, stuck in traffic, and/or park your car.
- Turn your cell phone off; sounds can still be heard on the vibration setting.
- Do not eat, chew gum, or smoke before or during your interview.
- Actively listen; take notes.
- Be mindful of your interaction and movements during the interview. Your body language, eye contact, handshake, smile, and manners are all being evaluated. Refer to Chapter 1 for more information.
- Show a genuine interest in the employer: Be courteous and respectful; say please, thank you, and you're welcome.
- Radiate friendliness: Greet everyone, including the receptionist, with warmth and a smile.
- Extend yourself: Offer a firm, strong handshake at the beginning and end of the interview.

As silly as it may sound, wearing a smile during your phone interview is important. Smiling improves your state of mind, gives your voice a cheerful boost, and shows enthusiasm and passion to the interviewer. You want to come across as friendly, amicable, and engaging in your phone interview. Did you know that talking with a smile creates a higher frequency in your mouth, changes to the tone of your voice, and provides reassurance to the listener (Westside Toastmasters, n.d.)?

In-Person Interview

Consider your interview as starting the second you step foot on the company's property. Professionalism should occur during every interaction, including with the parking attendant, the person in the lobby, and the secretary (Boxes 12-10 and 12-11).

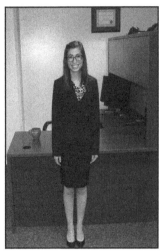

Figure 12-1. Professional interview dress—female.

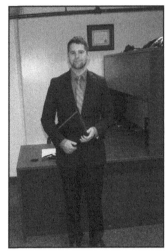

Figure 12-2. Professional interview dress—male.

What to Wear

As discussed in Chapter 2, portraying a professional image is an essential part of being a professional. As if being prepared for a job interview is not daunting enough, choosing your attire can also be challenging.

Attire for Women

Professional interview attire for women typically includes a suit jacket with either trousers or a skirt (Figure 12-1). The rule with a skirt is that the hemline should be no more than 1 inch above the knee. Color suggestions include black, navy, grey, and brown. In the summer months, a lighter color is fine. Patterns and "busy" designs should be avoided. You can choose to add a splash of color with a scarf or subtle jewelry. Keep heels at a sensible height, no greater than 2 inches. Make sure your shoes are clean and polished as this shows attention to detail. Makeup and jewelry should be subtle.

Attire for Men

Suit (black, navy, or grey) with a collared shirt that is pressed; belt worn in belt loops; dress shoes with socks (Figure 12-2). Make sure your dress shoes are clean and polished. Avoid patterns on shirts and ties that are too "busy" and may be distracting to the interviewer (Figure 12-3).

Interview in a Group Setting/Panel Interview

It is not unusual for more than one company representative to interview a candidate to provide a variety of opinions on the individual being interviewed, especially if the new hire will play a key role in the organization. In fact, sometimes these meetings are carried out simultaneously through the use of a panel interview, which is conducted by the hiring manager as well as two to four other members of the management team or work group. Employers respect and like job candidates who look professional and are relaxed, polite, and confident. Preparing for your interview will help you to relax and be confident. Get the correct name, credentials, and titles of all individuals whom you interview with. An easy way to do this is to ask for a business card. Know ahead of time, if possible, whom you will be interviewing with. With this knowledge, you can tailor specific questions to certain individuals to show that you have prepared yourself and done your research.

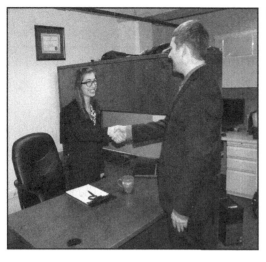

Figure 12-3. Professional interview scenario.

For example, if you are meeting with a middle-level manager, your questions may be geared towards day-to-day operations and how a typical work day goes. On the other hand, questions to a senior-level administrator may be more geared toward leadership style and how you can contribute to the mission of the organization.

Other: Academic Job Interview

The interview process in the academic world is much different than that in clinical practice. Though it varies by discipline and institution, the typical interview process in higher education is facilitated by a "search committee." This is a group of faculty (and sometimes a student representative) who have been charged with structuring and coordinating the recruitment and interview process. A search committee typically consists of four to six members who are internal and external to the department or division you are applying to. These individuals are responsible for leading the search process and formally make the decisions of which candidates will be asked to progress through the academic interview process.

The first step in this process is typically a phone interview with the search committee. This is the preliminary step which allows the search committee to gain an initial impression of the candidate's fit for the job and institution. The next step is an on-campus interview. This is typically an all-day process, which involves the candidate meeting with various individuals and groups on campus such as the search committee, department head, dean, and higher administrators (the provost or head of academics affairs). Furthermore, the on-campus interview typically requires that the candidate deliver a professional presentation to the search committee and/or faculty-body. This presentation is an opportunity for the search committee to experience the candidate's teaching style, as well as potentially learn more about their scholarship trajectory, if appropriate.

In preparing for an academic interview, it is critical to learn about each department you interview with. You can obtain such information from the institution's website. It is beneficial to have a good understanding of the institution's mission, curriculum philosophy, and overall approach to education. Second prepare your presentation thoroughly. Choose your topic wisely and be sure that your presentation expresses your interest and enthusiasm in the topic and teaching as a whole. After the presentation, you may be asked questions from the audience. Plan ahead and prepare answers to questions you may be asked regarding topics such as your scholarly interests, experience in teaching, and work history, as well as professional associations and activities you are involved in.

Box 12-12

COMPONENTS OF A THANK-YOU NOTE

- Begin by expressing gratitude; "Thank you for the opportunity to interview for ... "
- Mention specific details of the interview, but keep it concise.
  - If you interviewed with multiple people, it is beneficial to mention key components of your individual conversations with each interviewer.
- Restate your interest in the position and why you are a good fit.
- Be mindful of the valediction you use. These are the words or phrases that come before you sign your name, such as Sincerely, Respectfully, or Best regards.

Box 12-13

SAMPLE THANK-YOU NOTE

Dear Ms. Jones:

Thank you for meeting with me yesterday to discuss the occupational therapy position you have available in your facility. I was very impressed by your dynamic therapy department. I greatly enjoyed observing the treatment session with OT practitioner Ms. Joan Smith, MS, OTR/L. She shared a lot of valuable information with me regarding the facility's treatment philosophy and how your supervisory structure has facilitated her professional growth as a new graduate.

I was especially excited to learn about the population you serve. During my Level II fieldwork at Burke Rehabilitation, I spent six weeks working with individuals who have sustained traumatic brain injuries. This challenging experience allowed me to integrate my clinical skills with my keen interest in cognitive rehabilitation. The knowledge I gained through my research project on remediating short and long term memory deficits would prove very helpful in this setting as well.

It would be an understatement to say that I am extremely interested in your position. Please let me know if there is any other information you would need before making a decision. I look forward to hearing from you.

Sincerely,

Susan Strom, OTS

After the Interview

Immediately after the interview, you should write a handwritten thank-you note to each person you interviewed with (Boxes 12-12 and 12-13). This is why it is important to get a business card from each person who you meet with. A handwritten thank-you note is more than just fulfilling bare minimum social obligations. It is an opportunity for us to connect to the people in our lives in a meaningful way, and to express gratitude for the interview opportunity. In an increasingly informal digital world, continuing to pull out pen and paper is a way to distinguish yourself. The handwritten thank-you note speaks volumes simply as a medium and sends the message that you care enough to invest yourself personally in acknowledging another person's actions.

Writing a handwritten thank-you note signals to your interviewer that you're serious about the position and went the extra mile with a personal touch. Be sure to proofread for spelling and grammatical errors and to make sure it is legible. Like your professional portfolio, this may be another "thing" that sets you apart from the other job candidates.

Follow-up

When the interview comes to a close, the interviewer may state when you should expect to hear from them again. If you are not contacted during that time frame, it would be appropriate to follow-up in a professional manner. For example, the prospective employer states that they "will be completing the search process within two weeks, and that they will contact you either way." If two weeks come and go and you have not heard back, you can follow-up via phone and/or email stating that you are still interested in the position and curious to know if there are any updates in the search process.

Dealing With Rejection

Rejection for a job or being denied an interview is an unfortunate but realistic part of the job search process. However, receiving rejection can be a positive way to develop your skills and expand your opportunities as a professional. When receiving a rejection, it is important to:

- Stay positive: Tell yourself it is not personal.
- Follow up with interviewer or contact person: Use it as an opportunity to learn and request feedback of why you were not considered for the position. Express appreciation for their assistance.
- Complete a self-assessment: Assess your résumé, self-presentation, and job search methods
- Develop an action plan: Address the concerns that you discovered during the self-assessment. Set goals, identify strategies and resources, and implement your plan.

NEGOTIATING AND ACCEPTING A JOB OFFER

You got an offer, so now what? Negotiating is not easy, regardless of the position or years of experience, for all parties involved. Studies done at Wharton Business School reveal what we already know—that negotiating triggers anxiety (Brooks & Schweitzer, 2011). Furthermore, this anxiety can be harmful to the negotiating process. It was found that people who are anxious receive lower first offers, respond more quickly to offers, exit the bargaining situation earlier, and ultimately realize lower salary and benefit outcomes (Boxes 12-14 and 12-15). The conclusion of this study reports that if an applicant can harness their anxiety and feel more comfortable with the negotiation process, they will achieve a better outcome.

A self-confident mindset helps you to establish yourself in the negotiating process and can translate into more successful salary negotiations. Remember that typically, as part of the application process, you may have had to disclose your current salary. Therefore, the prospective employer already has that information when providing your offer. When given an offer that you are comfortable with, don't say "yes" on the spot (Brooks & Schweitzer, 2011). Ask for a couple of days to think it over. Then, take the time to evaluate the job offer so you are making an informed decision and you're sure you want the job. Consider the entire job offer including job responsibilities, salary, benefits, perks, hours, company culture, work environment, flexibility, the commute, and the other factors that matter most to you when you think about what you'd like to be doing in your next job. Make a list of the pros and cons—writing it down can help clarify whether this is the right job for you. Does it match your career goals? Are there opportunities for mentorship? Does the

---

Box 12-14

TIPS FOR NEGOTIATING LIKE A PROFESSIONAL

- Be evidenced-based. Use the AOTA Salary Workforce Survey (or Faculty Workforce Survey, if looking at academic positions) to procure salary data based upon experience, geographic area, and practice setting (AOTA, 2010, 2015).

- Be open and honest with potential employers. Help them understand why you deserve what you are requesting.

- Be prepared for tough questions. If you enter into negotiation, prospective employers may ask questions such as "Do you have other offers?" "Are we your top choice?" "What salary do you have in mind?"

- Keep records. Get the terms of your final offer in writing.

- Know when to negotiate ... and when to not. Asking for "too many changes" could make the employer rescind their offer.

Box 12-15

HOW SOCIAL MEDIA CAN HELP (OR HURT) THE JOB SEARCH

Social media plays a key role in the job search process today. Sites like Facebook, Twitter, and Instagram allow employers to get a glimpse of who a candidate is outside of his or her résumé, cover letter, and interview. More than one-third of employers used these sites in their hiring process.

Be mindful of your privacy settings, your profile pictures, pages that you "like" and visit, and hashtags (#) that you use. Remember that these social networks are public forums.

---

prospective employer support professional development and continued competence? Do you get that warm and fuzzy feeling of "that's a place I want to work." If there are some things that you're not happy with on the list, consider whether there is room to negotiate. Therefore, salary should not be the only variable you are considering. Most large corporations offer a salary and benefit package based upon experience. A company may offer the same rate to all new graduates because they are coming in with entry-level experience at the generalist-level.

SUMMARY

From start to finish, the job search process is intense and time-consuming. Take the time to prepare yourself, become knowledgeable about the position and company you are interviewing with, and be yourself. Know and believe in your value. Be professional above all else, in all forms including your overall presentation, communication, and actions.

LEARNING ACTIVITIES

1. Review your personal social media accounts. Are they portraying a professional image? Are the privacy settings appropriate? How can they be improved?

2. Do you own clothing and attire appropriate for a professional job interview? If not, identify two to three clothing items necessary to wear to a job interview.

3. Answer the sample interview questions provided within this chapter. What do you think the purpose of each of these questions is?

4. Review the AOTA workforce salary survey and identify the median salary for an occupational therapy position in the setting and geographical area for your upcoming fieldwork sites.

REFERENCES

American Occupational Therapy Association. (2010). Faculty workforce survey. Retrieved from http://www.aota.org/-/media/corporate/files/educationcareers/educators/oteddata/2010%20faculty%20survey%20report.pdf

American Occupational Therapy Association. (2015). *Salary & workforce survey.* Bethesda, MD: AOTA Press

Brooks, A. W., & Schweitzer, M. (2011). Can Nervous Nelly negotiate? How anxiety causes negotiators to make low first offers, exit early, and earn less profit. Retrieved from http://opim.wharton.upenn.edu/risk/library/WPAF2011-04_AWB,MS_NervousNelly.pdf

Elkins, K. (2015). The perfect time to show up for an interview. Retrieved from http://www.businessinsider.com/the-perfect-time-to-show-up-for-a -job-interview-2015-3

Equal Employment Opportunity Commission. (n.d.). Prohibited employment policies/practices. Retrieved from https://www.eeoc.gov/laws/practices/

Job Interview. (2016, April 26). In Wikipedia. Retrieved from https://en.wikipedia.org/wiki/Job_interview

Sundberg, J. (n.d.). How interviewers know when to hire you in 90 seconds. Retrieved from http://theundercoverrecruiter.com/infographic-how-interviewers-know-when-hire-you-90-seconds/

Wayne State University. (2017). Behavioral interview techniques—The STAR approach. Retrieved from http://careerservices.wayne.edu/behavioralinterviewinfo.pdf

Westside Toastmasters. (n.d.). The power of charm on the telephone. Retrieved from http://westsidetoastmasters.com/resources/power_of_charm/chap40.html

13

Continued Competence and Professional Engagement

Elizabeth D. DeIuliis, OTD, OTR/L

INTRODUCTION

Professional development and acquiring clinical and technical knowledge of the profession does not end after graduation, or even after getting your first position. As previously indicated, occupational therapy professionals are expected to be lifelong learners and embrace a professional responsibility to the field throughout their career. This chapter will discuss components of professionalism that exist within practice including continued competence, advanced competency and specialization, and expectations for engaging in professional service.

KEY WORDS

Competence: The quality or state of being functionally adequate or having sufficient knowledge, judgment skill or strength

Competency: The ability to do something successfully or meet necessary standards

Continued Education: Structured educational experiences beyond entry-level academic degree work that are intended to provide advanced or enhanced knowledge in a particular area

Continuing Education Unit: A unit of credit equal to 10 hours of participation in a professional learning program designed for professionals with certificates or licenses to practice various professions and secure credentials

Professional Development Unit: A unit of measure for professional learning and development to meet professional body requirements such as National Board for Certification in Occupational Therapy recertification

Professional Service: The act of helping, volunteering, or serving the profession

DeIuliis, E.D.
Professionalism Across Occupational Therapy Practice (pp 299-307).
© 2017 Taylor & Francis Group.

OBJECTIVES

By the end of reading this chapter and completing the learning activities, the reader should be able to:

1. Discuss the professional responsibility of continued competence in the occupational therapy profession

2. Explain how engaging in professional service is a professional responsibility

3. Identify resources available at the professional level such as service and volunteerism that can assist in the development of professionalism.

COMPETENCE

As indicated in previous chapters, health care providers, including occupational therapy practitioners, play a critical role in ensuring the physical and mental well-being of society and are often held to high standards. A health care professional's competence, or the application of knowledge, skills, and abilities, is a key part of professionalism. Competence refers to the use of knowledge, skills, judgement, attitudes, values, and beliefs to perform in a given role or situation. Competence is multifaceted and a professional's responsibility to maintain, as indicated in the *Occupational Therapy Code of Ethics* as part of Principle 5, Veracity (American Occupational Therapy Association [AOTA], 2015). Continued competence is a commonly recognized value of the occupational therapy profession, and is defined as a "dynamic, multidimensional process in which an occupational therapist or an occupational therapy assistant develops and maintains the knowledge, performance skills, interpersonal abilities, critical reasoning skills, and ethical reasoning skills necessary to perform his or her professional responsibilities" (AOTA, 2006). Continued competence is of the utmost importance to a wide range of stakeholders including the public, other health care providers, regulatory bodies, employers, insurers, and professional associations. If you ask occupational therapy consumers, such as clients and patients, if they value continued competence in their occupational therapy service provider the answer will be unanimously "Yes!" Maintaining your competence as an occupational therapy practitioner is critical to your career, the profession, and the public.

Why is continuing competence important?

1. Patients have the right to assume that their health care provider's credentials to practice provide assurance of his or her professional competence.

2. Clinicians themselves want assurance that those with whom they practice possess and use current knowledge and skills and are fully competent.

3. Continued competence is required to meet credential requirements (i.e., track continuing education and requirements for licensure and National Board for Certification in Occupational Therapy [NBCOT] recertification).

Continuing competence ensures that a professional is able to perform in a changing environment, contributes to occupational therapy practice, and increases public confidence in the profession.

The AOTA's Standards for Continuing Competence define continuing competence as a process involving the examination of current competence and the development of capacity for the future (AOTA, 2005). It is a component of ongoing professional development and lifelong learning.

Box 13-1

Tips to Get PDUs/CEUs

1. Develop a professional relationship with occupational therapy educational programs and accept fieldwork and doctoral students

2. Seek out a formal mentor and document your mentor relationship for NBCOT PDUs

3. Participate in and document professional service (see "Professional Engagement and Service")

Continued Competence

The Commission on Continued Competence and Professional Development is a body of the AOTA Representative Assembly (RA) that develops and maintains the Standards for Continuing Competence. The Commission on Continued Competence and Professional Development provides guidelines and tools that support the ongoing professional development of practitioners, including the AOTA Professional Development Tool (AOTA, 2003). It is also the body that researches the feasibility of developing board or specialty certifications that, if approved by the AOTA Representative Assembly, are then implemented by the Board for Advanced and Specialty Certification. To meet professional competence standards, professionals should plan for, track, manage, and assess their competence throughout their career.

Plan for

Professionals are responsible for being knowledgeable about the competency requirements of their work facility or institution, state regulatory board, advanced certification boards, and the NBCOT. Many health care professions, including occupational therapy, are regulated professions that heavily rely on continuing education to fulfill continuing competence credits. A continuing education unit (CEU) is a measure of the time involved in the continuing education activity. Many professions use CEUs to establish requirements for licensure and certification renewal, as well as standards for approving continuing education activities and providers. Another unit of measurement is a Professional Development Unit (PDU). For example, NBCOT requires 36 PDUs every three years to renew your certification. Additionally, many state licensure boards and regulatory bodies are dictating a need for proof of continued competence for licensure renewal. For example, in Pennsylvania, evidence of 24 continuing competence credits is required every two years to renew your occupational therapy license (Box 13-1).

Besides planning for and meeting NBCOT and state licensure competency requirements, a component of being a professional is pursuing a life-long learning perspective. Although your occupational therapy education program prepares you to be a generalist in clinical practice, there are various options to pursue advanced clinical practice or clinical mastery (Box 13-2).

Track/Manage

Occupational therapy practitioners and professionals are responsible for managing the various criteria and requirements necessary to maintain and renew licensure, certification, and registration. Professionals can use a portfolio as a strategy to organize, maintain and secure evidence of continuing competence, see "Professional Portfolio" in Chapter 11. Professionals are expected to produce evidence of competency, on demand, if a professional and/or regulatory body requests verification of your continued competency. Be sure to keep record of each PDU and CEU that you receive and store neatly in your professional portfolio.

Box 13-2

ADVANCED COMPETENCY

The AOTA offers opportunities for professionals to expand their clinical knowledge, skills, and professional knowledge with Board Certification and Specialty Certification.

Board Certification is offered in the areas of Gerontology, Mental Health, Pediatrics, and Physical Rehabilitation.

Specialty Certification is offered in Driving and Community Mobility, Environmental Modification, Feeding, Eating and Swallowing, Low Vision, and School Systems.

Additionally, there are other, non-AOTA advanced certifications that practitioners can pursue in their specialty areas, such as Certified Hand Therapist, Certified Lymphedema Therapist, Certified Psychiatric Rehabilitation Practitioner, Certified Brain Injury Specialist, and Assistive Technology Provider.

If you are interested in attaining more information about Board and Specialty Certification, refer to AOTA certification at AOTA.org.

Assess

This text has emphasized that self-reflection can be an important step to both personal and professional development. The NBCOT has designed a number of tools to help you self-assess your skill level across multiple areas of occupational therapy practice. Use them to:

- Document strengths in a specific practice area
- Identify professional growth opportunities
- Link current skills and abilities to critical job skills and performance plans
- Assess learning needs prior to re-entering the workforce after a prolonged absence
- Assess learning needs prior to transitioning from one area of practice to another
- Form the framework for a professional development plan

NBCOT Self-Assessment

Each self-assessment is divided into sections based on the domain areas of occupational therapy as outlined in the NBCOT (2012) Practice Analysis Study. Within each domain section, individuals can rate their perceived skill level for a variety of tasks. Upon completion, the assessment is scored, enabling the individual to better understand their competencies. The score report contains links to professional development activities appropriate to the practice area. These areas include:

- General Practice
- Physical Disability
- Pediatrics
- Older Adult
- Mental Health
- Orthopedics
- Community Mobility

NBCOT Navigator Tools

The NBCOT Navigator is a new virtual platform housing a web-based assessment delivery engine and certificant dashboard (NBCOT, 2016). The platform is designed to interface with a series of tools and resources to support certificants' continued competency. Through the platform, certificants can identify and access resources related to specific practice areas, receive feedback and track performance on an array of assessment tools, and organize documentation of completed professional development. The tool suite also enables occupational therapy professionals to earn Competency Assessment Units toward their next certification renewal. These interactive tools are also designed to help employers facilitate the ongoing competency assessment and professional development of their occupational therapists and occupational therapy assistants (NBCOT, 2016). At the end of every tool, customized feedback and a recommended reading list is provided, based on practice areas that the professional did not answer correctly. Examples include "edutainment-like" learning activities such as

- Virtual case simulations
- Mini-practice quizzes
- Evidence-based practice activities such as PICO Builders
- Orthotic builder
- Balloon match games

View more details at www.nbcot.org/navigator-tools.

Summary

New graduates may be under the impression that their education as an occupational therapy practitioner comes to an end after graduation and successful completion of the NBCOT examination. However, continued competency is an expectation of all occupational therapy practitioners, no matter what their experience level is. Professional development and continued competency allows occupational therapy generalists to build and create advanced clinical skills, and develop and refine many professional skills. Regulatory bodies and organizations such as the AOTA and NBCOT have developed pathways and tools that allow professionals to pursue, evaluate, and document their continued competency. Occupational therapy professionals are responsible for planning, tracking, and managing their continued competency to promote the provision of the best quality of services for our clients, as well as to advance the overall values of the profession.

PROFESSIONAL ENGAGEMENT AND SERVICE

Service is a key component of being a professional; it is the action of helping or doing work for someone. It typically occurs via volunteerism, and the purpose is to contribute to the welfare of others. As occupational therapy practitioners, we know that volunteerism is an important component of the occupation of work. Volunteer exploration and volunteer participation contributes to an individual's health, well-being, and quality of life (AOTA, 2014). Therefore, engaging in service-oriented activities assists in the development of an individual's professional identity as an occupational being. The AOTA's Centennial Vision challenges the profession to become more occupation-based. By creating more occupational-functioning individuals, we have the capacity to influence society as a whole to be more occupation-based. Engaging in service and increasing one's civic-mindedness can have this influence as well.

As an occupational therapy student, you may be involved in a student occupational therapy association through your occupational therapy education program. The student occupational therapy association can be a great way to learn more about the profession, educational curriculum of your institution, and engage in professional development opportunities as well as philanthropic efforts such as volunteering or fundraising. Professional service is the contribution to the welfare of the profession, including that of your colleagues. It shows a high level of commitment and dedication to the organization and/or profession which you are contributing to. In occupational therapy, service can occur across a wide range of activities such as participation and volunteering at your work site; within the community; or via your regional, state, and/or national organizations. Participation in volunteer and service activities has the potential to facilitate skill acquisition and adaptive strategies to enhance an individual's professionalism (Black & Living, 2004; Musick & Wilson, 2007). By engaging in professional and community service, an individual can enhance professionalism skills such as communication, flexibility, and teamwork. Professional service can be integrated in the work setting, regional, state and/or national platforms or in the community.

Professional Service in the Work Setting

As previously discussed, an occupational therapy clinician has a wide range of responsibilities outside of patient care. Various professional characteristics of an occupational therapy clinician are service-oriented. Here are some examples:

- Being a fieldwork educator or mentor to Level I, II, or doctoral occupational therapy student

- Allowing prospective occupational therapy students an opportunity to shadow you in practice

- Attending and actively participating in department meetings

- Volunteering for and participating in department quality or process improvement teams; e.g., there could be an intradepartment working group looking at best practices in upper extremity splinting, or improving clinical pathways for occupation-based intervention status-post joint replacement surgery

- Becoming involved in facility-wide committees, such as fall prevention or infection control

- Serving as a mentor to novice or junior staff members

Occupational therapy professionals need to serve as role models for their colleagues in engaging in professional service at their work setting. Active participation, timeliness, good interpersonal communication, and organization skills are important extrinsic qualities of professionalism to display during professional service. When your supervisor, manager, or administrator suggests or requests you to become involved in a work group or committee at your work site, instead of thinking about it as being extra work or an additional responsibility, embrace it and consider it an opportunity to develop yourself as a professional. Participation in these activities leads to advancement at your work setting by making you more valuable and marketable to your department. Each of these examples noted above will create opportunities to develop skills as a professional, as well as contribute to the work setting, clientele, and current and future colleagues of your profession.

Professional Service at the Professional Level

Did you know that many major entities and organizations within the occupational therapy profession function through a high level of support from volunteers? State and National Organizations such as NBCOT and the AOTA have elected positions, yet also rely heavily on volunteers (Table 13-1). Regionally, your state occupational therapy association most likely has a local district, which may have opportunities for volunteer work. Contact your regional executive officer to learn more about these potential opportunities. Does your geographic area have a fieldwork consortium? A fieldwork consortium is made up of a group of academicians, typically academic fieldwork coordinators, and clinicians who are fieldwork educators. You can consult the AOTA website or your local occupational therapy programs to learn if there is a local consortium, and what opportunities may be available for service within it.

TABLE 13-1 TYPES OF PROFESSIONAL SERVICE INVOLVEMENT	
Informal	Voting for officers of your local, state, or national organization
	Informing your state officers of your concerns
	Responding to requests for feedback
	Keeping informed of current events and issues
Formal	Attending state and local association meetings
	Informing your state representative of your desire to volunteer
	Responding to "call for volunteer" notices
	Serving on a committee
	Helping out at a conference
	Running for a state or local office

Adapted from American Occupational Therapy Association. (n.d.). Why be involved? Retrieved from https://www.aota.org/-/media/Corporate/Files/Practice/OTAs/OTA-Leadership/Benefits/20%20-%20Why%20Be%20Involved.pdf

Throughout the AOTA, many key committees are made up by volunteer positions. As an AOTA member, you are encouraged to set up a volunteer-service profile via the Coordinated Opportunities for Online Leadership (COOL) system. COOL is an online database maintained through AOTA where individuals can create a profile that matches them with volunteer opportunities according to their area(s) of expertise, years of experience, time available for volunteering, and other criteria. Service roles available through COOL include but are not limited to conference proposal reviewer, special interest section reviewer, *OT Practice* reviewer or editor, and various roles on the professional committees found within the AOTA and ACOTE. Professional service can occur informally or formally. See Table 13-2 for further information.

Lastly, the NBCOT has a growing list of volunteer opportunities for occupational therapy practitioners such as:

- **Item Writer Program:** Help to develop examination items for the OTR or COTA examinations
- **Certification Examination Validation Committee:** Serve on a committee that reviews and validates the OTR or COTA examinations
- **Simulation Question Development Committee (occupational therapy practitioner only):** Serve on a committee that develops, reviews, and validates clinical simulation test items for the OTR examination
- **Continuing Competency Project Development Taskforce (occupational therapy practitioner only):** Serve on a committee that develops products for the continuing competency program

Interested volunteers are encouraged to submit a volunteer application, which you can find on nbcot.org.

TABLE 13-2			
SUMMARY OF CEUS/PDUS EARNED FROM PROFESSIONAL SERVICE			
NBCOT PROFESSIONAL DEVELOPMENT ACTIVITIES	NBCOT PDU VALUE	MAXIMUM UNITS	DOCUMENTATION FOR AUDITS
Volunteering for ... • Organizations • Populations • Individuals ... that adds to the overall development of one's practice roles.	5 hours= 1 unit	18 for occupational therapy role 18 for professional role	Verification of hours via letter from organization, or report describing the hours and outcomes of services provided along with a completed NBCOT volunteer service form
Delivering professional presentations at state, national, or international ... • Workshops • Seminars • Conferences	1 hour = 2 units	36 for occupational therapy role 18 for professional role	Copy of presentation or program listing
Serving as adjunct faculty teaching an occupational therapy-related course. Must not be your primary employment role; counted once per topic; time spent in preparation is not counted.	1 credit hour = 6 units	36 for occupational therapy role 18 for professional role	Date, title of academic course or lecture, name of institution, letter from instructor regarding time spent, course or lecture goals and objectives

Adapted from American Occupational Therapy Association. (n.d.). Why be involved? Retrieved from https://www.aota.org/-/media/Corporate/Files/Practice/OTAs/OTA-Leadership/Benefits/20%20-%20Why%20Be%20Involved.pdf

SUMMARY

While it may appear on the outside to be a lot of committee work and meetings, program building, and philanthropic endeavors, engaging in professional service as an occupational therapy practitioner is much more than it seems. Professional service creates opportunities for networking with other professionals, potential mentors, and leaders within the profession. It allows you to make yourself more marketable and sustainable in the profession. Furthermore, professional engagement in service may create opportunities to advance your career.

LEARNING ACTIVITIES

1. Check out COOL on aota.org, and create your volunteer profile

2. Visit your state occupational therapy association's Web page and find your regional district; identify the names and contact information for the executive officer, secretary, and treasurer

3. Create and plan out some type of service project that would promote the occupational therapy profession, and involve student occupational therapy association club members at your program

4. Find out if your regional geographic area has a fieldwork consortium. To do this, check out the "fieldwork" tab at aota.org

REFERENCES

American Occupational Therapy Association. (n.d.). Why be involved? Retrieved from https://www.aota.org/-/media/Corporate/Files/Practice/OTAs/OTA-Leadership/Benefits/20%20-%20Why%20Be%20Involved.pdf

American Occupational Therapy Association. (2003). Professional development tool. Retrieved from http://www.aota.org/education-careers/advance-career/pdt.aspx

American Occupational Therapy Association. (2005). Standards for continuing competence. *American Journal of Occupational Therapy, 59*(6), 661-662.

American Occupational Therapy Association. (2006). AOTA fact sheet: Continuing competence in the occupational therapy profession. Retrieved from https://www.aota.org/-/media/corporate/files/advocacy/state/resources/cont-comp/ccfact.pdf

American Occupational Therapy Association. (2014). Occupational therapy practice framework: Domain and process. *American Journal of Occupational Therapy, 68*(Suppl. 1), S1-S48.

American Occupational Therapy Association. (2015). Occupational therapy code of ethics. Retrieved from http://www.aota.org/-/media/corporate/files/practice/ethics/code-of-ethics.pdf

Black, W., & Living R. (2004). Volunteerism as an occupation and its relationship to health and wellbeing. *British Journal of Occupational Therapy, 67*(12), 526-532.

Musick, M.A., & Wilson, J. (2007). *Volunteers: A social profile.* Bloomington, IN: Indiana University Press.

National Board for Certification in Occupational Therapy. (2012). 2012 practice analysis of the occupational therapist registered: Executive summary. Retrieved from http://www.nbcot.org/assets/candidate-pdfs/2012-practice-analysis-executive-otr

National Board for Certification in Occupational Therapy. (2016). NBCOT Navigator tool suite. Retrieved from http://www.nbcot.org/navigator-tools

14

Professionalism and Scholarly Writing

Elizabeth D. DeIuliis, OTD, OTR/L

INTRODUCTION

Scholarship is an important process of validating, empowering, and enhancing the practice and profession of occupational therapy. This text is not a research-methods resource; however, there are elements of scholarly writing that require a strong foundation of professionalism. Whether a professional is seeking to create, write, and/or present a scholarly product, professional and scholarly writing is crucial to the product's success.

KEY WORD

Dissemination: The act of spreading or dispersing something, such as a presentation or publication

OBJECTIVES

By the end of reading this chapter and completing the learning activities, the reader should be able to:

1. Identify why scholarly writing is different from other types of writing
2. Understand the elements of a professional PowerPoint presentation
3. Understand the elements of a professional poster presentation

DeIuliis, E.D.
Professionalism Across Occupational Therapy Practice (pp 309-319).
© 2017 Taylor & Francis Group.

Box 14-1

ACCREDITATION COUNCIL FOR OCCUPATIONAL THERAPY EDUCATION (ACOTE) STANDARDS RELATED TO SCHOLARLY WRITING

Standard B.8.8

- OTA: Demonstrate the skills to read and understand a scholarly report.

- OTR (MOT/MSOT): Demonstrate skills necessary to write a scholarly report in a format for presentation or publication.

- OTD: Write scholarly reports appropriate for presentation or for publication in a peer-reviewed journal. Examples of scholarly reports would include position papers, white papers, and persuasive discussion papers.

Adapted from Accreditation Council for Occupational Therapy Education. (2012). 2011 Accreditation Council for Occupational Therapy Education standards. *American Journal of Occupational Therapy, 66*(Suppl. 1), S6-S74.

SCHOLARLY WRITING AND OCCUPATIONAL THERAPY PRACTICE

The purpose of writing is to clearly communicate ideas and information to readers. Scholarly writing is innately different than what you may have previously experienced in a creative writing course. In creative writing, it is common to use many words to express opinions, feelings, and beliefs, as well as to use the first person. The goal of scholarly writing is to clearly, concisely, and accurately communicate information or data. Scholarly writing typically does not involve sharing one's opinions or beliefs without the support from resources or experts, also known as evidence. Writing and professional written communication are important skills for both occupational therapy students and occupational therapy professionals throughout their career. Although professional writing is heavily emphasized in occupational therapy education programs, competence with scholarly writing may not be accentuated as greatly in clinical practice.

STYLE/FORMATTING OF PROFESSIONAL WRITING

Professionals are expected to be knowledgeable about the accepted style and format of scholarly work that is to be disseminated (Box 14-1). The accepted style and formatting for the occupational therapy profession is published by the American Psychological Association (APA). APA style consists of rules or guidelines that an author/publisher observes to ensure clear and consistent presentation of written material. APA style rules and guidelines are found in the sixth edition of the *Publication Manual of the American Psychological Association* (APA, 2009). It concerns uniform use of elements such as:

- Selection of headings, tone, and length
- Punctuation and abbreviations
- Presentation of numbers and statistics
- Construction of tables and figures
- Citation of references
- Other elements that are a part of a manuscript

Box 14-2

RESOURCES IN LEARNING TO WRITE A CONFERENCE PROPOSAL

At their annual conference, the AOTA routinely offers a workshop or session on "How to Submit a Conference Proposal." These sessions cover the steps necessary for submitting an AOTA conference proposal, information that the reviewers evaluate, and explain the review process as a whole.

If you are submitting an abstract, proposal, or professional manuscript for dissemination, APA style is not the only norm with which you must comply; there are also other professional writing characteristics to attend to as well.

How to Write an Abstract/Proposal for a Professional Conference

When a conference is announced or a publication is launching a special edition issue, the organizers or editors will put out a "call for papers," a formal announcement to prospective presenters, contributors, and/or attendees (Box 14-2). This announcement typically includes the conference/ publication name, theme, and deadline for abstract submissions (Froude & Clemson, 2013).

1. Decide on the focus and presentation format. Is there a theme of the conference/publication to which you are submitting? What factors do the reviewers consider when rating the proposal, and is their proposal reviewer form available for you to look at? Generally speaking, there are two main types of format that your presentation may take.

   a. Poster Session: A more visual format for dissemination, a poster session allows for more informal discussion with attendees. A poster is not simply a research paper tacked onto a board. The authors illustrate their findings by displaying graphs, photos, diagrams, and a small amount of text on the poster. The authors will then hold discussions with the registrants who are circulating among the poster boards. Many authors find it helpful to present a brief introduction to answer the obvious questions and allow the remainder of the time for more in-depth discussions.

   b. Platform Presentation, Workshop, or Institute: Presented formally, typically in lecture format, with use of audio-visual equipment such as PowerPoint or Prezi. These can vary in length from 50 minutes to 1 hour and 50 minutes, all the way up to 3 or more hours, depending on the conference.

2. Prepare the abstract. Review the call for paper guidelines and abstract submission information. It is critical to follow the submission guidelines; you must stay within the word or character limit, use the headings outlined, and submit by the indicated deadline. Consider your audience and level of expertise of your topic. Don't use abbreviations. Incorporate evidence when appropriate, and cite using APA format. Also, don't forget to check your calendar. Are you available to attend the conference to present, if accepted? Make sure you know these things in advance.

3. Proofread multiple times. Have a peer review your abstract prior to submission for content and mechanical errors.

Box 14-3

COMPOSING SLIDES

- Include a slide with your objectives
- Keep the design very basic and simple
- Pick an easy-to-read font face
- Carefully select font sizes for headers and text
- Leave room for highlights, such as images or take-home messages
- Follow APA format and style for citing text and images

Box 14-4

USING CONSISTENCY

- Consistently use the same font and size on all slides
- Do not use a font size smaller than 24 point
- Match colors

Box 14-5

USING CONTRAST

- Use contrasting colors for text and background
- Light text on a dark background works best
- Patterned backgrounds can reduce the readability of text

View a sample conference abstract proposal form in Appendix A. If your abstract is accepted, congratulations! Now you need to create your professional presentation. The use of a PowerPoint presentation, or other applications such as Prezi, can be a great way to support a speech, visualize complex concepts, or focus attention on certain subjects (Boxes 14-3 to 14-9).

Box 14-6

APPLY BRILLIANCE AND ANIMATION CAREFULLY

- Carefully use color to highlight your message and create an impact.
- Avoid the use of flashy transitions such as text fly-ins, or special effects such as animation and sounds. These features may seem impressive at first, but are distracting and can affect your credibility.
- Use good quality images that reinforce and complement your message. Ensure that your image maintains its impact and resolution when projected on a larger screen.
- To test the readability of your font and font size, stand 6 feet from the monitor and see if you can read the slide.

Box 14-7

THINK SIMPLE

- Limit the number of words on each screen. Use key phrases and include only essential information.
- Limit punctuation.
- Avoid putting words in all capital letters.
- Limit the number of slides; presenters who constantly "flip" to the next slide are likely to lose their audience. A good rule of thumb is one slide per minute.

Box 14-8

HAVING A TAKE-HOME MESSAGE

- Connect with the learning objectives.
- Keep your audience in mind; what do they expect from this presentation?

Box 14-9

PRACTICE

- Rehearse for someone who has never seen your presentation. Ask them for honest feedback about colors, content, and any effects or graphical images you've included.
- Know your slides inside out.
- Speak freely.
- Speak with confidence; be loud and clear.
- Don't speak too fast.

continued

Box 14-9 (CONTINUED)

PRACTICE

- Maintain eye contact with the audience.
- Be aware of your body language and posture.
- Smile!

Box 14-10

STEPS TO BUILD A POSTER TEMPLATE IN POWERPOINT

1. Open a blank PowerPoint slide.
2. Go to "Page Setup."
3. Create a custom size; e.g., 56" width, 42" height.
4. Select "Landscape" for the slide orientation.
5. Select a slide theme or just leave it blank.
6. Go under "View" to "Master" to "Slide master"; here, you can designate the font size, type, color, and type of bullets used for the textboxes. It is much easier to make these changes in the slide master than to change the text manually for each text box you create.
7. Go back to "View," then to "Normal."
8. You can now add your individual textboxes and/or graphics.
9. Because this is a formal and professional presentation, posters should not contain arts and craft items such as glitter, handwritten or hand-colored items, pictures cut out of a magazine, and so forth.

PROFESSIONAL POSTER

Most scholars will create a template for a professional poster using PowerPoint. This template is then used to print a full-size poster (Box 14-10). A poster is usually a mixture of brief text along with tables, graphs, pictures, and other presentation formats. At a conference, the author(s) stand(s) by the poster display while other attendees come and view the presentation, as well as interact with the author(s).

Basic Poster Layout

Be sure to proofread your poster prior to its final printing to ensure it is free from typos and formatting errors. Additionally, attend to the poster size dimensions indicated in the author guidelines from the conference. Prior to the conference, it is a professional's responsibility to be knowledgeable of the author instructions. Do you need push pins to hang your poster? Do you need to remain by your poster board for the entire duration of the session? Are you expected to post or

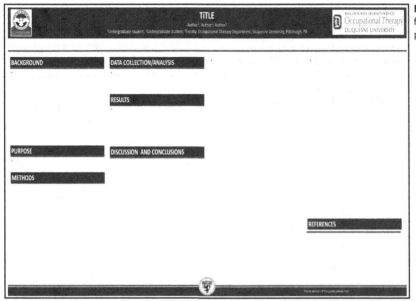

Figure 14-1. Template for professional poster presentation layout.

Box 14-11
TIP
Poster presenters and speakers at most professional conferences get discounted registration fees, as well as professional development units.

provide handouts? At the conference, arrive early and be sure to check the room/area where your presentation will be occurring. Professional dress is a given. Make sure all equipment works, and always start on time (Figure 14-1; Box 14-11).

SUMMARY

Participation in scholarly projects, service, and clinical practice are expectations of occupational therapy practitioners. In order to participate in professional conferences as a speaker or presenter, occupational therapy professionals must demonstrate competence in scholarly writing. Being knowledgeable of APA style and format, and attending to conference proposal guidelines are very important rules for scholarly writing success.

LEARNING ACTIVITIES

1. Find and read the author guidelines for the journal *OT Practice*

2. Find and read the author guidelines for an occupational therapy conference proposal

3. Seek out your State Occupational Therapy Association Annual Conference website and find their call for papers/abstract submission guidelines. Draft a potential abstract for a presentation, following these guidelines.

REFERENCES

Accreditation Council for Occupational Therapy Education. (2012). 2011 Accreditation Council for Occupational Therapy Education standards. *American Journal of Occupational Therapy, 66*(Suppl. 1), S6-S74.

American Psychological Association. (2009). *Publication manual of the American Psychological Association* (6th ed.). Washington, DC: American Psychological Association.

Froude, E., & Clemson, L. (2013). Writing for publication. *Australian Occupational Therapy Journal, 60*(4), 229.

APPENDIX A: SAMPLE CALL FOR PAPERS

2017 ANNUAL STATE OCCUPATIONAL THERAPY CONFERENCE

Proposal deadline: March 31, 2016

Proposals can be submitted at any time until **midnight March 31, 2016**

For each proposal submitted, you will be asked to choose from one of the following session types:

☒ **50 min. & 1 hour 50 min. Sessions**
This level of session allows for presentation of information that is usually in lecture format, but may involve other teaching methods.

☐ **Institute (2 hour 50 min.)**
This level of session provides an in-depth exchange of professional information. This session should include a variety of teaching methods and opportunities for audience participation.

☐ **Poster Session**
The Poster Session allows for a visual presentation of information. NOTE: At least one presenter is required to be present for the entire duration of the Poster Session.

The online form will prompt you to include the following:

Title (8 words or less)

Academia as an Occupational Therapy Practice Setting?

Choose a primary Content Focus
☐ Children & Youth; ☒ Education/Fieldwork; ☐ Emerging Practice; ☐ General; ☐ Health & Wellness; ☐ Mental Health; ☐ Productive Aging; ☐ Rehab & Disability; ☐ Research; ☐ Work & Industry

Abstract
The abstract (40 words or less) is printed in the program, and should articulate the purpose and content of the session.

Being an Occupational Therapy educator is an exciting option for practitioners who are eager to share their knowledge as they teach and mentor the next generation. Come listen to three unique perspectives of successfully transitioning from the clinic to the classroom.

Program Description/Learning Objectives/References (300 words or less)
The program description is a well written, well organized narrative which includes the purpose, intent, methods, and content of the presentation. The Program Description should be 300 words or less. Two or three Learning Objectives which are clear, behavioral, and relevant to occupational therapy are required. Learning objectives describe the knowledge and/or skills participants will acquire as a result of attending the session. References should be current and support the information presented in the Program Description. References are not included in the 300-word count and will be listed in a separate reference box.

The occupational therapist (OT) role is multifaceted, including practitioner, fieldwork educator, consultant, entrepreneur, researcher, and educator.[1] The role of an educator is a practice area that can be assumed in full-time, part-time, or adjunct positions. However, transitioning to a faculty role can be challenging, even for a seasoned clinician. With the changing health care environment and the profession's impending move to an entry-level doctorate, there is a high demand for OTs to practice in the academic setting. The field of occupational therapy is expected to increase faster than other professions at least through the year 2022.[2] ACOTE Standards mandate that at least half of full-time faculty must hold doctoral degrees.[3] As the number of academic programs in occupational therapy is steadily increasing, the ready pool of faculty members to staff these existing and new programs is insufficient. According to the AOTA Faculty Workforce Survey, the median age among occupational therapy faculty is 50, program directors is 52, and the average projected year for retirement is 2022.[4] The faculty shortage is an issue that must be addressed if the profession is to continue to grow and thrive. One way to combat this issue is to recruit from the profession's greatest resource: clinicians. OT practitioners by trade are natural teachers. Within the clinical context, OTs initiate interventions with clients that involve teaching valuable ways to increase occupational performance. Many of the skills and processes needed to excel in clinical practice resemble those that an occupational therapy educator must demonstrate. This presentation will: 1) Explore the complexity of the transition from practitioner to faculty member 2) Compare and contrast the role and workplace experience of a OT practitioner and an OT educator 3) Identify challenges and rewards for OTs considering the move from the clinic to the educational setting.

References:
1. Fisher, Thomas. (2014). Roles of Occupational Therapist. In Jacobs, K, MacRae, N. & Sladyk, K. (Eds). *Occupational Therapy Essentials for Clinical Competence* (2nd Ed., pp. 693-704). Thorofare, NJ: SLACK Incorporated
2. U.S Department of Labor, Bureau of Labor Statistics. (2012). Occupational therapist, assistants and aides. *Occupational outlook handbook.* Retrieved March 23, 2015 from http://www.bls.gov/ooh/healthcare/occupational-therapists.htm
3. Accreditation Council (2011). Accreditation Standards for a Master's-Level-Degree Educational Program

for the Occupational Therapist (OT). *American Journal of Occupational Therapy. 66, (6), S6-S74.*

4. American Occupational Therapy Association. (2007). *2007 Faculty Workforce Survey.* Bethesda, MD: AOTA

NOTE: No author names or any type of identifying information should appear in the program description

Primary Speaker Qualifications/Short Bio
The Primary Speaker Qualifications/Short Bio provides describes the experience and expertise of this speaker in presenting this information

Elizabeth D. DeIuliis is an Assistant Professor and the Academic Fieldwork Coordinator at Duquesne University and Elena Donoso Brown is an Assistant Clinical Professor at Duquesne University. The presenters share a unique experience in transitioning into the academic setting from clinical practice.

All proposals will be peer reviewed. Proposals that meet the submission requirements outlined above will be given priority review. Review will consider the following:

- Organization (objectives are clearly stated, overall plan is clear, concise and logical)

- Content (based on acceptable concepts of practice, education, research and/or theory)

- Appeal (timely and recommend proposal's inclusion in this year's program)

Neither names nor affiliations are provided to the reviewers. All submissions are given equal opportunity, and names of both submitter and reviewer remain anonymous. Written notification of proposal acceptance or rejection will be provided by the end of May, 2015.

_____

Important notes:

1. **Proposals submitted by a student must include a faculty mentor/co-presenter.**

2. **As per policy, all speakers must register for conference. Speakers are eligible to receive reduced conference registration fees as follows:**

- For a 50 minute **SHORT PRESENTATION**: 2 presenters are eligible for a reduced registration
- For a 1 hour, 50 minute **PRESENTATION**: 2 presenters are eligible for a reduced registration
- For a 2 hour, 50 minute **PRESENTATION**: 3 presenters are eligible for a reduced registration
- For a **POSTER** presentation, 2 presenters are eligible for a reduced registration

15

Professionalism and Ethics in Research

Andrea D. Fairman, PhD, OTR/L, CPRP

INTRODUCTION

"Ethical research depends on the knowledge and integrity of the investigator. Everyone who undertakes an investigation assumes a moral responsibility to abide by commonly accepted ethical standards"

—Kielhofner, 2006, p. 469

Professional responsibility, conduct, and competency are expectations of all occupational therapy practitioners, regardless of their roles. Practitioners who are scientists, researchers, and scholars are also morally and legally bound to comply with ethical and professional practices. The generation of research is critically important to advancing occupational therapy and ensuring the viability of the profession. This chapter will discuss recognized standards of research practice and highlight ethical and professional responsibilities of issues relevant to conducting rehabilitation research, with examples specifically related to the occupational therapy profession. Issues include protection of human subjects, authorship, responsible use of research funding, conflict of interest policies, reporting to funding sources, and other forms of dissemination.

KEY WORDS

Autonomy: Self-directing freedom; the state of existing or acting separately from others

Beneficence: Ethical principle encompassing the doing of active goodness

Conflict of Interest: A situation in which the concerns or aims of two different parties are incompatible

DeIuliis, E.D.
Professionalism Across Occupational Therapy Practice (pp 321-333).
© 2017 Taylor & Francis Group.

Control Group: A group of research participants who receive either no intervention or standard care intervention in order to provide a baseline comparison for the outcomes of experimental intervention

Exempt from Institutional Review Board Review: The least rigorous level of institutional review board examination, occurring when research poses no more than minimal risk to participants and falls into one of six categories as defined by federal regulations

Expedited Institutional Review Board Review: Occurs when research does not pose more than minimal risk to participants, and falls into one category for expedited review as defined by federal regulations

Informed Consent: Permission granted by a participant to a researcher for their participation in a study, given with knowledge and understanding of implications to the individual that participation will entail

Institutional Review Board: Institution-affiliated entities formed to protect the best interests and rights of persons involved in research; institutional review boards may also review research proposals for scientific merit, the competence of the researcher(s) involved, and the feasibility of the study being proposed

Justice: Ethical principle encompassing the equitable treatment of people

Risk-Benefit Ratio: The ratio between risks and benefits of a given action, such as participation in research, provided that risk is an inherent factor encountered in everyday life

OBJECTIVES

By the end of reading this chapter and completing the learning activities, the reader should be able to:
1. Describe the need for ethical oversight of research studies involving humans
2. Explain ethical principles that guide research
3. Describe important documents relevant to research
4. Identify and discuss ethical issues arising in research

PROTECTION OF HUMAN SUBJECTS

Ethical behavior with respect to research and scholarly activities is a complex matter involving the responsibility that researchers have to the persons under study (also called research subjects), other researchers, and society as a whole (Kellehear, 1993; Kimmel, 1988). In many instances, unethical behavior in research is very clearly identified. Researchers and clinicians alike understand that it is unethical to engage in practices that put their patients, clients, or subjects in danger or at risk for potential harm. However, there are also many gray areas in which it is hard to know the best course of action to take in a given situation when circumstances require the ability to interpret ethical guidelines and specific policies put in place by institutions.

One of the most notorious research projects to take place in the United States illustrating these gray areas was the Tuskegee Syphilis Experiment (Emanuel, Abdoler, & Stunkel, n.d.).

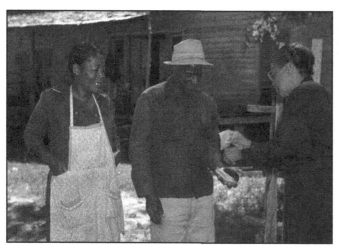

Figure 15-1. Photo of Tuskegee study from Centers for Disease Control and Prevention website. (Reprinted from www.cdc.gov/tuskegee/timeline.htm)

Box 15-1

TEACHING RESOURCE: MOVIE TO WATCH AND DISCUSS

The "Miss Evers' Boys" (Berstein & Sargent, 1997) film was produced for the HBO cable network; this docudrama explores the social and ethical issues at the heart of the infamous "Tuskegee Study of Untreated Blacks with Syphilis." The film presents the events from the viewpoint of Eunice Evers (actress Alfre Woodard), a local nurse who participated as a researcher and was aware of the study's true nature. As a health care professional, Miss Evers also displayed great kindness and compassion to the men participating in the study. She devoted her life to caring for the men as they suffered physical and mental disabilities secondary to the long-term effects of their untreated syphilis and eventually died (See Learning Activity using the "Miss Evers' Boys" film listed at the end of this chapter).

The Tuskegee study provides numerous examples of how clinicians and researchers can find themselves in situations where what is best for the individual or for society is unclear. The researchers involved in the Tuskegee study had initially sought to draw the attention of the United States government to impoverished black men who could not afford medical care for the treatment of syphilis, with hopes that funding would be allocated to help this population. Originally, the study was established to record the natural history and progression of syphilis, to provide evidence justifying treatment programs. The Tuskegee study began in 1932, before many of the regulations that govern the conduct of research were put into place. Additionally, when the study began, there was no known cure for syphilis and the course of the disease was not well understood. Many of the research participants were undereducated, and to try and make it more relatable for them, their condition was explained as "bad blood." The study provided the participants with free exams, treatments used at the time, and some financial incentives. The study continued for 40 years (1932-1972), and more became known about syphilis. Penicillin was used by clinicians outside the study to effectively treat the disease. However, this knowledge and intervention was withheld from the Tuskegee study research participants (Emanuel et al., n.d). One may wonder how such unethical behavior could be rationalized. Placed into the context of lack of funding and other resources, we can begin to understand how these ethical dilemmas evolve (Figure 15-1; Box 15-1).

In addition, there may have been a component of racism guiding the negative turn of the Tuskegee study, which was also seen in the human experimentation that was conducted

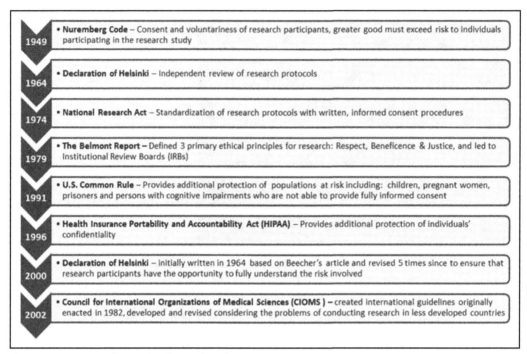

Figure 15-2. Timeline of research polices and guidelines.

in Nazi Germany. The atrocities that occurred under the guidance of Nazi physicians, where they used prisoners in concentration camps to conduct medical experiments, are some of the most horrific examples of unethical behavior that has occurred in the name of research. Out of the instances of misuse of power and authority in the name of science has evolved the guidelines that govern the protection of human subjects today. Specifically, the following regulations and codes were developed over the years and continue to guide ethical clinical research today (Figure 15-2).

Fischer (2006) provides a summary of many of the important documents that serve as guidelines in conducting clinical research. However, together these guidelines do not provide a comprehensive guide to ethical conduct; at some points, they may even seem to contradict one another. The next section will examine several of the guiding principles that occupational therapy professionals should apply to occupational therapy research.

RESEARCH POLICIES AND GUIDELINES

Research in occupational therapy does not necessarily conjure up images of a mad scientist performing cruel acts involving human experimentation. In fact, even past instances where unethical treatment of persons involved in human experimentation has occurred, many of the researchers involved identified motivations for contributing to the "greater good." The Nuremberg Code (National Institutes of Health, 1949) was one of the first set of guidelines established in reaction to the horrific acts of human experimentation that occurred in the Nazi concentration camps (Box 15-2). The principles of beneficence (do good) and nonmaleficence (do no harm) require investigators to minimize the harm and enhance benefits to the study population posed by their participation.

The principle of justice requires that persons be treated in an equitable manner. This means that no specific individual or group of persons either more greatly benefits or bears a larger burden than others. The principle of autonomy requires us to treat subjects as autonomous individuals

---

Box 15-2

THE NUREMBERG CODE (1947) HAS 10 PRIMARY POINTS:

1. All persons have the right to exercise free power of choice—no coercion

2. The research study should be well-designed to yield results that will benefit society

3. Animal trials should be conducted before human experiments occur whenever possible or appropriate

4. Research methods should or seek to decrease any level of suffering (pain, fatigue, distress)

5. No experiment that has the known result of injury death should ever be conducted

6. The importance of the research for the humanitarian importance, or greater good, should always exceed potential risk to individuals participating in the study

7. Facilities and preparations should be made to protect research participants from risk and any remote possibility of injury, disability, or death

8. Research should only be conducted by qualified personnel

9. Participants must be free to withdraw from a research study at any time

10. If at any time it appears that continuation of the research study is likely to result in injury, disability, or death, the study must be immediately terminated

---

whose welfare and rights need to be respected. Written, informed consent is necessary prior to involving subjects in any research activities (Box 15-3).

Sometimes, subjects may complete screening questions or tasks before being officially enrolled into a study. In addition, the confidentiality and privacy of research subjects must be respected and protected. In instances where the data being gathered is part of the individual's protected health information, Health Insurance Portability and Accountability Act (HIPPA) regulations apply and documentation must be maintained. In all instances, gathered data need to be handled with the utmost care to protect the welfare and confidentiality of research participants.

The Declaration of Helsinki called for the independent review of research protocols to apply eight basic principles: (1) collaborative partnership, (2) social value, (3) scientific validity, (4) fair subject selection, (5) favorable risk-benefit ratio, (6) independent review, (7) informed consent, and (8) respect for human subjects (World Medical Association, 2013). To ensure that the application of these principles protect the best interests and rights of persons involved in research, Institutional Review Boards (IRBs) were established in the mid-1900s at academic and medical institutions. Members of the IRB may also review research proposals for scientific merit, the competence of the researcher(s) involved, and the feasibility of the study being proposed. Special attention is paid to research studies conducted on vulnerable populations to ensure their rights are not violated and that informed consent is truly obtained.

As a professor of anesthesiology, Henry Beecher (1966) engaged in human research at Harvard's Massachusetts General Hospital. Appalled by what was discovered through the Nuremberg trials of the actions of Nazi scientists, Beecher noted some similarities in the actions of American scientists. In particular, he noted these researchers were exploiting persons, especially those from vulnerable populations. Beecher began lecturing and publishing articles to increase public awareness of this problem. Beecher's best known article is his 1966 essay in *The New England Journal of Medicine* entitled "Ethics and Clinical Research."

Box 15-3

BASIC REQUIREMENTS OF INFORMED CONSENT

1. Statement that the study involves research, an explanation of the purposes of the research and the expected duration of the subject's participation, a description of the procedures to be followed, and identification of any products that are experimental.

2. Description of any reasonably foreseeable risks or discomforts to the subject.

3. Description of any benefits to the subject or to others that may reasonably be expected from the research.

4. Disclosure of appropriate alternative procedures or courses of treatment, if any, that might be advantageous to the subject.

5. Statement describing the extent, if any, to which confidentiality of records identifying the subject will be maintained and that notes the possibility that external regulatory agencies, such as the U. S. Food and Drug Administration, may inspect the records.

6. For research involving more than minimal risk, an explanation as to whether any compensation and/or medical treatments are available if injury occurs and, if so, what they consist of, or where further information may be obtained.

7. Explanation of whom to contact for answers to pertinent questions about the research and research subjects' rights, and whom to contact in the event of a research-related injury to the subject. This requirement contains three components, each of which should be specifically addressed. The consent document should provide the name of a specific office or person and the telephone number to contact for answers to questions about the research study itself, research subjects' rights, and research-related injury.

8. Statement that participation is voluntary, that refusal to participate will involve no penalty or loss of benefits to which the subject is otherwise entitled, and that the subject may discontinue participation at any time without penalty or loss of benefits to which the subject is otherwise entitled.

Adapted from University of California Office of Research. (2015). Required Elements of Informed Consent. Retrieved from http://www.research.uci.edu/compliance/human-research-protections/irb-members/required-elements-of-informed-consent.html

---

Vulnerable populations include children, pregnant women, persons who are incarcerated, and persons with cognitive deficits that do not allow them to make decisions for themselves. All human research participants must volunteer and not be coerced in any way to participate. Once it can be determined that the individual understands all aspects of the study, including activities, potential risks, and benefits, informed consent must be obtained in writing before any research activities occur. The subject should clearly understand the purpose, nature, and duration of the study. It must be made clear that research subjects are free to cease participation in a study at any time, upon request, without any negative impact in the services they may be receiving from the investigator or institution. Death and/or disability should never be directly anticipated as a result of participating in any aspect of the research study.

Some individuals do not have the legal or cognitive capacity to provide fully informed consent. In such instances, the person's legal guardian or family member can provide consent. Children under the age of 18 years or persons who require legal guardianship because of their inability to

---

Box 15-4

BOOK REVIEWS: EXAMPLE OF VULNERABLE POPULATIONS

Acres of Skin: Human Experiments at Holmesburg Prison is a 1998 book by Allen Hornblum.

This book describes the practice of non-therapeutic medical experiments on prison inmates at Holmesburg Prison in Philadelphia, Pennsylvania, from 1951 to 1974. These experiments were conducted under the direction of dermatologist Albert Klingman.

ISBN-13: 978-0415923361

ISBN-10: 0415923360

The Plutonium Files was written by Eileen Welsome in 2000 to describe the shocking scientific trials related to atomic energy research conducted in the United States from the 1930s to the 1990s.

ISBN-13: 978-0385319546

ISBN-10: 0385319541

---

make informed decisions for themselves, or limitations due to cognitive, emotional, or physical incapacitation, also require written consent. For consent, a signature must be obtained from the parent, guardian, or person serving as Power of Attorney of the person being sought to participate in the study on the assent form in addition to, or instead of the consent form for an individual who is unable to consent. Often times, occupational therapy research is conducted on vulnerable populations. Special efforts need to be made to ensure these persons are not being coerced, feel obligated, or are unwillingly forced to participate in a research study regardless of the perception of risk (Box 15-4).

As previously noted, special care must be taken when conducting research with vulnerable populations that are often necessary for occupational therapy studies. Emancipatory research allows an approach to research with older, disabled populations that can also minimize conflicts when dual researcher roles exist (Good, 2001).

RANDOMIZATION

Situations may arise in which a researcher or clinician may feel compelled to move a client to the intervention, control, or alternative group despite randomized assignment. At times, the desire to provide the best possible care for one's client with the strong belief that the intervention will help may override the research protocol. However, the purpose of conducting the research study is to help establish the clinical efficacy of the intervention. If it were known that the intervention is effective, then it would not be necessary to conduct the study. As in the Tuskegee study, if the intervention truly has been established as the most effective in treating a condition, it would be unethical to withhold this intervention. In some instances, it is permissible to withhold treatment for a brief period or provide alternative treatment without any potential harm to the research subject. Research studies with these types of methodologies can help to establish baseline measures to understand the best frequency or duration of interventions, and/or to compare new interventions or assessments that may prove to be more effective or efficient.

Box 15-5

ILLUSTRATIVE CONFLICTS OF INTEREST*

1. Accepting financial gratuities or special favors from companies or individual parties that may affect judgment.

2. Engaging in research activities where immediate family has a financial, managerial, or ownership interest.

3. Providing special access to information to an entity to which a political or financial relationship exists.

4. Purchasing goods or services from a company in which there is a significant financial stake or other interest using research or other findings from one's institution.

5. Influencing negotiation of contracts between one's primary institution and outside organizations in which there is a significant financial or other relationship.

In July 1995, National Science Foundation ("NSF") "Investigator Financial Disclosure Policy" (now changed to "Conflicts of Interest Policies") and Public Health Service ("PHS") published final rules (PHS: http://grants2.nih.gov/grants/guide/notice-files/not95-179.html and NSF: http://www.nsf.gov/bfa/cpo/gpm95/ch5.htm#ch5-6) which in large part, parallel the NIH regulations.

*The University of Pittsburgh's Conflict of Interest (COI) Office (website: http://www.coi.pitt.edu/index.htm) provides a wealth of information and resources relevant to the successful management and adherence of regulations related to research operations.

Adapted from University of Pittsburgh. (2016). COI Summary for Consultants. Retrieved from http://www.coi.pitt.edu/Forms/StandardCOIMgmtPlan-HSR.htm

---

CONFLICTS OF INTEREST

There are many situations in which a conflict can arise that may potentially bias the researcher in a manner which could either decrease objectivity in how the data is interpreted or the dissemination of research findings the investigator may view as negative. Government legislation, such as the Bayh-Dole Act introduced by U.S. Congress in 1980, has encouraged entrepreneurship of researchers at universities (Shane, 2004). The Bayh-Dole Act recognizes the public service mission of universities in the form of economic development by accelerating the transfer of new technology to the marketplace, clinical, or diagnostic practice. Many institutions encourage faculty members, staff, and students to explore means of commercializing the inventions developing through their research through existing or new and independent companies. As a result, researchers and their institutions often enter into a variety of relationships with industry, such as sponsored research agreements or paid consultant roles. Conflicts of interest (COI) can arise when researchers find themselves in dual roles. A potential or actual COI arises when commitments and obligations to one's primary role or widely recognized professional norms are likely to be compromised by other interests or commitments, especially economic, particularly if those interests or commitments are not disclosed.

The opportunity for researchers to receive financial or other personal rewards from relationships such as these with commercial companies is not intrinsically unacceptable. However, it is crucial that such relationships do not in any way adversely affect the objectivity, integrity, or professional commitment to their role as a researcher. As a result, most academic institutions have very specific COI policies in place to ensure there is no threat to the integrity of the research as well as a variety of other factors (Box 15-5).

A clinician or researcher who decides to commercialize an invention or market a treatment technique for personal financial gain cannot also be a primary investigator on studies that determine efficacy or clinical utility of their creation. The specifics of these policies can vary from institution to institution, but generally include language that describes what is considered Significant Financial Interest, which is an external financial interest. Typically, as required by IRBs, all investigators are required to complete a COI training module on appointment and/or prior to submission of a proposal for external funding.

PUBLICATION BIAS

Negative results are equally as important to report as positive results, and should not be viewed as a failed study. All well-designed and executed studies are important to informing and guiding clinical practice. Sharing discoveries that interventions are not effective is just as valuable as studies that support the efficacy of clinical interventions. However, publication bias has been demonstrated with regard to clinical research (Easterbrook, Gopalan, Berlin, & Matthews, 1991). Easterbrook and colleagues (1991) found that clinical research studies with greater statistical significance had more publications in higher impact journals. Therefore, it is extremely important that journals such as the *American Journal of Occupational Therapy* include articles describing well-designed clinical research studies that do not demonstrate statistically significant results. The insightful evidence-based practitioner will closely examine the rigor of the research study's design in determining whether the intervention is likely to have the same clinical impact with his or her clients.

AUTHORSHIP

The value of publications in the academic arena cannot be underestimated. Success in securing additional funding, as well as growing and evolving one's career, can often largely depend on the quality and number of publications an academic is able to produce; therefore, affecting his or her field. The weight placed on publications can create a competitive environment. Order of authorship is to be determined according to the level of effort and time of each contributor. The occupational therapy profession has adopted the American Psychological Association's practices including formatting of manuscripts and citations. The American Psychological Association requires that any publication provide adequate citations to support claims, to appropriately disseminate information, to exercise ethical practices in accepting funding, and to use ethical decision making. This includes appropriately acknowledging contributors and listing order of authorship in accordance with these contributions (American Psychological Association, 2009). It is important to discuss and establish order of authorship early in the process. In academia, a great deal of weight is placed on the ability to be productive with respect to publications. Faculty members who successfully produce quality publications in high-impact journals are more likely to be eligible for promotion and tenure where applicable in institutions of higher education. In conjunction with promotion, financial incentives often occur as salary increases as well as other "perks," such as a larger or nicer office; these can be highly motivating as well. Likewise, faculty members who are unsuccessful in securing tenure within a given time frame risk losing their faculty appointments, and often, their jobs. There is a great deal at stake that can create hard feelings among research collaborators when there is disagreement regarding order of authorship. It is critical to determine in advance who is required to contribute to various aspects of the research project and writing to earn their place in the order of authorship. Depending on the venue, the most notable position of authorship is generally first or last. This typically depends on the area of research and profession.

Furthermore, investigators must only publish data that was gathered ethically (Research Advisory Council of the American Occupational Therapy Foundation, 1988). Researchers who break these ethical codes of conduct are "black listed" by the National Institute of Health and other federal grant funding agencies. The Office of Research Integrity via the U.S. Department of Health and Human Services publicly disseminates a list of researchers who have violated the Federal Research Misconduct Policy (Office of Research Integrity, 2011). Likewise, these researchers are often fined and cannot pursue future public (state or federal) funding, which significantly limits their ability to continue to pursue a successful career in academia.

Intellectual Property

Intellectual Property can be a very complex matter for persons who are employed by or are students at larger institutions. Generally speaking, if you use the resources of an organization or company to help develop your idea or invention, the institution retains ownership or partial ownership. Larger institutions generally have policies in place to make sure any monies generated by such ideas or inventions are credited back to the institution. The copyright law of the United States (Title 17, Section 107) governs the making of photocopies and the reproduction of copyrighted materials. Under certain conditions specified in the law, libraries and archives are authorized to furnish a photocopy or other reproduction. One of these specified conditions is that the photocopy is not to be used for any purpose other than private scholarship or research. If a user makes a request for, or later uses, a photocopy for purposes in excess of "fair use" that user may be liable for copyright infringement.

Summary

The emphasis on the use of research to inform practice, support intervention planning, and assist with reimbursement of services is stronger than ever in health care. Educators are responsible for teaching the future of the occupational therapy profession's best practice guidelines regarding ethical decision making with the use of evidenced-based practice and research (ACOTE, 2012). Occupational therapy students are responsible for ethically applying data to support their learning in academic programs in ways such as avoiding plagiarism and adhering to principles of academic integrity. Practitioners are responsible for being knowledgeable of how to search for, critique, and apply evidence to support their practice. In summary, knowledge and compliance of ethical practice in research is a professional obligation and responsibility of all occupational therapy practitioners.

Learning Activities

1. Read the following case study and complete the following prompts:

An assessment called the Standardized Touchscreen Assessment of Cognition (STAC) was initially developed in 2013 and is still undergoing validity testing (Cognitive Innovations, 2013b). The inventors of the STAC are Simon Carson, occupational therapist, and Heather Coles, speech language pathologist, who are both primarily employed at the University of Rochester, New York. The STAC differs from other cognitive assessments because it was designed to be appropriate for a wide range of individuals with cognitive deficits and etiologies, rather than just for concussion and dementia management. The STAC is a criterion-referenced test that assesses cognitive and linguistic functions. Similar to frequently used paper-and-pencil assessments of cognitive abilities, the STAC consists of theoretically validated tasks to assess attention, memory, visual and auditory memory, as well as executive function skills. The results that the assessment generates give the clinicians both quantitative and qualitative information about a person's cognitive abilities. Quantitative information includes accuracy of performance and speed of response. Qualitative information relates to the type and pattern of errors made. Different from other paper-and-pencil tasks, the STAC is self-administered using an application on an iPad, which eliminates examiner bias and administration (Cognitive Innovations, 2013b).

Given the STAC's potential use to evaluate cognition in multiple populations of adults with cognitive deficits, it should be compared to cognitive assessments that are similarly appropriate for a wide range of potential populations with cognitive impairments. This validity testing is important data to gather to best understand the clinical utility of an assessment tool as well as its accuracy of determining cognitive impairments resulting from multiple etiologies. Prior to making comparisons in clinical populations, evaluation of neurotypical adults was conducted in a research study by non-biased investigators at Duquesne University. Such research is critical to begin to validate the STAC for use in research and clinical practice (Cognitive Innovations, 2013a).

Download the trial version of the STAC onto an iPad. Administer first the STAC, and then the electronic version of the Montreal Cognitive Assessment to another person. The Montreal Cognitive Assessment is available for free at http://www.mocatest.org/, but you will need to register to access the assessment. Analyze and compare the results. Now, consider how you might be influenced if you had significant financial stake in the STAC—and answer the following discussion questions:

    a. How might your financial interest in the STAC affect your administration of the Montreal Cognitive Assessment?

    b. What are some ways to decrease or eliminate bias in a research study determining the validity of the STAC?

    c. How might the results reported for a study be influenced if the data was gathered, analyzed, or the overall study was funded by an individual or organization?

    d. Thinking about your response to the question above, how might such information influence your thoughts as a consumer of research?

2. Watch the movie "Miss Evers' Boys" (Bernstein & Sargent, 1997) and answer the following discussion questions.

    a. What does Miss Evers' opening recitation of the nurse's pledge do for the story?

    b. In scene I, the men appear to be wary of participating in a government study. Why?

    c. What was Miss Evers' initial reason for participating in the study?

    d. Were the men unable to understand the course of their illness and treatment? Explain your answer.

    e. What argument does Dr. Douglas use with Dr. Brodus to allow the study to continue?

    f. What was the reason that syphilis was not considered worthy of government research funds?

    g. In scene six, what is Ms. Evers' objection to the proposed study? How is it overcome by both doctors?

    h. Why didn't the "boys" receive penicillin when it became available? How did Dr. Douglas defend his refusal to allow government patients to receive penicillin?

    i. Why isn't the study terminated even when the results are absolutely clear?

    j. What is Brodus' answer when he is accused of not helping his own race? Is there any validity to his position?

REFERENCES

Accreditation Council for Occupational Therapy Education. (2012). 2011 Accreditation Council for Occupational Therapy Education (ACOTE) standards. *American Journal of Occupational Therapy, 66*(Suppl. 1), S6-S74.

American Psychological Association. (2009). *Publication manual of the American Psychological Association.* Washington, DC: American Psychological Association.

Beecher, H. K. (1966). Ethics and clinical research. *The New England Journal of Medicine, 274*(24), 367-372.

Bernstein, W. (Producer), & Sargent, J. (Director). (1997). *Miss Evers' Boys* [Motion picture]. United States: HBO.

Cognitive Innovations. (2013a). A cutting-edge cognitive evaluation tool. STAC: Standardized Touchscreen Assessment of Cognition. Retrieved from http://www.cognitive-innovations.com/info.html

Cognitive Innovations. (2013b). iPad-based cognitive assessment. STAC: Standardized Touchscreen Assessment of Cognition. Retrieved from http://www.cognitive-innovations.com

Copyright Law of the United States, 17 USC §107. Retrieved from http://www.copyright.gov/title17/circ92.pdf

Council for International Organizations of Medical Sciences. (2002). International guidelines for biomedical research involving human subjects. Retrieved from http://www.cioms.ch/publications/guidelines/guidelines_nov_2002_blurb.htm

Easterbrook, P. J., Gopalan, R., Berlin, J. A., & Matthews, D. R. (1991). Publication bias in clinical research. *The Lancet, 337*(8746), 867-872.

Emanuel, E., Abdoler, E., & Stunkel, L. (n.d.). Research ethics: How to treat people who participate in research. Retrieved from http://bioethics.nih.gov/education/FNIH_BioethicsBrochure_WEB.PDF

Fischer, B. A. (2006). A summary of important documents in the field of research ethics. *Schizophrenia Bulletin, 32*(1), 69-80.

Good, G. A. (2001). Ethics in research with older, disabled individuals. *International Journal of Rehabilitation Research, 24*, 165-170.

Kellehear, A. (1993). *The unobtrusive researcher.* Sydney, Australia: Allen and Unwin.

Kielhofner, G. (2006). *Research in occupational therapy: Methods of inquiry for enhancing practice.* Philadelphia, PA: F. A. Davis.

Kimmel, A. J. (1988). *Ethics and values in applied social research.* Newbury Park, CA: Sage.

National Institutes of Health. (1949). The Nuremberg code. Retrieved from https://history.nih.gov/research/downloads/nuremberg.pdf

Office of Research Integrity. (2011). Federal research misconduct policy. Retrieved from http://ori.hhs.gov/federal-research-misconduct-policy

Research Advisory Council of the American Occupational Therapy Foundation. (1988). The foundation: Ethical considerations for research in occupational therapy. *American Journal of Occupational Therapy, 42*(2), 129-130.

Shane, S. (2004). Encouraging university entrepreneurship? The effect of the Bayh-Dole Act on university patenting in the United States. *Journal of Business Venturing, 19*(1), 127-151.

University of California Office of Research. (2015). Required Elements of Informed Consent. Retrieved from http://www.research.uci.edu/compliance/human-research-protections/irb-members/required-elements-of-informed-consent.html

University of Pittsburgh. (2016). COI Summary for Consultants. Retrieved from http://www.coi.pitt.edu/Forms/StandardCOIMgmtPlan-HSR.htm

World Medical Association. (2013). World Medical Association Declaration of Helsinki: Ethical principles for medical research involving human subjects. *Journal of the American Medical Association, 310*(20), 2191-2194.

RESOURCES

1964: Declaration of Helsinki was developed by the World Medical Association as a statement of ethical principles for medical research involving human subjects, including research on identifiable human material and data. (Can be found online at: http://www.wma.net/en/30publications/10policies/b3/17c.pdf)

Late 1970s: Council for International Organizations of Medical Sciences (CIOMS) (2002) is an international nongovernmental organization founded under the auspices of the World Health Organization and the United Nations Educational, Scientific and Cultural and Organization. CIOMS undertook its work on ethics in relation to biomedical research in the late 1970s. CIOMS provides international ethical guidelines for biomedical research involving human subjects. (Book can be found online at http://www.recerca.uab.es/ceeah/docs/CIOMS.pdf.) Current version from 2002, but is updated periodically.

INTERNET RESOURCES

Committee on Publication Ethics (COPE). (2016): www.PUBLICATIONETHICS.org

National Commission for the Protection of Human Subjects of Biomedical and Behavioral Research. (1979). The Belmont Report: Ethical principles and guidelines for the protection of human subjects of research. Retrieved from www.hhs.gov/ohrp/humansubjects/guidance/belmont.html

The Nuremberg Code: history.nih.gov/research/downloads/nuremberg.pdf

Financial Disclosures

Dr. Elizabeth D. DeIuliis has no financial or proprietary interest in the materials presented herein.

Dr. Leesa M. DiBartola has not disclosed any relevant financial relationships.

Dr. Andrea D. Fairman has no financial or proprietary interest in the materials presented herein.

Dr. Sarah E. Wallace has no financial or proprietary interest in the materials presented herein.

Index

Silents, 17
simulation, 117–118, 127–128
situational learning, 119
skill acquisition model, 8, 9
skills. *See also* communication skills
　　hard, 242, 246, 283, 287–288
　　soft, 242, 243, 246, 283, 286
slides, composing, 312
SMART boards, 125
smart devices, 35–36, 146–148
SMART goals, 133
social distance, 32
social media, 36
　　in classroom, 147　148
　　guidelines for, 34
　　in job search, 296
　　privacy and confidentiality in, 36
　　professional boundaries on, 36
　　professional image on, 36–37
　　unprofessional use of, 150
social networking, in classroom, 147–148
social responsibility, 69
specialty certification, 302
speech-language pathology
　　education accreditation and requirements
　　　for, 73
　　intraprofessional roles of, 74
　　professional development tools and
　　　measures of, 75
　　professional organization of, 72
　　professionalism documents in, 75
　　professionalization of, 72
　　regulatory body and practice credentials
　　　for, 73–74
　　scope of practice of, 73
　　terminology of, 74–75
Standards of Practice in Occupational Therapy,
　　233
STAR approach, 287–288
state licensure, 232
student dress code, 141–145
student evaluation
　　of fieldwork experience, 188–198
　　of fieldwork performance, 181–187
student/fieldwork educator weekly review, 199
student response systems, 125
supervision

definition of, 164
direct, 164, 172–174
fieldwork, 171–178, 203
guidelines for, 98
indirect, 164
professionalism and, 203
regulatory oversight and, 173–178
synchronous learning, 107, 124–125

tardiness, 151
teaching philosophy statement, 240, 251, 280–
　　281
team-based care, 76–84
team-based learning, 125–126
teamwork, 33
technology
　　clinical uses of, 35
　　unprofessional use of in class, 150–151
　　use policy for, 146–148
telehealth, 43, 47–48
thank-you note, 294–295
theoretical frameworks, 8–9, 9–12
therapeutic modes, 101–102
time management, 25–26
TLSI 3.1, 123
Traditionalists, 17, 22–23
transdisciplinary approach, 80
transformation, 117
Tuskegee Syphilis Experiment, 322–324

unprofessional behavior
　　for fieldwork educators, 225–227
　　for fieldwork students, 223–225, 227

Vark Questionnaire, 123
volunteer work, 304–305, 306
vulnerable populations, 326–327
Vygotsky, Lev, 115

white papers, 97–98, 110
work rules, 11
work experience skill sets, 243
World Federation of Occupational Therapy,
　　Code of Ethics of, 96